Leading and Managing Health Services

Second edition

A combination of skills and aptitudes in management and leadership is required to build a successful career in the health industries. Including perspectives from across health sectors, *Leading and Managing Health Services* considers the fundamental skills students need to successfully navigate change and innovation in health service settings.

This second edition reflects changes to the health services industry in recent years. Two new chapters, on empathic leadership and leading and managing in the digital age, cover concepts such as compassionate care, digital health, artificial intelligence and telehealth. Each chapter includes definitions of key terms for easy reference; contemporary case studies to provide relevant industry perspectives; and end-of-chapter questions for deep student engagement through reflection and self-analysis.

Written by leading academics and industry experts, *Leading and Managing Health Services* provides students with practical skills to lead and manage in a wide range of healthcare settings, regardless of where they are in the organisational structure.

Gary E. Day is Deputy Dean (Programs) and Professor of Health Services Management at ECA – College of Health Sciences, and Adjunct Professor – Health Services Management at Queensland University of Technology.

Sandra G. Leggat is Emeritus Professor, Health Services Management at La Trobe University.

Cambridge University Press acknowledges the Australian Aboriginal and Torres Strait Islander peoples of this nation. We acknowledge the traditional custodians of the lands on which our company is located and where we conduct our business. We pay our respects to ancestors and Elders, past, present and emerging. Cambridge University Press is committed to honouring Aboriginal and Torres Strait Islander peoples' unique cultural and spiritual relationships to the land, waters and seas, and their rich contribution to health and society.

Cambridge University Press acknowledges the Māori people as tangata whenua of Aotearoa New Zealand. We pay our respects to the First Nation Elders of New Zealand, past, present and emerging.

Leading and Managing Health Services

Second edition

Edited by
Gary E. Day
Sandra G. Leggat

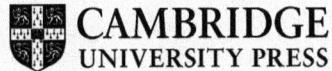

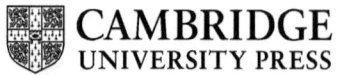

Shaftesbury Road, Cambridge CB2 8EA, United Kingdom

One Liberty Plaza, 20th Floor, New York, NY 10006, USA

477 Williamstown Road, Port Melbourne, VIC 3207, Australia

314–321, 3rd Floor, Plot 3, Splendor Forum, Jasola District Centre, New Delhi – 110025, India

103 Penang Road, #05–06/07, Visioncrest Commercial, Singapore 238467

Cambridge University Press is part of Cambridge University Press & Assessment, a department of the University of Cambridge.

We share the University's mission to contribute to society through the pursuit of education, learning and research at the highest international levels of excellence.

www.cambridge.org
Information on this title: www.cambridge.org/highereducation/isbn/9781009540087

© Cambridge University Press & Assessment 2025

This publication is copyright. Subject to statutory exception and to the provisions of relevant collective licensing agreements, no reproduction of any part may take place without the written permission of Cambridge University Press & Assessment.

First published 2015
Second edition 2025

Cover designed by Marianna Berek-Lewis

Typeset by Integra Software Services Pvt. Ltd.

A catalogue record for this publication is available from the British Library

A catalogue record for this book is available from the National Library of Australia

ISBN 978-1-009-54008-7 Paperback

Additional resources for this publication at www.cambridge.org/highereducation/isbn/9781009540087/resources

Reproduction and communication for educational purposes
The Australian *Copyright Act 1968* (the Act) allows a maximum of one chapter or 10% of the pages of this work, whichever is the greater, to be reproduced and/or communicated by any educational institution for its educational purposes provided that the educational institution (or the body that administers it) has given a remuneration notice to Copyright Agency Limited (CAL) under the Act.

For details of the CAL licence for educational institutions contact:

Copyright Agency Limited
Level 12, 66 Goulburn Street
Sydney NSW 2000
Telephone: (02) 9394 7600
Facsimile: (02) 9394 7601
E-mail: memberservices@copyright.com.au

Cambridge University Press & Assessment has no responsibility for the persistence or accuracy of URLs for external or third-party internet websites referred to in this publication and does not guarantee that any content on such websites is, or will remain, accurate or appropriate.

Please be aware that this publication may contain several variations of Aboriginal and Torres Strait Islander terms and spellings; no disrespect is intended. Please note that the terms 'Indigenous Australians', 'Aboriginal and Torres Strait Islander peoples' and 'First Nations peoples' may be used interchangeably in this publication.

For EU product safety concerns, contact us at Calle de José Abascal, 56, 1°, 28003 Madrid, Spain, or email eugpsr@cambridge.org.

For Elizabeth, Alex, Emily, Georgia, Ryley and Ruby

For Will, Evan, Sarah, Geoffrey and Zoe, Piper, Ava, Spencer and Flynn

Contents

List of contributors	page xvii
Acknowledgements	xx

Part 1 Introduction — 1

1 Concepts of leadership and management in health services — 2
Sandra G. Leggat

Introduction	3
Definitions	3
Organisations	3
Management	4
Leadership	6
Power and skills	7
Functions	10
Summary	11
Reflective questions	12
Self-analysis question	12
References	12

2 Leading and managing: Frameworks and theories — 15
Gary E. Day

Introduction	16
Definitions	16
Leadership theories	16
Management theories	21
Summary	24
Reflective questions	25
Self-analysis question	25
References	25

Part 2 Leads Self — 29

3 Leading ethically — 30
Gian Luca Casali and Gary E. Day

Introduction	31
Ethical decision-making	31

Influential factors	32
Frameworks for ethical decision-making	36
Future ethical considerations for health managers	37
Summary	37
Reflective questions	37
Self-analysis question	38
References	38

4 Self-management — 40
John Adamm Ferrier

Introduction	41
Definitions	42
Intelligence	44
Critical thinking	45
Motivation	46
Social learning	47
Aids for self-management	49
Summary	50
Reflective questions	51
Self-analysis questions	51
References	51

5 Emotional intelligence and self-awareness — 54
Leila Karimi and Jiri Rada

Introduction	55
Definitions and new developments	55
Characteristics of emotional intelligence	56
Models of emotional intelligence	58
Leadership and emotional intelligence	61
Healthcare and emotional intelligence	61
Summary	62
Reflective questions	63
Self-analysis question	63
References	63

6 Exploring values — 66
Eleanor Milligan and Jennifer Jones

Introduction	67
Definitions	67
Personal values	68
Professional values	69
Leadership and values	70
Summary	74
Reflective questions	74

Self-analysis questions	75
References	75

7 Ambiguity and leadership   77
Mark Avery

Introduction	78
Definitions	78
Healthcare	79
Management and ambiguity	81
Leadership and ambiguity	83
Summary	85
Reflective questions	85
Self-analysis questions	85
References	86

8 Leadership and critical reflective practice   87
Ahmad Saedisomeolia

Introduction	88
Definitions	88
Types of reflection	89
Leadership and critical reflective practice	91
Strategies for developing critical reflection	93
Summary	95
Reflective questions	96
Self-analysis questions	96
References	96

9 Empathic leadership   99
Sandra G. Leggat

Introduction	100
The loss of compassionate care	101
Workspace spirituality theory	102
Summary	105
Reflective questions	105
Self-analysis question	105
References	105

Part 3 Engages Others   109

10 Communication leadership   110
Mark Keough

Introduction	111
Definitions	111

Essential elements of communication 112
Healthcare and communication 114
Leadership and communication 116
Communication and learning 118
Communication and marginalised groups 118
Summary 120
Reflective questions 120
Self-analysis questions 121
References 121

11 Leading interprofessional teams 122
Katrina Radford and Janna Anneke Fitzgerald

Introduction 123
Definitions 123
Teams with professional boundaries 124
Teams with role-related boundaries 125
Leadership of interprofessional teams 126
Management of interprofessional teams 127
Summary 129
Reflective questions 129
Self-analysis question 129
References 129

12 Clinical governance 131
Cathy Balding

Introduction 132
History 132
Leading effective clinical governance into the future 137
Summary 138
Reflective questions 139
Self-analysis questions 139
References 139

13 Partnering with stakeholders 142
Sharon Brownie and Audrey Holmes

Introduction 143
Definitions 143
The importance of stakeholder partnerships 143
Stakeholder groups in healthcare 145
Success factors in stakeholder partnerships 148
Management and stakeholder partnerships 148
Leadership and stakeholder partnerships 150
Summary 151

Reflective questions	151
Self-analysis questions	151
References	151

14 Power and political astuteness
Nicola McNeil

155

Introduction	156
Definitions	156
Authority	156
Sources of power	157
Use of power	160
Influence tactics	162
Increasing power	164
Summary	164
Reflective questions	165
Self-analysis questions	165
References	165

15 Influencing strategically
Mark Avery

167

Introduction	168
Definitions	168
Using influence	169
Frameworks for influencing strategically	170
Summary	174
Reflective questions	175
Self-analysis questions	175
References	175

16 Networking
John Rasa

177

Introduction	178
Definitions	178
Leadership and networking	181
Personal networking	181
Operational networking	183
Strategic networking	183
Interorganisational networking	184
Intraorganisational networking	186
Summary	187
Reflective questions	187
Self-analysis questions	187
References	187

Part 4 Achieves Outcomes — 189

17 Holding to account — 190
Ged Williams and Linda Fraser

Introduction	191
Definitions	191
Leadership and holding to account	192
Frameworks for holding to account	193
Summary	197
Reflective questions	198
Self-analysis questions	198
References	198

18 Critical thinking and decision-making — 200
Richard Baldwin

Introduction	201
Critical thinking	201
Barriers to critical thinking	202
Developing critical-thinking skills in decision-making	203
Decision-making	204
Biases and errors in decision-making	205
Evidence-based management decision-making	206
Summary	207
Reflective questions	207
Self-analysis questions	208
References	208

19 Managing and leading staff — 210
Godfrey Isouard

Introduction	211
Human resources	211
Skills utilisation	212
Organisational behaviour and culture	212
Leadership and management	213
Effective health teams	216
Summary	217
Reflective questions	217
Self-analysis questions	218
References	218

20 Project management — 221
Zhanming Liang

Introduction	222
Definitions	222
Frameworks	223

Core components and development	224
Evaluation and learning	226
Management of projects	229
Summary	231
Reflective questions	231
Self-analysis question	231
References	231

21 Financial management — 233
Christine Dennis

Introduction	234
Types of budgets	234
Healthcare funding	237
Casemix	237
Reforms in funding	239
Management and financial performance	240
Costs	240
Variance	240
Budget development	241
Controlling and monitoring a budget	245
Summary	246
Reflective questions	246
Self-analysis questions	246
References	246

22 Negotiating — 248
Sandra G. Leggat

Introduction	249
Concepts	249
Frameworks for negotiating	249
Management and negotiation	252
Negotiation skills improvement	253
Summary	253
Reflective questions	253
Self-analysis questions	254
References	254

Part 5 Drives Innovation — 257

23 Creativity and visioning — 258
Godfrey Isouard

Introduction	259
Definitions	259
Organisations	259

Management and innovation	261
Leadership and innovation	264
Summary	265
Reflective questions	265
Self-analysis questions	266
References	266

24 Evidence-based practice 268
Sandra G. Leggat

Introduction	269
Use of evidence	269
Frameworks for evidence-based management	270
The role of knowledge management	273
Summary	273
Reflective questions	273
Self-analysis question	274
References	274

25 Successfully managing conflict 276
Gary E. Day

Introduction	277
Types and origins of conflict	277
Is all conflict bad?	278
Management of conflict	279
Approaches to conflict resolution	281
Considerations when managing conflict	284
Summary	285
Reflective questions	285
Self-analysis questions	285
References	285

26 Building positive workplace cultures 287
Gary E. Day and Kirsty Marles

Introduction	288
Definitions	288
Typology of workplace cultures	289
Measuring workplace culture	290
Organisational implications of different workplace cultures	291
Management imperatives in building positive workplace cultures	292
Leadership imperatives in building positive workplace cultures	293
Managing stress and burnout: Strategies for health managers	295
Summary	297
Reflective questions	297
Self-analysis questions	297
References	298

27 Leading and managing change — 301
Gary E. Day

Introduction	302
Definitions	302
Management of change	302
People and change	304
Frameworks for change management	306
Mentoring and coaching staff through change: Key success factors for health managers	309
Cultural considerations in managing change with First Nations peoples	311
Summary	312
Reflective questions	313
Self-analysis questions	313
References	313

28 Healthcare quality and service improvement — 316
Mohamed Khalifa

Introduction	317
History of healthcare quality and improvement	317
The modified 12-domains model for healthcare quality and improvement	319
Summary	326
Reflective questions	326
Self-analysis question	326
References	326

29 Leading and managing in the digital age — 330
Mark Keough and James Boyd

Introduction	331
Key benefits	332
Definitions	332
Challenges of health care in the digital age	334
Data analytics in health care	335
Artificial intelligence and machine learning: Implications for health service delivery	337
Telemedicine	338
Implications for health managers in a digital age	339
Summary	341
Reflective questions	341
Self-analysis questions	341
References	342

Part 6 Shapes Systems — 343

30 Workforce planning — 344
Ged Williams and Ben Archdall

Introduction	345
Definitions	345

Australia's healthcare workforce: Demand and supply	346
Framework for workforce planning	348
Management and workforce planning	354
Summary	355
Reflective questions	355
Self-analysis questions	356
References	356

31 Strategic planning and sustainability — 358
Sandra G. Leggat

Introduction	359
Use of strategic planning	359
Framework for strategic planning	360
Summary	365
Reflective questions	366
Self-analysis question	366
References	366

32 Health service planning — 369
Chaojie Liu and John Adamm Ferrier

Introduction	370
Definitions	370
Population-based planning	370
Health service planning: Considerations for Indigenous populations	370
Institutional-based planning	371
Reasons for planning	372
Management and health service planning	373
Frameworks for health service planning	376
Technology use in health service planning	380
Summary	381
Reflective questions	381
Self-analysis questions	381
References	381

Index — *386*

Contributors

Editors

Gary E. Day RN, EM, DipAppSc (Nurs Mgt), BNurs, MHM, DHSM, FCHSM, FGLF

Deputy Dean (Programs) and Professor of Health Services Management at ECA – College of Health Sciences, and Adjunct Professor – Health Services Management at Queensland University of Technology.

Professor Gary E. Day is a senior executive with over 35 years' experience as a consultant, project manager, director and chief executive officer, and as a clinician, academic, researcher and author. Gary has worked in both the for-profit and the not-for-profit healthcare sectors across Australia and internationally, and in the higher education sector. He has played leading roles in major infrastructure and change-management projects, and organisation-wide roles in workforce development and learning, in medical education and in clinical governance and quality.

Sandra G. Leggat MHSc, MBA, PhD, FCHSM

Emeritus Professor, Health Services Management at La Trobe University.

Emeritus Professor Sandra G. Leggat has worked as a senior health executive in management and in consulting roles, both in Australia and Canada. She has studied healthcare systems around the world, focusing on human resource management and leadership. Sandra has written many journal publications and book chapters, and she has editorial experience with the *Australian Health Review* and the *Asia Pacific Journal of Health Management*. Sandra chairs of the board of a regional hospital in Australia.

Authors

Ben Archdall RN
Manager, Workforce Mapping, Analysis, Planning, Projections, Department of Health, Queensland Government.

Mark Avery PhD, MBus (Res), BHA, FCHSM, FIML, FAICD, CHE
Senior lecturer, Health Services Management, School of Applied Psychology, Griffith University.

Cathy Balding MBus, PhD, FCHSM, GAICD
Adjunct Professor, James Cook University; Founder and Director, Qualityworks Pty Ltd.

Richard Baldwin RN, AssDipNursAdmin, BHlthAdmin, MBA, PhD, FCHSM
Former chief examiner, Australasian College of Health Service Management; former Director of Health Services Management, Faculty of Health, University of Technology Sydney.

James Boyd BSc(Hons), PhD
Professor and Chair of Digital Health and Innovation, School of Psychology and Public Health, La Trobe University.

Sharon Brownie RN, RM, BEd, MEd Admin, M Hth S Mgt, GAICD, FCNA, DBA
Director of Health Strategy & Partnerships in the School of Health Science, Swinburne University.

Gian Luca Casali BBA, MBA, PhD
Associate professor, School of Management, Queensland University of Technology.

Christine Dennis BNsg, MHlthServMgmt, DBA, LMFCHSM, FGIA
Associate Professor Health Service Management, Flinders University; board director roles in acute care, aged care and disability services.

John Adamm Ferrier CertGenNurs, DipAppSci (P&O), GradCertNurs (Periop), GradDipNurs (Periop), RN, PGradDipHSM, MHA, FCHSM MACN
Senior lecturer, China Health Program and MHA Course Coordinator, School of Psychology and Public Health, La Trobe University.

Janna Anneke Fitzgerald RN, GradDipAdultEd (VET), MClinPrac, PhD
Emeritus Professor, Griffith Business School, Griffith University.

Linda Fraser FACHSM, MBA, MAdvPrac (Critical Care), BHSc, RN
Lecturer (Health Services Management), Griffith University.

Audrey Holmes BA, MA
Former adjunct research fellow, Population and Social Health Research Program, Griffith Health, Griffith University.

Godfrey Isouard BSc, MHA, PhD, MLE, FCHSM, FACBS
Adjunct Professor, Health Services Management, School of Health, University of New England.

Jennifer (Jenny) Jones BA (Hon 1st class), PhD
Clinical ethicist (retired), member Queensland Children's Hospital Clinical Ethics Consultation Service.

Leila Karimi PhD (OrgPsych), MAPS
Professor, Psychology Discipline, Health Sciences Department, RMIT University.

Mark Keough DComm, GradCert (Mediation), BA, Cert IV TAE
Principal, Mark Keough Consulting; adjunct academic (Education), Flinders University.

Mohamed Khalifa MBBS, MSc, PhD, FAIDH
Course Coordinator, ECA Higher Education College of Health Sciences, Fellow of the Australian Institute of Health Innovation, Macquarie University, and Visiting Fellow, School of Psychology and Public Health, La Trobe University.

Zhanming Liang MSc, MBBS, PhD, FCHSM
Associate Dean and Associate Professor, College of Business, Law and Governance, James Cook University.

Chaojie (George) Liu MB, MPH, PhD
Professor and Associate Dean, School of Psychology and Public Health, La Trobe University.

Kirsty Marles DBA, GradCert Health Services Management, GradDip Public Health.
Independent Management Consultant, Sensemaking.

Nicola McNeil BCom (Hons), LLB, PhD
Associate Professor in Management, School of Business, Law and Entrepreneurship, Swinburne University of Technology.

Eleanor Milligan Grad Dip Ed, BA (Hons, 1st class), PhD
Chair, Griffith University Human Research Ethics Committee and Chair, Student Misconduct Committee; Deputy Chair, North West Hospital and Health Board; Deputy Chair, Queensland Voluntary Assisted Dying Review Board.

Jiri Rada BA, BPHE, MSc, PhD
Senior lecturer, RMIT University.

Katrina Radford BPsych (Hons), GradDip Higher Ed, MHRM, PhD
Associate professor, Griffith Business School, Griffith University.

John Rasa BA, GD (Industrial Law and Industrial Relations), MHP, MAICD, LMFCHSM
Affiliate associate professor, MBA (Healthcare Management), Deakin University.

Ahmad Saedisomeolia PhD
Associate professor, College of Health Sciences; Dean (Scholarship and Research), Education Centre of Australia; Research scientist affiliate, School of Human Nutrition, McGill University.

Ged Williams AO, RN, RM, CritCareCert, GradCertPSM, BachAppSc (Adv Nurs), GradCertLaw, LLM, MHA (UNSW), MAICD, FACN, FACHSM, FAAN
Nursing and allied health consultant, SEHA: Abu Dhabi Health Service Company; Professor of Nursing, Griffith University; Chief Nursing Officer, Alfred Health.

Acknowledgements

Cambridge University Press and the authors would like to acknowledge the feedback provided by peer reviewers of the draft manuscript, including Judith Anderson, Paula Bowman, Nicolie Jenkins, Matylda Howard, Jennifer Kosiol, Shaun Larkin, David Lim, Andrew Mathieson, Rebekkah Middleton, Luke Molloy, Melanie Murray, Jayne Porter, Paul Preobrajensky and Morgan Smith. Their feedback and comments were invaluable to the development of this edition.

The authors and Cambridge University Press would like to thank the following for permission to reproduce material in this book.

Figure 10.1: © 2011 NSW Ministry of Health / New South Wales and South Australian Department of Health. Reproduced under CC BY 4.0, https://creativecommons.org/licenses/by/4.0/deed.en; **Figure 20.1, 20.2:** © 2019 Taylor & Francis. Reproduced with permission.; **Figure 24.1:** © CSIRO Publishing. Reproduced with permission.; **Figure 30.1:** © 2023 Australian Public Sector Commission. Reproduced under CC BY 4.0 (https://creativecommons.org/licenses/by/4.0/); **Figure 30.2:** © 2010 World Health Organization. Reprinted with permission.

Part 1
Introduction

1 Concepts of leadership and management in health services

Sandra G. Leggat
With acknowledgement to Mindaugas Stankunas

Learning objectives

How do I:

- define management and leadership in healthcare organisations?
- distinguish between top, middle and first-line managers?
- understand how power is used in management and leadership?
- identify areas for personal skills development?

Introduction

Intense debate surrounds the differences between the roles, functions and even the differences between leaders and managers (Lease, 2006). Leadership is not wholly different from management; indeed, it is a component of management and a responsibility of management, especially of senior managers. Effective managers need to be effective leaders, and the most effective leaders are also good managers.

Definitions

When people are asked to explain what management is, they tend to give different answers. Some say that it is a science, while others argue that it is an art and still others claim it is a practice. People often give examples of successful entrepreneurs, like Jack Welch, or international companies like Apple.

It is tough to explain differences between management and leadership. In some languages there is no term for leadership. This suggests that common words like 'management' and 'leadership' have confused meanings, depending on the geographic setting. Therefore, it is important to discuss definitions and functions of management and leadership in context.

Organisations

Why do we need management? Let's say that someone has been asked to prepare a health promotion project highlighting the dangers of skin cancer. If they decide to do everything by themselves, most likely they will not need to think about the division of tasks such as planning, organising and controlling. However, the situation changes if colleagues join them in the project. The person will need to plan activities and organise who will do what so that they can monitor the process. In this case, they become a manager. The management function normally appears only within **organisations**.

Researchers have identified many different types of organisations (McKenna, 1998), for example, a hunting tribe in Papua New Guinea, a primary healthcare unit in the Northern Territory, a university in Aotearoa New Zealand, a cancer research institute in France and the World Health Organization. What do these organisations have in common? First, they have one or more objectives, which gives the activity direction and purpose. The research institute may wish to better understand cancer and its treatment. The tribe has a mission to hunt for food and survive. The university trains specialists and health professionals. Second, all of these organisations have two or more members. Third, the members are organised. The primary healthcare centre has doctors, nurses, a receptionist and a practice manager. These people have different responsibilities, targeted at achieving a common goal. The World Health Organization has a sophisticated organisational structure, with different specialists and functions.

Organisation: A group of individuals who interact with each other to achieve a common goal

Organisations are platforms for management. All organisations (from tribes to international corporations) have similar structures, presented in Figure 1.1. All organisations produce results, or outcomes. For example, results for a tribe will be hunted game; for a hospital, healthy patients; for a pharmaceutical company, a new drug to treat hypertension. However, these desired results do not occur without someone doing something; processes are used to achieve results. For a hospital, processes may be the examination, treatment and rehabilitation of patients; for a university, the teaching of students; and for a non-governmental organisation, running a project to reduce smoking.

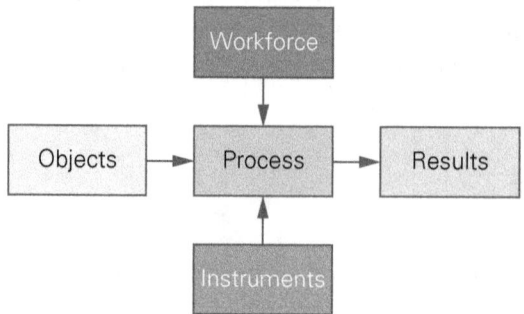

Figure 1.1 Structure of an organisation

These processes (the core of any organisation) are possible if we have objects, people and tools. Hospital patients are defined as objects. Little will happen to these patients if there are no health specialists (workforce). The workforce ensures processes within the organisation. Doctors, nurses and allied health specialists care for patients. In addition, for most of the processes, tools or instruments are required. Doctors and nurses would not be able to do much without facilities, technologies and drugs. These instruments help the workforce in the process towards achieving the common goals or outcomes.

A disorganised group of people will not achieve their organisation's goals. Management aims to help a group work effectively and in a shared direction.

Management

Management: Planning, organising, leading and controlling resources to achieve an organisation's goals

Health management: Planning, organising, leading and controlling resources to promote, restore or maintain health

Health system: Combined activities whose primary purpose is to promote, restore or maintain health

There are many definitions of **management**. However, the main principle is the same in all definitions and lies in the classic works of French mining engineer Henri Fayol, known for his theory on the fundamental functions of management. According to Fayol (1917), every manager plans, organises, commands (or leads), coordinates and controls. This definition of management is generic: it should be suitable for all industry sectors.

Health management occurs in health organisations. According to the World Health Organization (2000), the organisations, institutions and resources that are devoted to producing health actions are components of a **health system**. Some authors use the terms 'healthcare management' or 'health services management'; these emphasise the organisation and delivery of services (Fulop, Allen, Clarke & Black, 2001). Health management covers the management and organisation of the health system and its various subsystems and components (Hunter & Brown, 2007).

However, health management has an unfortunate reputation. It is often regarded as an unnecessary activity that, at best, diverts resources from the frontline activities of providing healthcare and preventing ill health (Green, Collins & Mirzoev, 2012). A 2013 systematic review suggested there is a positive correlation between the performance of healthcare systems and their organisation and management practices, leadership and manager characteristics (Lega, Prenestini & Spurgeon, 2013), and there is evidence of good management practices influencing employee outcomes (Pham, 2021), especially under the working conditions associated with a global pandemic (Gadolin, Skyvell Nilsson, Larsman, Pousette & Törner, 2022). However, there is little robust evidence to clearly show a positive effect of good health managers on patient, organisational and health systems outcomes. There are so many confounding factors in complex health systems that it is difficult to establish a strong correlation, and thus further research is required.

Health management is a social process that reflects national social, political and cultural values. It cannot be transferred easily from one country to another. Most likely, successful health management practices in Aotearoa New Zealand will not work in Tajikistan. This is not because of ineffectiveness in New Zealand's principles; simply, these two countries have different histories of development.

WHAT KINDS OF MANAGERS DO HEALTH SYSTEMS NEED?

The World Health Organization's (1999) regional office for Europe has identified the most important functions of public health managers. Although these principles apply to the European region, they are relevant in the Australasian context, and while the focus is public health, the need to understand an organisation's or service's target market is an essential skill for managers in the private sector as well.

> Essentially what is needed are public health managers, with the skills to manage partnerships and coordinated multisectoral action within alliances. They must … be trained in population-based analysis of health problems, be grounded in the approaches to deal with problems of lifestyles, the environment and health care, and be capable of the advocacy and networking needed to bring many partners together. They must also be skilled in creating excellent public health information for the general public, professionals and politicians.
>
> Within the health service itself they must be trained in policy and programme planning, including target-setting, outcome measurement and evaluation, and instrumental in shaping the pattern of services provided. They must be able to help plan, monitor and evaluate broad health development programmes, defined by disease category or client group, making scientifically informed judgements about the balance to be struck … between health promotion, disease prevention, therapy and rehabilitation.

All organisations have formal managerial positions, such as chief executive officer, director, president, vice-chancellor and director of nursing. A 2011 survey found that 22 400 managers were employed in all health services in Australia (Martins & Isouard, 2014), and this number had increased by 15.6 per cent since 2006.

For many years, there was a common understanding that management functions should be delegated to formal managers with the power to manage organisations, and their departments and units. However, new approaches suggest that these responsibilities should not be concentrated in formal positions but shared within the organisation (e.g. see Czabanowska, Smith, Stankunas, Avery & Otok, 2013). This means that more people in organisations should have the opportunity to participate in decision-making and the running of organisations.

Leadership

New approaches to management have inspired discussion on the importance of leadership. According to the classic work of Abraham Zaleznik (1977) managers are reactive, and while they are willing to work with people to solve problems, they do so with minimal emotional involvement. On the other hand, leaders are emotionally involved and seek to shape ideas instead of reacting to others' ideas.

Moreover, leadership is not locked to formal positions in organisations. This means that everybody can be a leader, and there can be more than one leader in an organisation. Many academics and managers emphasise the growing importance of leadership in healthcare (Beaglehole, Bonita, Horton, Adams & McKee, 2004; Simpson & Calman, 2000). According to the literature, every healthcare organisation should be engaged in developing leaders at every level, and in creating collaborative organisational cultures (Czabanowska et al., 2013).

> **Leadership:** 'A process whereby an individual influences a group of individuals to achieve a common goal' (Northouse, 2013, p. 5)

What it is **leadership**? Researchers mostly define it according to their individual perspectives and the aspects of the phenomenon that most interest them (Yukl, 2013), leading to many and varied views. Ralph Stogdill (1974, p. 7) reviewed over 3000 studies directly related to leadership and found many different definitions. We use the Northouse (2007) definition of leadership, which emphasises the key elements of leadership: it is a process, it entails influence, it occurs within a group setting or context and it involves achieving goals that reflect a common vision.

According to Rowitz (2003, as cited in Stankunas et al., 2012, p. 582), health leadership 'includes commitment to the community and the values it stands for'. Grainger and Griffiths (1998, as cited in Stankunas et al., 2012, p. 582) argue that 'health leaders differ from leaders in other sectors, as they are required to balance corporate legitimacy, while also existing outside the corporate environment'. Kimberly (2011, as cited in Stankunas et al., 2012, p. 582) suggests that a flatter, 'more distributed and collaborative world will require a new generation of leaders in public health with new mind sets, an appetite for innovation and interdisciplinary collaboration and a strong dose of political savvy'. Koh (2009, as cited in Stankunas et al., 2012, p. 582) believes that a health leader 'must be the transcendent, collaborative "servant leader" who knits and aligns disparate voices together behind a common mission, pinpoints passion and compassion, promotes servant leadership, acknowledges the unfamiliarity, ambiguity, and paradox, communicates succinctly to reframe, and help understand the "public" part of public health leadership'. Another study emphasises that health leaders must be 'exceptional "networker–connectors" capable of "putting the pieces of the jigsaw together"; they combine administrative excellence with a strong sense of professional welfare and actively develop the profession, articulate its shared values and build for the future' (Day et al., as cited in Stankunas et al., 2012, p. 582).

This brief discussion of health leadership reveals that most authors agree on the presence of Northouse's (2007, p. 3) leadership elements in health leadership. However, they also emphasise specific characteristics, such as a servant leader approach to community and specific orientation to public health values, which make it unique and important in the health sector (Stankunas et al., 2012, p. 582).

Challenges

The health sector creates many challenges for leadership. McAlearney (2006) suggests two main challenges in developing leadership in healthcare settings: environment and organisation. Environmental challenges arise because healthcare organisations are faced with a myriad of regulatory influences, some largely out of their control. Therefore, provider organisations rarely have power or influence over some areas – for example, the reimbursement of hospital and doctor services.

McAlearney (2006, p. 968) suggests that 'multiple hierarchies of professionals, on both the clinical and administrative sides of the organization, generate special challenges for directing the organization and coordination of work in healthcare. Often noted is the cultural chasm between administrators and clinicians'. McAlearney also says that the healthcare industry is behind other sectors in implementing new leadership and management methods. This suggests there is a need for competent managers and leaders in healthcare organisations.

Power and skills

Both leadership and management are about influencing people to achieve organisational goals. The outcome (effectiveness) of the influence process depends largely on the **power** of the leader or manager over their followers or staff. Two major types of power have been identified: positional and personal (Rahim, 1988). Positional power is based on legitimate authority and control over resources, rewards, punishments, information and the physical work environment. Personal power comes from task expertise, friendship and loyalty. Gary Yukl (2010) claims that personal and positional power have different subpowers, brief descriptions of which are presented in Table 1.1.

Power: An agent's ability to influence the target

Table 1.1 Types of powers

Power	Subpower	Description
Position	Legitimate	Formal authority and the right to set rules and directions for followers
	Reward	The right to control resources and give rewards to followers
	Coercive	The right to enforce punishments, penalties and sanctions
	Information	The right to control important information
	Ecological	The right to control the physical environment and organisation of work
Personal	Referent	Control through followers' positive feelings about the leader
	Expert	Control through competency in the particular field

Source: Adapted from Yukl (2010).

Power studies suggest that expert and referent power are more effective (e.g. see Schriesheim, Hinkin & Podsakoff, 1991). However, other powers do not show any positive correlation with followers' satisfaction and performance. It could be concluded that leaders use more expert and referent power to influence followers, while managers use more positional power (see Figure 1.2).

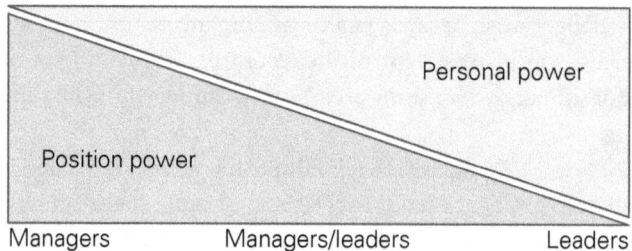

Figure 1.2 Power distribution between managers and leaders

How much power do managers and leaders need? The most common answer would likely be 'as much as possible'. However, more power is not always better. More power is necessary in organisations in which major change is required. Managers with too much 'position power may be tempted to rely on it instead of developing personal power and using other approaches' (e.g. consultation or coalitions) (Yukl 2013, p. 199).

It is important to have the skills necessary to use available power. These can reduce the need to have a lot of power. Robert Katz (1955) suggests that effective management is based on three types of skills. Technical skills come from specific knowledge in a particular area of work, human skills involve working and communicating with people, and conceptual skills help in developing ideas and vision, and in understanding economic principles.

Three levels of management can be identified in healthcare organisations, and this classification presents the most common hierarchical management structure found in organisations (see Figure 1.3). Top-level (executive or senior) managers such as chief executive

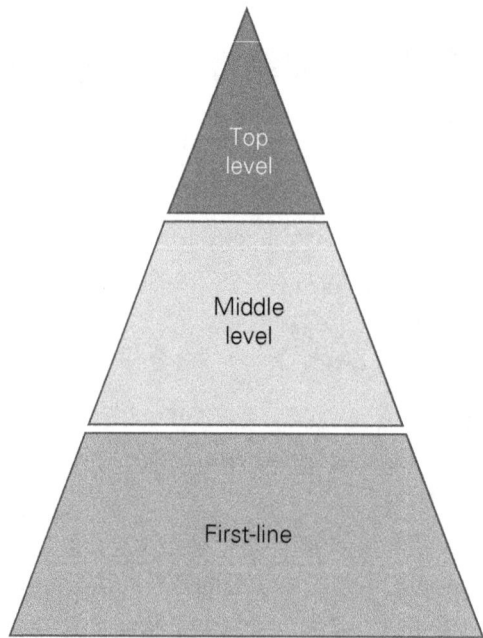

Figure 1.3 Levels of management within an organisation

officers are responsible for the performance of all departments and the organisation. Middle-level managers (e.g. director of obstetrics and gynaecology) supervise first-line managers and non-managerial employees. Finally, first-line managers (e.g. the nurse manager in the obstetrics department) are responsible for the daily supervision of nurses and non-managerial employees.

Liang and Howard (2010) identify four tiers of top-level managers in the health sector in New South Wales: directors-general, deputy directors-general, department of health division directors and chief executive officers of area health services. The Australian Bureau of Statistics (ABS, 2013) uses a different classification, identifying four groups of managers in the health sector: chief executive officers and general managers, specialist managers (who work in areas such as finance, human resources, information technology, medical and other clinical services, nursing and allied health services), service managers (who are concerned with catering, cleaning, maintenance and other support services) and managers not further defined. Australian Census 2011 data show that 12.3 per cent of all health managers in Australia are chief executive officers and general managers, 68.3 per cent are specialist managers, 15.2 per cent are service managers and 4.1 per cent are not defined (ABS, 2013).

The management skills identified earlier in this chapter are required in different proportions depending on the manager's position within the organisation (see Figure 1.4). First-line managers need more technical skills, while top-level managers need more conceptual skills than other managers. However, human skills are important at all levels.

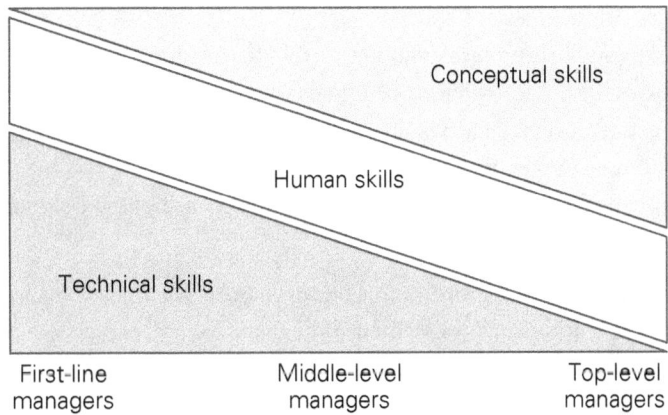

Figure 1.4 Katz's three-skills approach to management in relation to management level

Source: Adapted from Katz (1955).

In an alternative approach, Mumford, Campion & Morgeson (2007) identify four types of management skills: cognitive, interpersonal, business and strategic. This work reinforces Katz's (1955) theory that management skills are important for all leaders and managers but in different proportions. According to Mumford et al. (2007), the seniority of the manager determines which skills are most important. For example, while human skills are important across organisational levels, strategic thinking tends to be more important for top-level managers. There is strong evidence that leadership and management skills can be enhanced through appropriately structured training (Leggat, Smyth, Balding & McAlpine, 2016; Ravaghi, Beyranyand, Mannion, Aryankhesal & Belorgeot, 2021).

Functions

As mentioned, an essential component of an organisation is the people, or workforce (see Figure 1.1). The group of staff that works directly with patients – such as doctors, nurses and allied health specialists – is called the direct group. Other groups provide support for the direct group, ensuring, for example, that doctors and nurses have adequate equipment and supplies, that facilities are cleaned, financial issues are taken care of and patient bookings are attended to, thereby freeing the direct group from these duties and responsibilities. The support groups may not have direct contact with patients but undoubtedly are valuable to the functioning of the organisation. Given the other groups' supportive roles, the direct group can focus on the care tasks. However, all direct and support staff need to be organised. They must know what, when, where and how to do tasks. Therefore, another group of staff in an organisation, which we can call the 'executive group', undertakes the main responsibilities of management and leadership in the organisation.

What is it that managers do? Fayol (1917) proposes five primary functions of management: planning, organising, commanding (or leading), coordinating and controlling. Later authors have added further functions, like staffing and decision-making (Longest, Rakich & Darr, 2000), or have merged some of the functions (Waddell, Devine, Jones & George, 2009). Following the definition of health management given on page 4, we can say that managers have four functions:

1. Planning: identifying the goals of the organisation and the courses of action that will best achieve these goals
2. Organising: establishing tasks and authority relationships that enable people to work together to achieve the organisation's goals
3. Leading: articulating a clear vision, energising, motivating and enabling staff so they can contribute to achieving the organisation's goals
4. Controlling: evaluating how well an organisation is achieving its goals and identifying ways to improve performance.

It would seem obvious that different managers have different roles: meaning that for each manager the relative importance (or daily use) of these four managerial functions depends on their position in the organisation. Results from studies show that the amount of time managers spend on planning and organising resources to maintain and improve organisational performance increases as they ascend the management hierarchy. Thus, first-line managers spend significantly less time on planning and organising, and more time on leading and controlling, than top-level managers (Gomez-Mejia, McCann & Page, 1985; Mahony, Jerdee & Carroll, 1965).

Some people use the terms 'management' and 'leadership' interchangeably, but this is not correct. While management has four main functions, leadership implements only one of these. It could be perceived that health leaders' roles and responsibilities are relatively glamorous (e.g. setting the vision for the organisation, inspiring and motivating people), while managers are required to undertake 'boring' and mundane tasks such as staffing and budgeting. However, Alvesson & Sveningsson (2003) have found that leaders often engage in passive, mundane activities, such as listening to employees, and that these activities are critical to the leaders' effectiveness.

According to John Kotter (1990), each system of action in an organisation has three main steps: (1) deciding what needs to be done, (2) creating networks of people and relationships that can accomplish the agenda, and (3) ensuring that those people actually do what needs to be done. Leaders and managers are involved in every step, but in different ways. For the first step, managers undertake planning and budgeting, while leaders set the organisation's direction. For the second, managers are concerned with organising and staffing, while leaders seek to align people. For the last step, managers do some controlling and problem-solving, while leaders seek to motivate and inspire people.

Louis Rubino (2011) contributes to this discussion by arguing that running healthcare organisations has two 'foci': external and internal, and that leaders usually have an external focus, while the focus of managers is more internal. 'Leaders tend to spend the majority of their time communicating and aligning with outside groups that can benefit their organisation (partners, community, vendors) or influence them (media, government, public agencies)' (Rubino 2011, p. 18). Meanwhile, managers are concerned with internal stakeholders (administrators, professionals, operators).

In summary, managers are concerned with the present and achieving targets, with a focus on control of the organisation. Leaders are more focused on the future, concerned with promoting direction, purpose and vision (Iles & Preece, 2006).

The Asia Pacific SHAPE Declaration, adopted in 2008, endorses five capabilities for health managers, developed from the literature and research (Briggs 2008, p. 12). These capabilities are:

1. Being trained and experienced to lead and manage in a range of differing health systems and organisational arrangements.
2. Possessing a deep contextual understanding of health systems, public policy, professional cultures and politics.
3. Being competent in organisational sensemaking as negotiators of meaning and as active participants, constructors, organisers and persuaders within health systems.
4. Having a range of backgrounds, including clinical and non-clinical experience and qualifications, and being able to demonstrate broad contextual health knowledge across more than one set of logic.
5. Understanding how clinical work should be structured and managed and working actively with clinicians and others to deliver coherent, well-managed health services (Briggs, Smyth & Anderson, 2012).

These capabilities go beyond the textbook definitions of leadership and management and recognise the inherent complexities in healthcare systems around the world.

Summary

- The main functions of managers are planning, organising, leading and controlling. Health management is about planning, organising, leading and controlling resources in order to promote, restore or maintain health.
- There are three levels of management in healthcare organisations: first-line, middle and top.

- Effective management is based on three types of skills: technical, human and conceptual.
- Leaders and managers use positional and personal power to influence followers.
- Leaders influence individuals to achieve a common goal. Health leadership has specific characteristics, including a servant leader approach to community and specific orientation to public health values.

Reflective questions

1. What comes to mind first when you hear the words 'leadership' and 'management'? Why?
2. Are leadership and management different from one another? If so, how?
3. What are the differences between the functions of leaders and managers?
4. Do you agree that everyone can be a leader? Explain your answer.
5. How can healthcare organisations select and develop effective leaders?

Self-analysis question

Think about the most effective leader you have ever worked with or observed closely or know well from the media or other sources. List the five key traits, skills or practices of this leader. Think about the person who, in your understanding, is the least effective leader you have encountered. List the five traits, skills or practices of this person that you think are most important in determining that they are a poor leader. Now, consider how they could develop, improve or change these characteristics to become more effective in their leadership.

References

Alvesson, M. & Sveningsson, S. (2003). Managers doing leadership: The extra-ordinarization of the mundane. *Human Relations, 56*, 1435–1459. https://doi.org/10.1177/00187267035612001

Australian Bureau of Statistics (ABS). (2013). *2011 census of population and housing* [Customised report]. ABS.

Beaglehole, R., Bonita, R., Horton, R., Adams, O. & McKee, M. (2004). Public health in the new era: Improving health through collective action. *Lancet, 363*, 2084–2086. https://doi.org/10.1016/S0140-6736(04)16461-1

Briggs, D. S. (2008). Shape declaration on the organisation and management of health services: A call for informed public debate. *Asia Pacific Journal Health Management, 3*(2), 10–13.

Briggs, D. S., Smyth, A. & Anderson, J. A. (2012). In search of capable health managers: What is distinctive about health management and why does it matter? *Asia Pacific Journal of Health Management, 7*(2), 71–78.

Czabanowska, K., Smith, T., Stankunas, M., Avery, M. & Otok, R. (2013). Transforming public health specialists into public health leaders. *Lancet, 381*, 449–450. https://doi.org/10.1016/S0140-6736(13)60246-9

Fayol, H. (1917). *Administration industrielle et générale: Prévoyance, organisation, commandement, coordination, contrôle* [French]. H. Dunod & E. Pinat.

Fulop, N., Allen, P., Clarke, A. & Black, N. (2001). Issues in studying the organisation and delivery of health services. In N. Fulop, P. Allen, A. Clarke & N. Black (eds), *Studying the organisation and delivery of health services: Research methods* (pp. 1–23). Routledge.

Gadolin, C., Skyvell Nilsson, M., Larsman, P., Pousette, A. & Törner, M. (2022). Managing health care under heavy stress: Effects of the COVID-19 pandemic on care unit managers' ability to support the nurses – A mixed-methods approach. *Journal of Nursing Management, 30*(8), 4080–4089.

Gomez-Mejia, L., McCann, R. C. & Page, R. C. (1985). The structure of managerial behaviours and rewards. *Industrial Relations, 24*, 147–154. https://doi.org/10.1111/j.1468-232X.1985.tb00986.x

Green, A., Collins, C. & Mirzoev, T. (2012). Management and planning for global health. In M. H. Merson, R. E. Black & A. J. Mills (eds), *Global health: Diseases, programs, systems, and policies* (3rd ed., pp. 653–706). Jones & Bartlett Learning.

Hunter, D. J. & Brown, J. (2007). A review of health management research. *European Journal of Public Health, 17*(Suppl 1), 33–7. https://doi.org/10.1093/eurpub/ckm061

Iles, P. & Preece, D. (2006). Developing leaders or developing leadership? The Academy of Chief Executives' programmes in the north east of England. *Leadership, 2*, 317–40. https://doi.org/10.1177/1742715006066024

Katz, R. L. (1955). Skills of an effective administrator. *Harvard Business Review, 33*(1), 33–42.

Kotter, J. P. (1990). What leaders really do. *Harvard Business Review, 68*(3), 103–111.

Lease, D. R. (2006). Management reviled: Is leadership just a good management repacked? Paper presented at the Academy of Business Education Conference, San Antonio, TX.

Lega, F., Prenestini, A. & Spurgeon, P. (2013). Is management essential to improving the performance and sustainability of health care systems and organisations? A systematic review and a roadmap for future studies. *Value in Health, 16*, S46–S51. https://doi.org/10.1016/j.jval.2012.10.004

Leggat, S. G., Smyth, A., Balding, C. & McAlpine, I. (2016). Equipping clinical leaders for system and service improvements in quality and safety: An Australian experience. *Australian and New Zealand Journal of Public Health, 40*(2), 138–43.

Liang, Z. & Howard, P. F. (2010). Competencies required by senior health executives in New South Wales, 1990–1999. *Australian Health Review, 34*, 52–8. https://doi.org/10.1071/AH09571

Longest, B. B., Rakich, J. S. & Darr, K. (2000). *Managing health services organizations and systems*. Health Professions.

Mahony, T. A., Jerdee, T. H. & Carroll, S. J. (1965). The job(s) of management. *Industrial Relations, 4*, 97–110. https://doi.org/10.1111/j.1468-232X.1965.tb00922.x

Martins, J. M. & Isouard, G. (2014). Health service managers in Australia: Progression and evolution. *Asia Pacific Journal of Health Management, 9*, 35–52. Retrieved from http://www.achsm.org.au

McAlearney, A. S. (2006). Leadership development in healthcare: A qualitative study. *Journal of Organizational Behavior, 27*, 967–82. https://doi.org/10.1002/job.417

McKenna, E. (1998). *Business psychology and organisational behaviour: A student's handbook*. Psychology.

Mumford, T. V., Campion, M. A. & Morgeson, F. P. (2007). The leadership skills strataplex: Leadership skill requirements across organizational levels. *Leadership Quarterly, 18*, 154–66. https://doi.org/10.1016/j.leaqua.2007.01.005

Northouse, P. G. (2013). *Leadership theory and practice* (6th ed.). Sage.

——— (2007). *Leadership: Theory and practice* (4th ed.). Sage.

Pham, T.N.M. (2021). The relationship between human resource management practices, work engagement and employee behavior: A case study in Vietnam. *The Journal of Asian Finance, Economics and Business, 8*(4), 1003–1012.

Rahim, M. A. (1988). The development of a leader power inventory. *Multivariate Behavioural Research, 23*, 491–502. https://doi.org/10.1207/s15327906mbr2304_6

Ravaghi, H., Beyranyand, T., Mannion, R., Aryankhesal, A. & Belorgeot, V.D. (2021). Effectiveness of training and educational programs for hospital managers: A systematic review. *Health Services Management Research, 34*(2), 113–126.

Rubino, L. (2011). Leadership. In S. B. Buchbinder & N. H. Shanks (eds), *Introduction to health care management* (pp. 17–38). Jones & Bartlett Learning.

Schriesheim, C. A., Hinkin, T. R. & Podsakoff, P. M. (1991). Can ipsative and single-item measures produce erroneous results in field studies of French and Raven's (1959) five bases of power? An empirical examination. *Journal of Applied Psychology, 76*, 106–114. https://doi.org/10.1037/0021-9010.76.1.106

Simpson, J. & Calman, K. (2000). Making and preparing leaders. *Medical Education*, *34*, 211–215. https://doi.org/10.1046/j.1365-2923.2000.0650a.x

Stankunas, M., Sauliune, S., Smith, T., Avery, M., Sumskas, L. & Czabanowska, K. (2012). Evaluation of leadership competencies of executives in Lithuanian public health institutions. *Medicina (Kaunas)*, *48*(11), 581–587.

Stogdill, R. M. (1974). *Handbook of leadership: A survey of theory and research*. Free.

Waddell, D., Devine, J., Jones, G. R. & George, J. M. (2009). *Contemporary management*. McGraw-Hill Australia.

World Health Organization (WHO). (2000). *The world health report 2000: Health systems; Improving performance*. WHO.

———— (1999). *Health21: The health for all policy framework for the WHO European region (European Health for All Series no. 6)*. Retrieved from http://www.euro.who.int/__data/assets/pdf_file/0010/98398/wa540ga199heeng.pdf?ua=1

Yukl, G. (2013). *Leadership in organizations* (8th ed.). Pearson Education.

———— (2010). *Leadership in organizations* (7th ed.). Pearson / Prentice Hall.

Zaleznik, A. (1977). Managers and leaders: Are they different? *Harvard Business Review*, *55*(3), 67–78.

Leading and managing: Frameworks and theories

2

Gary E. Day
With acknowledgement to Melanie Bish

Learning objectives

How do I:

- determine the most appropriate leadership style or approach to a given work situation?
- learn about how management theory has changed over time?
- consider the best way to develop my own leadership and management skills?
- integrate knowledge of leadership and management theory to inform future practice?

Introduction

Effective leadership and management can have a 'strong positive influence on workplace empowerment, increase nurses' job satisfaction and decrease the frequency of adverse patient outcomes' (Boamah, Laschinger, Wong & Clarke, 2018, p. 180). Healthcare professionals must understand the main theories of leadership and management and how these approaches translate into improving work practices so that they might develop their own work capacity. This chapter presents leadership and management theories used by healthcare professionals to inform their practice.

Definitions

Definitions that locate the concepts of leadership and management in a healthcare context are important. Leadership in healthcare receives attention from government, policy-makers, organisational managers, clinicians and researchers (Kean & Haycock-Stuart, 2011). To be effective, leadership must be appropriate for healthcare in its broadest sense, and issues must be addressed in their political, social, policy and economic contexts (Swearingen, 2009). Gopee and Galloway (2014, p. 65) identify four possible meanings of the term **leadership**:

1. the activity of leading
2. the body of people who lead a group
3. the status of the leader
4. the ability to lead.

Leadership: 'A process whereby an individual influences a group of individuals to achieve a common goal' (Northouse, 2013, p. 5)

The definition of leadership used in this book is 'a process whereby an individual influences a group of individuals to achieve a common goal' (Northouse, 2013, p. 5).

Management focuses on the organisation of people's endeavours as they work to achieve agreed goals that contribute to ensuring an organisation functions effectively and efficiently. A preference for approaches that emphasise employee empowerment is clear in current management practices, evidenced by a move away from hierarchical structures and the adaptation of contemporary leadership techniques.

Management: Planning, organising, leading and controlling resources to achieve an organisation's goals

Leadership theories

Evolvement

Leadership is a complex and multi-dimensional phenomenon that has 'taken on [even] greater importance in today's fast-paced and increasingly globalised world' (Benmira & Agboola, 2021, p. 3). Early **theories** focus on the characteristics and behaviours of successful leaders. In later theories, consideration of the role of followers and the context for leadership is evident. While many of the early theoretical constructs focus on an individualistic viewpoint of leadership and discuss the concept in relation to one person's actions (Bolden, Gosling, Marturano & Dennison, 2003; Martin, 2007), in recent years consideration of leadership concepts has moved to a shared, collective and collaborative approach (Benmira & Agboola,

Theory: An idea or group of ideas based on a set of principles to explain a phenomenon, account for a specific situation or underpin an approach to future actions

2021). Most of the research generated may be categorised into one of four main approaches (Yukl, 1989, as cited in Rowden, 1999, p. 30):

1. trait approaches
2. situational approaches
3. power–influence approaches
4. behavioural approaches.

Table 2.1 offers an overview of the evolution of leadership theories.

Table 2.1 Evolution of leadership theories

Era	Period	Theory	Leadership focus
Trait	1840s 1930s–1940s	Great man trait	The innate qualities of the leader Identifying attributes and features of effective leaders
Behavioural	1940s–1950s	Behavioural	The expertise and accomplishments of the leader
Situational	1960s	Contingent and situational	The leader's adaptability to different scenarios in the work setting
'New' leadership	1990s 1990s 2000s	Transactional Transformational Shared Collaborative Collective Servant Inclusive Complexity Adaptive Values-based	Leadership as a cost–benefit exchange Leadership that improves the skills, attitudes, aptitudes, capacity and achievements of employees Sharing power and influence with staff Leading staff across functions and organisational boundaries Leadership that brings together a range of skilled staff to meet organisational objectives Leadership that focuses on the needs of staff before that of the leader Diverse input of employees to help shape strategy, work systems and values Leadership that focuses on the complex relationships and interactions within an organisation Leadership that can distinguish between, and apply solutions, to adaptive and technical problems Leadership that draws on the shared beliefs, assumptions and values of the leader and the followers

Source: Adapted from Benmira & Agboola (2021).

Leadership theories in contemporary health care

'Healthcare organisations are social systems in which human resources are the most important factor. Leadership plays a key role, affecting outcomes for professionals, patients and work environment' (Specchia et al, 2021, p. 1). The COVID-19 pandemic of 2020–2022 stress-tested traditional leadership and management models. 'Traditional models of health leadership are characterized by top-down structures dependent on hierarchy – which emerged historically from military models. With supporting evidence, many of today's leaders are now working hard to shift their organizations to models of empowered teams ... with the hopes of inciting a broader cultural shift' (Smith & Bhavsar, 2021, p. 332). These components are essential in assisting all professionals to navigate their work in the complexities of the healthcare delivery context. Healthcare leaders may utilise a mixture of theories, models and conceptual **frameworks** to guide their conduct.

> **Framework:** A comprehensive resource to support and sustain practices by identifying parameters, creating a common language, including guiding principles and providing a prescriptive approach within which to work

Servant leadership

'Servant leadership is a form of moral-based leadership where leaders tend to prioritize the fulfillment of the needs of followers, namely employees, customers and other stakeholders, rather than satisfying their personal needs. Although the concept is not new among both academics and practitioners, it has received growing consideration in the last decade, due to the fact that it can positively affect a series of individual and organizational outcomes, such as job satisfaction and organizational commitment.' (Canavesi & Minelli, 2022, p. 267)

Servant leadership places emphasis on 'leadership as service' (Parris & Peachey, 2013; Sendjaya, Sarros & Santora, 2008; van Dierendonck, 2011), which relies heavily on 'relationship-orientated behaviours' (Northouse, 2009). Yoshida, Sendjaya, Hirst and Cooper (2013, as cited in Orazi et al., 2014, p. 39) describe it as 'a holistic approach to leadership that encompasses the rational, relational, emotional, moral, and spiritual dimension of the leader–follower relationship such that followers enhance and grow their capabilities', which results in the development of a greater sense of self-worth. This approach is suitable for leading multidisciplinary teams through change processes, as it relies on the establishment and maintenance of 'mutual trust and empowerment of followers' (Howatson-Jones, 2004, p. 22). Servant leadership supports the role of a values-based approach to leadership, as it promotes positive organisational and individual outcomes.

Transactional leadership

Transactional leadership remains useful as an approach to meeting short-term goals and completing tasks (Richards, 2020, p. 46). Characteristics of this approach are focused on the activities taking place at a daily operations level, with employee motivation being achieved through financial remuneration in exchange for services (Bass & Avolio, 1990).

A task-orientated style of leadership can have a positive influence on performance specifically, as an increased quality of internal communication through goal-setting, monitoring and feedback ensures that knowledge is generated to improve effectiveness and increase efficiencies (Bryant, 2003). The degree to which the leader and followers agree on the transactional aspects of the work equates to the level of the leader's positive influence on performance and organisational commitment, and on the degree of trust in the leader (Whittington, Coker, Goodwin, Ickes & Murray, 2009).

Transactional leaders operate well in structured environments, where goal-setting and efficient routines can lead to positive outcomes. Transactional leadership is effective in crisis situations, when a clear direction is needed for the common good and deviance is not tolerated (Orazi et al., 2014).

Transformational leadership

'Transformational leaders use various behaviors to produce organizationally beneficial behaviors (e.g., better task performance and helping behaviors) through ignition of followers' work engagement. That is, employees who inspired by transformational leadership are more likely to immerse themselves in the work, and, in turn, this is likely to result in better task performance and helping behaviors' (Lai, Tang, Lu, Lee & Lin, 2020, p. 1).

During times in which retaining and attracting suitable staff are critical to organisational success and patient care, transformational leadership is positively correlated to worker job satisfaction, reduced burnout, staff retention and increased patient safety (Perez, 2021; Hussain & Khayat, 2021; Robbins, 2020; Bosak, Kilroy, Chênevert & Flood, 2021; Ree & Wiig, 2019). Leaders who use a transformational style of leadership engage peers across periods of change and prioritise the provision of resources needed to achieve goals (Hocker & Trofino, 2003), which makes the approach suitable in organisations requiring change, development, initiative and creativity in turbulent and uncertain environments (Bass & Avolio, 1990). During the COVID-19 pandemic, 'anxiety weakened the influence of core transformational leadership behaviors and intellectual stimulation on well-being'; however, transformational leadership practices proved to have resilient effects on staff (McCombs & Williams, 2021, p. 1254). Collaborative decision-making, mentoring, a patient focus and the use of ethical frameworks are all supported by transformational leadership (Hocker & Trofino, 2003).

The approach of the transformational leader encourages an evolvement of the basic values, beliefs and attitudes of followers in ways that inform their approach to work, which result in a greater level of empowerment to achieve the vision and mission of the organisation. The benefits are visible in a greater level of productivity, heightened employee morale and positive personal and professional growth (Gopee & Galloway, 2014).

Charismatic leadership

In early studies of charismatic leaders, charisma was defined as the particular persona of an individual that sets them apart and, as a consequence, sees them treated as the host of some exceptional qualities (Weber, 1947). The qualities credited to charismatic leadership may also be attributed to transformational leadership, and include refined interpersonal skills, self-confidence, courage, the ability to imagine different and better futures, the ability to communicate vision, and a willingness to take risks (Taylor, 2007a). Charismatic leaders demonstrate a preference for relationship-oriented behaviours (Northouse, 2009). They are highly motivated leaders characterised by a confidence in their skills and a disposition that projects determination and inspires followers to cope in times of uncertainty. In this sense, charismatic leaders are entrepreneurial, make sacrifices and take risks to achieve what they believe is the most beneficial outcome for the organisation (Orazi et al., 2014).

A leadership style that often emerges in times of crisis, charismatic leadership has the capacity to generate excitement, enthusiasm and loyalty while exhibiting the skills required to carry out the identified tasks (Taylor, 2007b). Charismatic leadership styles have also been shown to motivate individuals to be more engaged and to exhibit more organisational citizenship behaviours (Horn, Mathis, Robinson & Randle, 2021). Given the investment required of those who opt for this leadership style, concern exists about their ability to retain its enchantment over a sustained period, strengthening the argument that organisations are more effective if they invest in the development of leadership capacity across all levels of staff (Conger & Kanungo, 1988).

Authentic leadership

Regarded as being in the formative phase of development and a newcomer to leadership research, authentic leadership is highly desirable in a period in which people are seeking genuine and trustworthy leaders (Northouse, 2013). It suggests that to be able to lead, individuals must be true to themselves and to their guiding values system, or set of principles, and must act in accordance with them in a consistent manner (Marquis & Huston, 2015).

Authentic leaders have distinguishing characteristics that include understanding of their own purpose through ongoing self-reflection, consistency between their beliefs and actions, genuine compassion for their followers, strong connections and practices of self-discipline through striving for professional and personal balance (Shirey, 2006). Authentic styles of leadership have been shown to have positive outcomes on hospital performance and patient care quality (Aboramadan, Alolayyan, Turkmenoglu, Cicek & Farao, 2021; Puni & Hilton, 2020). A high level of self-knowledge, commitment to enhancing their own leadership capacity and engagement in an interpersonal process with colleagues to nurture skills in others feature in this style of leadership (Northouse, 2013; Shirey, 2006).

Clear benefits of authentic leadership are the inspiration and excitement it can generate in others to achieve a level of performance that is regarded as success. Such success confers benefits at the individual and organisational levels. It results in favourable personal outcomes that may include feelings of self-efficacy and job satisfaction, which create increased organisational commitment, with the positive organisational outcomes verified by growth, meeting of financial targets and fulfilment of a service need (Shirey, 2006). Staff benefit from authentic leaders who show transparency in their leadership and display a commitment to their espoused values, actions and behaviours (Luthans & Avolio, 2003).

E-leadership

The introduction of advanced information technology in healthcare organisations is changing the approach to healthcare leadership (Avolio & Kahai, 2003) and, given the continuing growth and application of information technology in the healthcare sector, theorists suggest that e-leadership will become routine rather than the exception in organisational leadership (Zaccaro & Bader, 2003). E-leadership and the rise of virtual teams became synonymous with the COVID-19 pandemic in 2020. Leaders had to adapt to the new ways of working and managing their teams. Kashive, Khanna & Powale (2022) argue that communication quality is critical for the relationship between internal and external leadership roles and trust. Additionally, for e-leadership to be successful, role clarity is essential in the relationship between external leadership roles and conflict. 'Internal and external leadership roles showed a significant effect on leadership effectiveness, which were further related to team performance in virtual teams' (p. 277).

> Thriving in remote work environments implies that [health] managers must adjust the organisation's structure, making them less hierarchical, and developing new abilities to establish a strong and trustworthy relationship with their employees to maintain their competitiveness, while retaining a genuine concern for their employees' well-being. Similarly, successful e-leadership must be able to consolidate and lead effective virtual teams to accomplish organisational goals. (Contreras, Baykal & Abid, 2020, p 135)

Leaders and followers have a greater level of access to information and to each other, which is changing the nature and content of their interactions. The purpose of e-leadership is to enhance the relationships among organisational members that are defined by an organisation's structure (Avolio & Kahai, 2003).

The challenges facing leaders who operate in circumstances in which communication is no longer an interaction in person extend to building trust, maintaining open lines of communication and being open to subtle cues of concern (Barr & Dowding, 2012). Leaders adopting this approach are encouraged to facilitate communication and provide opportunities for shared learning (Avolio & Kahai, 2003).

Management theories

Skilled management has significant positive effects on productivity, profitability and the ability of organisations to adapt and change to meet emerging challenges. To achieve this in healthcare services, approaches to management need to be based on investment in skills, opportunities for employee engagement in the workplace and quality positions that provide incentives for employees to contribute (Orazi et al., 2014). In their practice, healthcare managers may use a combination of the theories discussed in this section.

Evolvement

During the Industrial Revolution, Frederick Winslow Taylor developed the four principles of scientific management that, if adhered to, would see productivity increase (see following). The works of Henri Fayol and Max Weber, produced in the late 19th and early 20th centuries, sought to combine theory with practice in addressing the fundamental issue of how organisations should be structured (Wren & Bedeian, 2009). The 'management functions of planning, organisation, command, coordination and control' were first identified by Henri Fayol (1925). These were expanded by Luther Gulick (1937) with the introduction of the seven activities of management: planning, organising, staffing, directing, coordinating, reporting and budgeting (Marquis & Huston, 2015).

A shift occurred during the 1920s, when the focus turned to people rather than equipment. Several theories were generated in the human relations era, including participative management, the Hawthorne effect, Theory X and Theory Y, and employee participation (Marquis & Huston, 2015).

The evolution of management approaches
Scientific management

A branch of the classical management perspective, scientific management theory proposes that efficiency and labour productivity are improved by scientifically determined jobs and management practices. Applying the four principles of management developed by Fredrick Winslow Taylor in the late 1800s, scientific management aims to improve the performance of individual workers using analytical procedures to increase workplace efficiency (Daft & Marcic, 2013). Taylor's (1911, pp. 12–77) four principles of management are:

1. Develop a science for each element of the job to replace the old rule-of-thumb method.
2. Scientifically select employees and then train, teach and develop them to do their jobs.
3. Supervise employees to ensure that the work is completed in accordance with the prescribed methods for doing their jobs.
4. Divide the work and responsibility almost equally between managers and employees.

Organisational behaviour

Contemporary views on motivation, leadership, trust, teamwork and conflict management are informed by research on organisational behaviour (Robbins, Bergman, Stagg & Coulter, 2011), which addresses individual, group and organisational processes in terms of the effect of the individual on the organisation and the effect of the organisation on the individual (Davidson & Griffin, 2006). Advocates of this approach believe that people are the most important asset of an organisation and should be managed accordingly. Theorists' work in this area has served as a foundation for management practices such as employee-selection procedures and employee-motivation programs (Robbins et al., 2011).

Hawthorne effect

A series of studies conducted in the 1920s and 1930s by the Hawthorne Works, at the Western Electric Company in Chicago, provide insight into individual and group behaviours (Mayo, 1953). Experiments established that psychological factors are important variables in worker output and that the need for social acceptance affects output more than financial incentive (Davidson & Griffin, 2006). There is some debate concerning the rigour of several of the studies, but there is consensus that their importance in stimulating interest in seeing employees as more than extensions of production machinery far outweighs how academically sound the research was (Daft & Marcic, 2013). The studies are viewed as having had a significant effect on management beliefs about the role of human behaviour in organisations (Robbins et al., 2011). They identified the need for a new paradigm of management thought and have led to managers being equipped to handle the human element in the workplace (Davidson & Griffin, 2006).

Human relations movement

Instigated by the findings of the Hawthorne studies, the human relations movement is based on the notion that a person has control over themselves, as opposed to an authoritarian approach (Daft & Marcic, 2013). The importance of employee satisfaction resulting in improved performance is advanced by the philosophies of Abraham Maslow and Douglas McGregor.

Maslow (1943) observed that individuals' problems often stem from an inability to satisfy their needs. He created a hierarchy of needs, starting with psychological needs and progressing to safety, belonging, esteem and self-actualisation needs. The theory remains influential in contemporary approaches to management (Daft & Marcic, 2013).

McGregor's (1960) work challenges the classical perspective and human-relations assumptions about human behaviour through Theory X and Theory Y, which specify the extreme attitudinal position held by managers. Theory X represents the negative view of workers consistent with scientific management, and Theory Y the positive approach, which aligns with the human-relations perspective. McGregor advocates a Theory Y approach to managing people (Davidson & Griffin, 2006).

Systems approach

In the 1960s, attention turned to analysing organisations from a **systems** perspective, generating a theory that focuses on systems and how they work and function within an organisation. The relationships between the parts are seen as equally important as the properties of the parts themselves (Davidson & Griffin, 2006).

Organisations are viewed as being composed of interdependent factors that include, but are not limited to, individuals, groups, attitudes, goals, motives, formal structure, status and authority. The approach argues that managers need to coordinate the work of various parts of their organisation and to ensure that all of its interdependent parts are working together so that the organisation's goals are achieved (Robbins et al., 2011). Managers are also encouraged to understand the synergy of the whole organisation rather than just its separate elements so that the organisation is managed as a whole (Daft & Marcic, 2013).

System: 'A set of interrelated and interdependent parts arranged in a manner that produces a unified whole' (Robbins et al., 2011, p. 56)

MANAGING A HOSPITAL WITH A SYSTEMS APPROACH: LESSONS FROM THE COVID-19 PANDEMIC

A large public hospital, dealing with an influx of acutely unwell COVID-19 patients, exemplifies how the systems approach to management is used. Consider the role of the hospital coordinator when a large number of unwell patients suffering acute 'flu-like symptoms arrive at the emergency department by ambulance and private vehicles. The assessments at triage reveal multiple patients in respiratory distress requiring admission. The intensive care ward is currently over capacity with ventilated COVID-19 patients, and the medical wards are full with less acute patients. In addition, there is a dwindling supply of PPE equipment and medical gases, the hospital is struggling to source enough suitably trained and qualified staff, rosters are being stretched to cover larger-than-usual occurrences levels of sick leave due to quarantine requirements, thus necessitating the redirection of non-COVID patients to other facilities, and there is pressure on the pathology, pharmacy and medical stores departments to provide timely results and medical supplies. To ensure the delivery of quality and safe care, the management of these patients will require the coordination of several departments. The hospital coordinator must understand the respective units throughout the organisation that will need to be engaged, and that:

- There must be enough vacant beds in the respective units (intensive care, cardiac care) to admit the patients.
- All non-critical patients need to be discharged or transferred to other suitable facilities so that acute COVID-19 patients can be accommodated.
- The operating suite will need to have a theatre vacant to deal with the emergency cases, and all non-urgent cases have to be rescheduled.

> ## MANAGING A HOSPITAL WITH A SYSTEMS APPROACH: LESSONS FROM THE COVID-19 PANDEMIC Continued
>
> - The necessary qualified staff must be on shift to care for the patients.
> - Additional training and support must be provided to nursing staff caring for ventilated patients in the general ward area.
> - Emotional support and leadership must be provided for stressed staff.
>
> This scenario also provides an example of how hospital units need to work together to achieve a common goal of safe care for patients and a safe working environment for staff. A hospital should be viewed, from a management perspective, as an entire integrated system, rather than as a series of independent departments.

Situational management

Situational management takes the position that there is no singular management theory that has universal application, as there are always numerous factors that are specific to each situation and that will directly influence organisational performance. As there is no optimal state in any organisation, the management approach used and its success are dependent upon the nature of the task that needs to be undertaken or the situation that needs to be dealt with at a particular point in time and under prevailing environmental circumstances (Gopee & Galloway, 2014). Known also as the contingency approach, this theory is widely adopted in the healthcare sector. Wu and colleagues (2020) outline perfectly the use of situational management during the COVID-19 pandemic, whereby the nursing management team 'effectively mobilized all available manpower [sic]; secondly, up-skilled and trained personnel within a very short period of time; thirdly, provided reliable logistical support for front-line protection equipments; and finally, motivated nurses during this very difficult time to make a significant positive contribution to the fight against pandemic' (p. 1).

Summary

- Leadership and management theories are broad constructs with variation in definitions to suit the context and purpose.
- The study of leadership has progressed from broad conceptualisations of traits and behaviours of leaders to an approach that focuses on the sphere of influence and the development of interdependent relationships to influence the culture of a workplace.
- The effectiveness and efficiency of services are influenced by the application of leadership and management theories.
- Healthcare professionals may use a combination of different leadership and management theories in their practice.

Reflective questions

1. Why is it so important to underpin practice with theory?
2. What do you think needs to feature in future leadership and management theory for them to be relevant to health professionals?
3. Based on the content of this chapter and your experience, what do you perceive to be the strengths and weaknesses of transactional leadership?
4. With which of the leadership theories presented are you aligned?
5. Can you identify the leadership theory that underpins the conduct of one of your colleagues?

Self-analysis question

How does your leadership style affect your colleagues? Provide examples.

References

Aboramadan, M., Alolayyan, M. N., Turkmenoglu, M. A., Cicek, B. & Farao, C. (2021). Linking authentic leadership and management capability to public hospital performance: The role of work engagement, *International Journal of Organizational Analysis*, *29*(5), 1350–1370. https://doi.org/10.1108/IJOA-10-2020-2436

Avolio, B. J. & Kahai, S. S. (2003). Adding the 'E' to E-leadership: How it may impact your leadership. *Organizational Dynamics*, *31*(4), 325–338. https://doi.org/10.1016/S0090-2616(02)00133-X

Barr, J. & Dowding, L. (2012). *Leadership in health care* (2nd ed.). Sage.

Bass, B. & Avolio, B. (1990). The implications of transactional and transformational leadership for individual, team and organizational development. In R. W. Woodman & W. A. Passmore (eds), *Research in organizational change and development* (Vol. 4, pp. 231–272). JAI.

Benmira, S. & Agboola, M. (2021). Evolution of leadership theory. *BMJ Leader*, 5:3–5.

Boamah, S. A., Laschinger, H. K. S., Wong, C. & Clarke, S. (2018). Effect of transformational leadership on job satisfaction and patient safety outcomes. *Nursing Outlook*, *66*(2), 180–189. https://doi.org/10.1016/j.outlook.2017.10.004

Bolden, R., Gosling, J., Marturano, A. & Dennison, P. (2003). *A review of leadership theory and competency frameworks* (Edited version of a report for Chase Consulting and the Management Standards Centre). Retrieved from: https://ore.exeter.ac.uk/repository/handle/10036/17494

Bosak, J., Kilroy, S., Chênevert, D. & Flood, P. C. (2021). Examining the role of transformational leadership and mission valence on burnout among hospital staff. *Journal of Organizational Effectiveness: People and Performance*, *8*(2), 208–227. https://doi.org/10.1108/JOEPP-08-2020-0151

Bryant, S. E. (2003). The role of transformational and transactional leadership in creating, sharing and exploiting organizational knowledge. *Journal of Leadership & Organizational Studies*, *9*(4), 32–44. https://doi.org/10.1177/107179190300900403

Canavesi, A. & Minelli, E. (2022). Servant leadership: A systematic literature review and network analysis. *Employee Responsibilities and Rights Journal*, *34*, 267–289. https://doi.org/10.1007/s10672-021-09381-3

Conger, J. A. & Kanungo, R. N. (1988). *Charismatic leadership: The elusive factor in organizational effectiveness*. Jossey-Bass.

Contreras, F., Baykal, E. & Abid, G. (2020). E-Leadership and teleworking in times of COVID-19 and beyond: What we know and where do we go. *Frontiers in Psychology, 11*. https://doi.org/10.3389/fpsyg.2020.590271

Daft, R. L. & Marcic, D. (2013). *Management: A new workplace*. South-Western Cengage Learning.

Davidson, P. & Griffin, R. W. (2006). *Management* (3rd Australasian ed.). Wiley.

Fayol, H. (1925). *General and industrial management*. Pittman.

Gopee, N. & Galloway, J. (2014). *Leadership & management in health care* (2nd ed.). Sage.

Gulick, L. (1937). Notes on the theory of the organisation. In L. Gulick & L. Urwick (eds), *Papers on the science of administration* (pp. 3–13). Institute of Public Administration.

Hocker, S. M. & Trofino, J. (2003). Transformation leadership: The development of a model of nursing case management by the army nurse corps. *Lippincott's Case Management, 8*(5), 208–213. https://doi.org/10.1097/00129234-200309000-00006

Horn, D., Mathis, C. J., Robinson, S. L. & Randle, N. (2021). Is charismatic leadership effective when workers are pressured to be good citizens? *Journal of Psychology, 149*(8), 751–774. https://doi.org/10.1080/00223980.2014.978253

Howatson-Jones, I.L. (2004). The servant leader. *Nursing Management, 11*(3), 20–24. https://doi.org/10.7748/nm2004.06.11.3.20.c1978

Hussain, M. K. & Khayat, R. A. M. (2021). The impact of transformational leadership on job satisfaction and organisational commitment among hospital staff: A systematic review. *Journal of Health Management, 23*(4). https://doi.org/10.1177/0972063421105504

Kashive, N., Khanna, V. T. & Powale, L. (2022). Virtual team performance: E-leadership roles in the era of COVID-19. *Journal of Management Development, 41*(5), 277–300. https://doi.org/10.1108/JMD-05-2021-0151

Kean, S. & Haycock-Stuart, E. (2011). Understanding the relationship between followers and leaders. *Journal of Nursing Management, 18*(8), 31–35. https://doi.org/10.7748/nm2011.12.18.8.31.c8843

Lai, F., Tang, H., Lu, S., Lee, Y. & Lin, C. (2020). Transformational leadership and job performance: The mediating role of work engagement. *Sage Open, 10*(1). https://doi.org/10.1177/2158244019899085

Luthans, F. & Avolio, B. J. (2003). Authentic leadership: A positive developmental approach. In K. S. Cameron, J. E. Dutton & R. E. Quinn (eds), *Positive organizational scholarship* (pp. 241–261). Berrett-Koehler.

Marquis, B. L. & Huston, C. J. (2015). *Leadership roles and management functions in nursing theory and application* (8th ed.). Wolters Kluwer.

Martin, A. (2007). The future of leadership: Where do we go from here? *Industrial and Commercial Training, 39*(1), 3–8. https://doi.org/10.1108/00197850710721345

Maslow, A. (1943). A theory of human motivation. *Psychological Review*, (July), 370–96.

Mayo, E. (1953). *The human problems of an industrial civilization*. Macmillan.

McCombs, K. & Williams, E. (2021). The resilient effects of transformational leadership on well-being: Examining the moderating effects of anxiety during the COVID-19 crisis. *Leadership & Organization Development Journal, 42*(8), 1254–1266. https://doi.org/10.1108/LODJ-02-2021-0092

McGregor, D. (1960). *The human side of enterprise*. McGraw-Hill.

Northouse, P. G. (2013). *Leadership: Theory and practice* (6th ed.). Sage.

——— (2009). *Leadership: Theory and practice* (5th ed.). Sage.

Orazi, D., Good, L., Robin, M., van Wanrooy, B., Butar, I., Olsen, J. & Gahan, P. (2014). *Workplace Leadership: A Review Of Prior Research*. Retrieved from: https://research.aib.edu.au/en/publications/workplace-leadership-a-review-of-prior-research

Parris, D. L. & Peachey, J. W. (2013). A systematic literature review of servant leadership theory in organizational contexts. *Journal of Business Ethics*, 113, 377–393. doi.org/10.1007/s10551-012-1322-6

Perez, J. (2021). Leadership in healthcare: Transitioning from clinical professional to healthcare leader. *Journal of Healthcare Management, 66*(4), 280–302. https://doi.org/10.1097/JHM-D-20-00057

Puni, A. & Hilton, S. K. (2020). Dimensions of authentic leadership and patient care quality. *Leadership in Health Services, 33*(4), 365–383. https://doi.org/10.1108/LHS-11-2019-0071

Ree, E. & Wiig, S. (2019). Linking transformational leadership, patient safety culture and work engagement in home care services. *Nursing Open, 7*(1), 256–264. https://doi.org/10.1002/nop2.386

Richards, A. (2020). Exploring the benefits and limitations of transactional leadership in healthcare. *Nursing Standard, 35*(12), 46–50. https://doi.org/10.7748/ns.2020.e11593

Robbins, B. (2020). Transformational leadership in health care today. *The Health Care Manager, 39*(3), 117–121. https://doi.org/10.1097/HCM.0000000000000296

Robbins, S., Bergman, R., Stagg, I. & Coulter, M. (2011). *Foundations of management* (Vol. 6). Pearson Education.

Rowden, R. W. (1999). The relationship between charismatic leadership behaviors and organizational commitment. *Leadership & Organizational Development Journal, 21*(1), 30–35. https://doi.org/10.1108/01437730010310712

Sendjaya, S., Sarros, J. C. & Santora, J. C. (2008). Defining and measuring servant leadership behavior. *Journal of Management Studies, 45*, 402–423. http://dx.doi.org/10.1111/j.1467-6486.2007.00761.x

Shirey, M. R. (2006). Building authentic leadership and enhancing entrepreneurial performance. *Clinical Nurse Specialist, 20*(6), 280–282. https://doi.org/10.1097/00002800-200611000-00007

Smith, K. & Bhavsar, M. (2021). A new era of health leadership. *Healthcare management Forum, 34*(6), 332–335. https://doi.org/10.1177/08404704211040817

Specchia, M. L., Cozzolino, M. R., Carini, E., Di Pilla, A., Galletti, C., Ricciardi, W. & Damiani, G. (2021). Leadership styles and nurses' job satisfaction. Results of a systematic review. *International Journal of Environmental Research and Public Health, 18*, 1552. https://doi.org/10.3390/ijerph18041552

Swearingen, S. (2009). A journey to leadership: Designing a nursing leadership development program. *Journal of Continuing Education in Nursing, 40*, 107–114. https://doi.org/10.3928/00220124-20090301-02

Taylor, F. W. (1911). *The principles of scientific management*. Harper & Row.

Taylor, V. (2007a). Leadership for service improvement (part 1). *Nursing Management, 13*(9), 30–34. https://doi.org/10.7748/nm2007.02.13.9.30.c4337

——— (2007b) Leadership for service improvement: Part 3. *Nursing Management, 14*(1), 28–32. https://doi.org/10.7748/nm2007.04.14.1.28.c4342

van Dierendonck, D. (2011). Servant leadership: A review and synthesis. *Journal of Management, 37*(4), 1228–1261. https://doi.org/10.1177/0149206310380462

Weber, M. (1947). *The theory of social and economic organization*. Free.

Whittington, J. L., Coker, R. H., Goodwin, V. L., Ickes, W. & Murray, B. (2009). Transactional leadership revisited: Self-other agreement and its consequences. *Journal of Applied Social Psychology, 39*(8), 1860–1886. https://doi.org/10.1111/j.1559-1816.2009.00507.x

Wren, D. A. & Bedeian, A. G. (2009). *The evolution of management thought* (6th ed.). Wiley.

Wu, X., Zheng, S., Huang, J., Zheng, Z., Xu, M. & Zhou, Y. (2020). Contingency nursing management in designated hospitals during COVID-19 outbreak. *Annals of Global Health, 86*(1):70, 1–5. https://doi.org/10.5334/aogh.2918.

Zaccaro, S. J. & Bader, P. (2003). E-leadership and the challenges of leading e-teams: Minimizing the bad and maximizing the good. *Organizational Dynamics, 31*(4), 377–387. https://doi.org/10.1016/S0090-2616(02)00129-8

Part 2
Leads Self

3 Leading ethically

Gian Luca Casali and Gary E. Day

Learning objectives

How do I:

- understand the importance of ethics in the health manager's decision-making process?
- understand the different perspectives of the four schools of moral philosophy and how they can influence a health manager's decision-making?
- understand the concepts of moral courage and whistleblowing?
- identify the main factors that influence ethical decision-making?
- identify the eight steps in the decision-making framework?

Introduction

This chapter explores the notion of ethics and ethical decision-making frameworks in leading and managing health services. Chapter 1 outlined the four sets of skills, or functions, that every manager should possess, which are usually summarised under the acronym POLC: planning, organising, leading and controlling. With leadership being one of the four functions of management, it is important to understand both the management and the leadership aspects of ethical decision-making.

Ethical decision-making

For managers, ethical decision-making incorporates the development and dissemination of frameworks to assist staff to make decisions in line with the organisation's direction and values, ensuring current staff understand these frameworks and recruiting staff who will work within the frameworks. For leaders, **ethical decision-making** is about taking action when it is needed, guiding others in working through difficult and complex decision-making processes and being a role model for other staff.

Ethical decision-making: Decisions that consider values, morals and norms

New managers in the healthcare system face multiple and sometimes competing frameworks that guide management practice. These may include managerial ethical frameworks, clinical decision-making frameworks and, in some cases, religious frameworks. All of these may come into play regarding single or multiple issues, increasing the complexity in finding an acceptable ethical solution that satisfies all of the competing values, including those of the patient.

Health managers face many challenges in today's work environment, which is characterised by rapid changes, globalisation, tough competition and higher demands for socially responsible healthcare provision. In such a complex and uncertain milieu, managers must make decisions affecting not only their organisation, their personal career, their patients and their families, but also the wider community. Achieving an understanding of how those decisions are made is vital.

Research has shown that the likelihood of making unethical decisions in the workplace is relatively high, particularly during the COVID-19 pandemic. In Australia and Aotearoa New Zealand, results from KPMG's (2020) fraud survey of senior executives found that:

- 83 per cent of respondents believed the organisation was vulnerable to fraud taking place in the new environment.
- Issues driving a rise in fraud and corruption during the COVID-19 era were distracted businesses not focusing on controls (75%); remote working (69%) and IT systems limitations (40%).
- 42 per cent of executives said their organisation had to delay fraud and corruption prevention programs due to COVID-19.
- The biggest threats to the organisation were suppliers (67%), employees (67%) and contractors (41%).

Even if these results reflect the actions of only a few bad managers or staff, those unethical behaviours were widely visible to others and were likely to have influenced decision-making within the organisational culture that allowed them to exist. These statistics present a challenge to those wanting to promote virtuous or ethical management behaviour in organisations.

Despite best efforts to address the problem by introducing so-called codes of ethics or codes of conduct into organisational cultures (St John, 2016), unethical practice can and does still occur. While good regulations and sound organisational practices are important, ethics goes beyond good rules and good practices; it involves the ability to make value-based judgements appropriate to personal and professional identities and situational contexts, both regular and irregular.

Creating and sustaining procedural uniformity when dealing with ethical issues in organisations is a near-impossible task. Ethical decision-making at the managerial level remains highly individualised work even when it necessitates collaboration, as the manager is often the one responsible for getting people together and facilitating groups to discuss problems, as well as for monitoring and evaluating outcomes. In completing their tasks, managers are subjected to a wide range of influences; they can react differently to diverse situations, and even if they are not guided by commitments to contrasting ethical principles, they may still prioritise them in varying ways.

A preference for a particular ethical approach is only one of the factors that can influence a decision-maker, and all the individual differences that arise from the variable influences of these factors can increase complexity and uncertainty in an organisation, especially when it comes to predicting behaviour. Recently, organisations have introduced codes of ethics and codes of conduct as tools to minimise the likelihood of staff engaging in unethical behaviours. However, just because organisations provide staff with codes of ethics or conduct, this is no guarantee that they will consider these documents in their decision-making (McNamara, Smith & Murphy-Hill, 2018; Casali & Perano, 2021). The mere introduction of a code of ethics without taking into consideration these individual differences, then, could be detrimental for the organisation. Instead of achieving a higher degree of consistency across the organisation when facing ethical situations, codes could create more conflict between staff, as they will inevitably differ in their interpretations of the codes and the situations to which they are to be applied. The factors influencing these differing responses are embedded in each individual manager and are open to investigation.

Influential factors

Heuristic: An individual procedure, guideline or rule of thumb developed to assist people in solving complex problems (Bazerman, 2012)

Individual responses in the decision-making process are the results of numerous factors that have contributed to the creation of the personality of the person making the decision, and more specifically to their particular predispositions (or **heuristics**). It is not possible, for example, to separate nationality from the individual. But then, an individual from a particular ethnic background could act differently from another individual from the same ethnic background because of other factors, in addition to cultural norms and values that have contributed to the development of the two individuals' characters.

Bazerman (2012) defines heuristics as individual procedures, guidelines or 'rules of thumbs' developed to assist people in solving complex problems. 'Management practitioners often preconsciously rely on simple heuristics when approaching ill-structured decision problems ... Practitioners in organisations often make decisions under high uncertainty and pressure to maintain legitimacy, professionalism and speed' (Stingl & Geraldi, 2021, para 88). As a result, when solving a problem, they tend to rely upon those principles and constructs that are embedded in them, rather than engaging in a totally new decision-making process. The various factors that contribute to people's predispositions and influence their decision-making are discussed in the sections following.

Ethical factors

The first group of factors that affect individuals' ability to make decisions can be described as ethical or moral – that is, beliefs about right and wrong. **Morality** can be taken to mean 'moral judgments, standards and rules of conduct' (Ferrell, Fraedrich & Ferrell, 2005, p. 5) or 'the principles, norms, and standards of conduct governing an individual or group' (Trevino & Nelson, 2007, p. 13).

In general, people hold different sets of values, morals and norms; however, they all involve a claim that one ought to act in a certain way. Due to this normative propensity, ethics and morality tend to be constructed of shared understandings, which are responsive to the demands of certain contexts. Being socially and historically embedded, the quest for shared understandings has led to the creation of various schools of moral philosophy. In everyday decision-making, we knowingly and unknowingly tend to draw on these philosophies.

Four major schools of moral philosophy have been used to profile the expression of morality in ethical decision-making: **egoism, utilitarianism, virtue ethics** and **deontology**. These cover a spectrum of ethical styles, from a focus on consequences (utilitarianism and egoism), through a focus on the moral traits within people that are developed from habit and education over time (virtue ethics), to a focus on universal principles and duties that ought to be applied in all like circumstances (deontology) (Ferrell, Fraedrich & Ferrell, 2008; Trevino & Nelson, 2007).

The main difference between utilitarian and egoistic philosophies is one of scope. Utilitarians are concerned with creating the greatest good for the greatest number, while egoists commit to maximising the good for themselves alone. A similar difference of scope could be said to apply to deontology and virtue ethics. Deontologists focus on universal rights and duties, while virtue ethicists focus on the embodiment of virtues in the individual. These traits are acquired through learning and habits.

In the past, the virtue ethics approach has been most closely aligned with professional life when practitioners are trained in groups under apprentice-like conditions (such as nurses and doctors) but go on to practise mainly as individuals. In such a setting, codes of ethics expressing universal principles are also important, but until recently greater emphasis has been placed on the character and integrity of the practitioner and their ability to interpret the application of those rules independently.

Morality: The standards, principles and rules that govern an individual's or a group's conduct

Egoism: A doctrine that maximises the greatest good or benefit for the individual

Utilitarianism: A doctrine that maximises the greatest good for the greatest number of people

Virtue ethics: A system that focuses on the embodiment of virtues in the individual

Deontology: An ethical theory that applies universal principles and duties in all similar circumstances

THE ETHICAL DILEMMA

An ethical dilemma emerges for a health manager steeped in egoism when facing a decision about patient prioritisation. The manager, driven by personal career ambitions, may be tempted to allocate resources disproportionately to high-profile cases that boost their department's success metrics and the manager's reputation. This egoistic approach conflicts with the ethical principle of patient equality. Balancing personal gains against equitable patient care requires the manager to confront their egoistic motives and consider the greater good. Upholding ethical standards demands that decisions prioritise patients based on medical need rather than personal career gains, navigating the fine line between self-interest and the ethical responsibility inherent in healthcare management.

There is animated debate in ethics over whether the focus should be on applying universal principles to all situations or on finding principles appropriate for each situation – in short, whether one should subscribe to an absolutist or a pluralist viewpoint. Both sides have strong supporting arguments.

A large portion of the current literature on ethical decision-making is based on Lawrence Kohlberg's (1979) cognitive moral development (or CMD) model (for example, Lind, 1995; Rest, 1979). Cognitive moral development is a theory that divides respondents into different categories based on their individual level of moral development. Typically, however, each respondent can belong to only one stage at any given time, reflecting the absolutist view. Thus, if a person strongly identifies with only one school of morality, or has reached a certain level of moral development, they will mostly adopt principles and criteria from that approach or level in reaching an ethical decision. The problem with this approach is the underlying assumption that individuals fit perfectly into only one level or school. In reality, it seems more plausible that individuals could belong to different levels or schools in different situations, or that even in the same situation they could act as a result of a combination of different levels or schools. With this approach, a person will reach an ethical decision by using a mix of principles from more than one school of moral philosophy or level of moral development. To reduce the likelihood of preconceived bias towards an absolutist approach, the framework for managerial ethical decision-making proposed later in this chapter has been developed in such a way that it is flexible enough to capture a continuum of responses, from absolutism to pluralism.

For health managers, insisting on what is right requires perseverance. An important concept that has been supported recently, particularly in the nursing literature, is that of **moral courage** (Sadooghiasl, Parvizy & Ebadi, 2016; Khoshmehr, Barkhordari-Sharifabad, Nasiriani & Fallahzadeh, 2020; Pajakoski, Rannikko, Leino-Kilpi & Numminen, 2021). In ancient Greek epics, the term 'courage' was explained as the bravery that a person possesses, and it was illustrated in heroes' fearlessness about death so long as their values were put first. In a less heroic but more professional context, moral courage can be displayed by managers who stand by their values despite there being a cost in doing so. Kidder (2005) defines moral courage as being at the intersection of three acts: applying values, recognising risks and enduring the hardship. The last of these is the essential component of moral courage.

Moral courage: A quality of mind that enables individuals to stand by their values despite personal or professional cost

A commonly understood example of moral courage is the concept of **whistleblowing**, the term used to describe the actions of employees who go outside their workplace to publicly disclose organisational malpractices such as fraud, theft, corruption, resource wastage, negligence (including medical negligence), misrepresentation and major safety violations. Whistleblowing demonstrates a high level of morale courage. Although whistleblowers are afforded protection under federal and state legislation, and while a whistleblower in a healthcare organisation may do the right thing by a patient or the organisation by revealing serious problems or breaches of policy or protocol, negative consequences to whistleblowers include occupational, legal, financial, socio-emotional and other (e.g. physical health, character assassination) harms (Lim, Zhang, Hussain & Ho, 2021).

Whistleblowing: Openly disclosing organisational malpractice

Personal factors

Personal factors that affect people's ability to make decisions are all those that are directly related to the individual decision-maker, including their ethnicity, age, gender identity, education, professional experience, ethical training, cognitive moral development and personal values. Ford and Richardson (1994) argue that these factors can be subdivided into two groups: individual factors related to birth (such as sex, ethnicity and age) and individual factors related to human development and interactions with others (such as religion, employment, cognitive moral development, education and professional experience). An individual may be influenced by numerous personal factors; however, not every factor will necessarily affect them to the same degree. In practice, when a person is put in a situation of making a decision, initially, the individual factors related to birth will shape the decision-making process, and the process will be further shaped by the individual factors related to human development and interactions with others.

Organisational factors

Organisational factors comprise those inherent to a particular enterprise that are in some degree able to influence individual decision-making. The most common organisational factors are codes of ethics and codes of conduct, rewards and sanctions, ethical climate and culture, industry type, organisational size, referent groups and training. Organisational factors can influence decision-making in different ways. Organisational culture, for example, can affect an individual decision-maker's judgement by emphasising certain values shared within the organisation.

But organisational values may come into conflict with values that individuals within the organisation usually hold and act upon outside the organisation. For example, Casali and Day (2010), researching problems that emerged from an investigation into hospital fatalities, have found that both the values of the staff and the espoused values of the organisation in question were similar and positive, whereas the values promoted by the organisational culture included bullying, fear, tokenistic consultation and power control.

External factors

External factors that affect people's ability to make decisions are those that belong neither to the individual nor to their organisation but nonetheless influence the decision-making process from the outside. They are also referred to by researchers as the general environment; they are seen as the background conditions in which an organisation operates. External factors can include significant others, business competitiveness, peer group pressure and the external environment (Casali & Perano, 2021).

External factors, even though they may not influence decision-making directly, can indirectly play an important role in shaping it. Some external factors may be within the control of the decision-maker, while others may not. For example, government health policy and funding are not within the direct control or influence of the health manager, but the health manager will still be required to make decisions within the confines of both the budget and the health policy. Additionally, government health policy may be at odds with the manager's personal ethics and values, but there is an expectation that the health manager will nevertheless make decisions in the best interests of the organisation.

Frameworks for ethical decision-making

Decision-making: A cognitive process that aims to choose a course of action from several options or alternatives

Decision-making is usually defined as a cognitive process that aims to choose a course of action between different alternative options (Bazerman, 2012). The word 'cognitive' is derived from a Latin word, *cognoscere*, which means to know; therefore, a cognitive process is a process that through knowledge and analysis of available information arrives at a final choice.

Drawing on 40 years of research on ethical decision-making, Casali & Perano (2021) argue that ethical decision-making is a multi-faceted phenomenon. They suggest that despite the diversity of approaches (e.g. influencing factors, models of ethical decision-making, adopted measuring scales), 'empirical research has also failed to generate cumulative results' (p. 615). One possible explanation for this is 'the general lack of consensus regarding the list of influencing factors and the degree to which each factor influences decision makers' (p. 615).

When it comes to decision-making, it is important to understand the cognitive processes that occur. Human information-processing occurs as a series of essential stages (conceptualisation, judgement, perception and reasoning), which need to be undertaken before a person can make a decision. At any one of the stages, if it is based on raw data and sensory inputs, a different decision may be made. For the experienced manager, past experiences and knowledge assist in framing the final decision (Kolasa, 1982; Maqsood, 2006). For the new manager, who may not have experienced similar inputs or situations, the reasoning process has to rely more heavily for guidance on available frameworks, procedures, protocols and guidelines.

In information-processing, the information is firstly recognised (perceived) and secondly compared with existing similar or inherent information (existing knowledge). Therefore, it is assumed that knowledge is not only created, used and reused throughout the process, but also heavily influenced by individual perceptions that, acting as catalysts, can affect every step of the process. More specifically, as discussed earlier, individual perceptions are affected by many factors including values, nationality, education, work experience and gender identity that ultimately underpin the overall process.

A well-accepted framework for decision-making is provided following. Its creators, Robbins and Coulter (2005), describe the decision-making process in a sequential series of eight steps. There are many frameworks like this one, but not all include the last two steps (Bazerman, 2012).

1. **Identify the problem.** Conduct a full analysis of the problem.
2. **Identify the decision criteria.** Create a list of criteria to assess the alternative options.
3. **Allocate weights.** Rate the criteria from the most important to the least important.
4. **Develop alternatives.** Generate alternative options to resolve the problem.
5. **Analyse alternatives.** Assess the alternative options against the weighted criteria.
6. **Select an alternative.** Choose the alternative with the highest score.
7. **Implement the alternative.** Plan how to act out the decision and inform the people responsible for implementing it.
8. **Evaluate the decision's effectiveness.** Conduct research to find out if the decision and its implementation have fixed the problem.

If health managers use heuristics as shortcuts in their decision-making process, it can be assumed that they may use them on every one of the eight steps in the decision-making framework. Managers should be able to recognise as many of the factors that influence them as possible in order to predict which heuristics they may use in reaching a decision. Understanding the cognitive process involved in decision-making is the theoretical foundation for the personal–structural element of the managerial ethical decision-making framework proposed here. The framework is flexible and enables attention to be given to a large number of different factors that have been found to be influential in ethical decision-making, as well as a step-by-step process that would enable the manager to consider ethical dimensions at each decision point.

For managers, the important steps to keep in mind to ensure decisions have a strong ethical underpinning include looking at issues from the perspective of all four schools of moral philosophy in order to evaluate all possible ethical angles and to minimise biases. It is important to remember that there are different types of factors that can influence decision-making and that managers have control over some (ethical and individual), less control over others (organisational) and no control over the rest (external). Using the decision-making framework helps managers to maintain consistency and to build self-confidence as decision-makers.

Future ethical considerations for health managers

With increased use of artificial intelligence (AI), machine learning and the digital transformation in healthcare, managers will face a growing number of ethical and moral considerations in its pervasive use, including in justice and fairness, freedom and autonomy, privacy, transparency, patient safety and cyber security, trust, beneficence, informed consent, anonymity, access control and data integrity (Li, Ruijs & Lu, 2023; Zakerabasali & Ayyoubzadeh, 2022).

Summary

- Unethical behaviours such as theft and fraud can be the results of unethical decision-making.
- There are four schools of moral philosophy (ethical egoism, utilitarianism, virtue ethics and deontology), each of which presents a different perspective on how a person may arrive at a decision.
- Decision-making is influenced by ethical, personal, organisational and external factors.
- Moral courage is a combination of applying values, recognising risks and being persistent.
- There are eight distinct steps that should be taken in the managerial ethical decision-making framework.

Reflective questions

1. Why is an understanding of ethics important to the health manager in the decision-making process?
2. How might age and social culture influence decision-making? Provide some examples.
3. How might organisational culture influence decision-making?

4. What is a code of conduct, and what is its role in ethical decision-making?
5. Why is analysing alternatives an important step in the decision-making process?

Self-analysis question

From the perspective of a health service manager, consider the strengths and weaknesses of the four schools of moral philosophy (ethical egoism, utilitarianism, virtue ethics and deontology) in relation to your workplace. What are the risks to your organisation of making decisions from the perspective of each of the schools?

References

Bazerman, M. H. (2012). *Judgment in managerial decision making* (8th ed.). Wiley.

Casali, G. L. & Day, G. E. (2010). Treating an unhealthy organisational culture: The implications of the Bundaberg Hospital Inquiry for managerial ethical decision making. *Australian Health Review*, *34*(1), 73–79. https://doi.org/10.1071/AH09543

Casali, G. L. & Perano, M. (2021). Forty years of research on factors influencing ethical decision making: Establishing a future research agenda. *Journal of Business Research*, *132*, 614–630.

Ferrell, O. C., Fraedrich, J. & Ferrell, L. (2008). *Business ethics: Ethical decision making and cases* (7th ed.). Houghton Mifflin.

——— (2005). *Business ethics: Ethical decision making and cases* (6th ed.). Houghton Mifflin.

Ford, R. C. & Richardson, W. D. (1994). Ethical decision making: A review of the empirical literature. *Journal of Business Ethics*, *13*(3), 205–221.

Khoshmehr, Z., Barkhordari-Sharifabad, M., Nasiriani, K. & Fallahzadeh, H. (2020). Moral courage and psychological empowerment among nurses. *BMC Nursing*, *19*(43). https://doi.org/10.1186/s12912-020-00435-9

Kidder, R. M. (2005). Moral courage, digital distrust: Ethics in a troubled world. *Business and Society Review*, *110*(4), 485–505. https://doi.org/10.1111/j.0045-3609.2005.00026.x

Kohlberg, L. (1979). *The meaning and measurement of moral development*. Clark University.

Kolasa, B. J. (1982). *Introduction to behavioural sciences for business* (3rd ed.). Wiley Eastern.

KPMG (2020). *COVID-19: KPMG Fraud Survey*. Retrieved from: https://assets.kpmg.com/content/dam/kpmg/au/pdf/2020/covid-19-fraud-survey-2020-infographic.pdf

Li, F., Ruijs, N. & Lu, Y. (2023). Ethics & AI: A systematic review on ethical concerns and related strategies for designing with AI in healthcare. *AI*, *4*, 28–53. https://doi.org/10.3390/ai4010003

Lim, C., Zhang, M. W. B., Hussain, S. F. & Ho, R. (2021). The consequences of whistle-blowing: An integrative review. *Journal of Patient Safety*, *17*(6), e497–e502. https://doi.org/10.1097/PTS.0000000000000396

Lind, G. (1995). The Meaning and Measurement of Moral Judgment Revisited. Paper presented at the American Educational Research Association, San Francisco, CA.

Maqsood, T. (2006). *The role of knowledge management in supporting innovation and learning in construction*. RMIT.

McNamara, A., Smith, J. & Murphy-Hill, E. (2018). Does ACM's code of ethics change ethical decision making in software development? *Proceedings of the 26th ACM Joint Meeting on European Software Engineering Conference and Symposium on the Foundations of Software Engineering*, (October), 729–733. https://doi.org/10.1145/3236024.3264833

Pajakoski, E., Rannikko, S., Leino-Kilpi, H. & Numminen, O. (2021). Moral courage in nursing – An integrative literature review. *Nursing & Health Sciences*, *23*(3), 570–585. https://doi.org/10.1111/nhs.

Rest, J. (1979). *Development in judging moral issues*. University of Minnesota.

Robbins, S. P. & Coulter, M. K. (2005). *Management* (8th ed.). Pearson / Prentice Hall.

Sadooghiasl. A., Parvizy, S. & Ebadi, A. (2016). Concept analysis of moral courage in nursing: A hybrid model. *Nursing Ethics*, *25*(1), 6–19. https://doi.org/10.1177/0969733016638146

Stingl, V. & Geraldi, J. (2021). A research agenda for studying project decision-behaviour through the lenses of simple heuristics. *Technological Forecasting and Social Change*, *162*, 120367. https://doi.org/10.1016/j.techfore.2020.120367

St John, E. (2016). *Despite codes of conduct, unethical behaviour happens: Why bother?* The Ethics Centre. Retrieved from: https://ethics.org.au/despite-codes-of-conduct-unethical-behaviour-happens-why-bother/

Trevino, L. K. & Nelson, K. A. (2007). *Managing business ethics: Straight talk about how to do it right* (4th ed.). Wiley.

Zakerabasali, S. & Ayyoubzadeh, S. M. (2022). Internet of Things and healthcare system: A systematic review of ethical issues. *Health Science Reports*, *5*, e863. https://doi.org/10.1002/hsr2.863

4 Self-management

John Adamm Ferrier

Learning objectives

How do I:

- ensure a plan for self-management that helps my integration into the workforce and facilitates lifelong learning?
- motivate myself to strive for continuous improvement through self-management?
- set personal and professional goals for self-management?
- plan to improve areas of intelligence that I have identified as not being as strong as needed?
- find and work with a mentor?

Introduction

The context in which health professionals help people has evolved: as evidence-based technologies are implemented to improve patient and consumer health outcomes, new roles, tasks, responsibilities and accountabilities develop as a consequence (Arntz, Gregory & Zierahn, 2016). The health industry is challenged with fundamental change, not only forcing health professionals to acquire new skills continuously (Hirschi & Koen, 2021), but also to contribute towards changing the environments in which health services are delivered. Demands on the individual have also changed, including the need for the individual to actively participate in and plan their personal development.

The focus has shifted from the employer having responsibility for workforce development to each individual needing to be aware of their own strengths and limitations and to take responsibility for their career development (Dachner, Ellingson, Noe & Saxton, 2021). In other words, self-management of personal development, in terms of acquiring new skills and setting goals, is fundamental to achieving professional growth. In doing so, the individual is likely to develop personal awareness, adaptability, agency and resilience, which can foster the trust and respect of peers. People who are deeply aware of their own strengths and opportunities for growth, and who have a genuine desire to pursue aspirational goals, are more likely to inspire others. It follows that self-management skills are fundamental for those aspiring to leadership roles. People have varying abilities, talents, life experiences, upbringings and opportunities that shape their lives. While self-management is a foundational philosophy of lifelong learning, it comes more naturally to some than to others.

Some of the literature discusses self-management from a management perspective (Markham & Markham, 1995); theorists come from a variety of backgrounds, including organisational development, psychology and sociology. An added complexity is the interchangeability of some of the terms found in the literature (self-management, self-leadership, self-control, self-efficacy, self-regulation and so on); for the sake of clarity, in this chapter the terminology is restricted so as to facilitate understanding while acknowledging that others may have different perspectives.

Patricia Benner (1982) describes the learning and acquisition of skills by nurses as they enter the workforce as occurring in five stages, and these can be applied to many professions. *Novices* are those entering the workplace with little or no experience, whereas *advanced beginners* 'demonstrate marginally acceptable performance' (p. 403) and need assistance in identifying priorities. The next stage, *competency*, requires 2 or 3 years of experience, in which the health professional 'begins to see his or her actions in terms of long-range goals' (p. 404). With continued application and practice, *proficiency* is gained, whereby the health professional 'perceives situations as a whole' rather than as a series of sequential or consequential steps (p. 405). With further development, the health professional attains the *expert* level and, with the body of practical knowledge and skills amassed over time, can rely on intuitive understanding of issues as they arise. This transition from novice to expert occurs with the active participation of the individual in a process of reflective self-management. The cycle of observation, planning, action and review is familiar to most students of health. People consciously and unconsciously monitor the external environment through their senses, process this information, make choices about how they will respond, and act (or not, as the case may be) in accordance with what might be the likely outcomes. They sense, think, act and react. If people practise a certain action sufficiently often, it may become habitual, thereby reducing cognitive demand – for example, experienced motor vehicle drivers may not recall actions that required intense concentration when they were learning to drive. The transition from student to the workforce is similar: tasks expected of new graduates that initially require significant concentration and guidance often need less conscious thought and planning over time as their proficiency grows.

Healthcare and health delivery are increasingly dependent upon teams within organisations, and organisations require effective communication within teams if they are to achieve their purpose.

> Organizations are [built] around people ... an environment of mutual understanding and trust fosters good interpersonal relationships and can be linked to improved productivity for organization and enhanced performance for individuals. (Saxena 2015, p. 134)

Definitions

Self-management: A behavioural process involving the exercise of choice in which the individual is aware of possible alternative actions and appreciative of the consequences (Manz & Sims, 1980; Markham & Markham, 1995)

Manz and Sims (1980) and Markham and Markham (1995) agree that **self-management** is a behavioural process involving the exercise of choice in which the individual is aware of possible alternative actions and appreciative of the consequences. Luthans and Davis (1979) suggest that self-control is dependent upon what people observe as being associated with consequential rewards or punishments; that learning is based on positive and negative experiences which shape the choices people make. Manz and Snyder (1983) note that individuals develop behaviours in three ways: through their own previous personal experience, through their observation of people around them and through what might be considered 'socially endorsed performance criteria' (p. 69).

Manz (1992) subsequently differentiated self-management from self-leadership, which aligns individuals into teams contributing to 'organisational strategic processes' (p. 1119). This is an important link, because the collective contribution of team members adds to departmental achievements, which in turn contribute to organisational outcomes. Self-management, therefore, is not only of concern to the individual, but also has an effect on organisational performance. Houghton and Neck (2002) conceptualise self-leadership as encompassing self-regulation, self-control and self-management (Figure 4.1) through a process of cognition (or awareness) and motivation. Lawrence (2023) suggests that wisdom is achieved through habitual reflective learning, about 'being open to having our basic beliefs about life challenged' (p. 20). Hassi and Storti (2023) consider wisdom an essential component of effective leadership.

If self-management is characterised by making optimal choices, it follows that a person adept at self-management will become more effective within, and valuable to, their workplace (Baum, 1998). This is of paramount interest to organisations. A high-quality organisation is one in which every employee knows what is expected of them, has the requisite skills and resources to achieve these expectations and is empowered so to do. Breevaart, Bakker & Demerouti (2014) note that those who are adept at self-management are most likely to be engaged with, and in control of, their immediate work environment, are secure in their resources, identify challenges and reduce workplace obstacles. Such people are often respected and considered leaders by their peers, even though they may not occupy a formal leadership or management position.

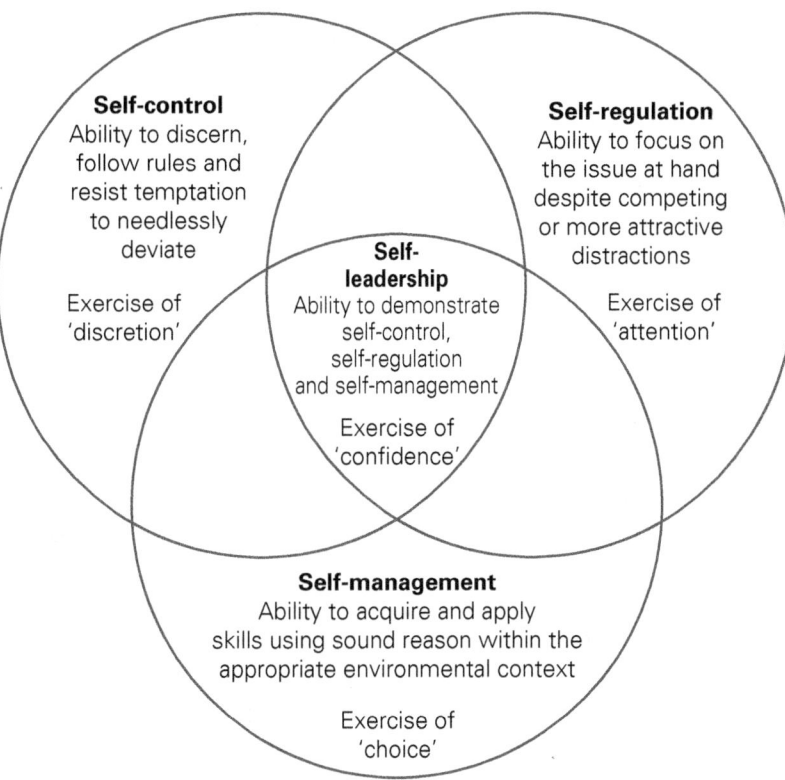

Figure 4.1 Relationships between self-control, self-regulation, self-management and self-leadership

Source: Adapted from Houghton & Neck (2002).

A DIFFERENT PERSPECTIVE?

Simon, an old colleague of mine, recently enrolled in the Master of Public Health program at the university where I teach. He called me in some distress regarding a subject with which he was struggling. 'I just can't seem to understand what this is all about. I *sailed* through my Master of Physiotherapy without any problem whatsoever.'

I sympathised and confessed that when I had studied this degree, I had experienced something similar. I asked Simon how he was approaching his learning in the subject. After some discussion, he admitted he was skimming over the detailed information provided in the lectures, relying on the tutorial notes alone, and not participating much in tutorials – if he attended at all. Simon defended this approach in that it 'worked when I was doing my physio masters [sic]'. I gently explained that refining existing skills built on existing knowledge was different to learning unfamiliar information, and that there was no short cut to *deeper* learning. Learning needs to be an active process that takes time and effort. Simon agreed that he would set aside an hour each day to review the background information and highlight the parts he did not understand before attending the tutorial each week. We then explored how he might arrange his time to prepare for the major assignment, to reflect on exactly what the assessment tasks required and to relate that back to the lecture materials and the recommended readings. I also pointed out that, since they were studying online,

> **A DIFFERENT PERSPECTIVE?** Continued
>
> participating in the tutorials helped students to develop a sense of belonging and fostered networks that could extend into his professional life.
>
> A few weeks later I met Simon on campus and asked how he was doing. He was beaming: he had *aced* that dreaded assignment. In revising his study practices, Simon also modified his work practices, taking time each day to plan his activities and to focus on the key tasks first.

Intelligence

Intelligence: The 'ability to learn from experience, and to adapt to, shape and select environments' (Sternberg, 2012, p. 503)

What role does **intelligence** play in self-management? Sternberg (2012, p. 503) defines intelligence as the 'ability to learn from experience, and to adapt to, shape and select environments' expressed as the individual changing to suit the circumstances (adaptation), the individual changing the circumstances (shaping) or, when these two strategies fail, opting for a new environment. The Greek philosopher Aristotle described three distinct applications of intelligence: understanding, action (praxis) and production. Aristotle was investigating excellence, whereas Sternberg's focus is on success (Tigner & Tigner, 2000). This may appear to be splitting hairs, except for one important point: excellence can be a subjective perspective, whereas success involves external or objective verification; in other words, it is relational. Sternberg's theory is by no means universally accepted: Gottfredson (2003) argues against its validity, citing a lack of data and the 'solid, century long evidentiary base' associated with psychometric approaches (p. 392).

Gardner states there is no single general intelligence (Sternberg, 2012) and describes a theory of *multiple* human intelligences, in that 'each human being is capable of seven relatively independent forms of information processing' (Gardner & Hatch, 1989, p. 4). Gardner's domains include interpersonal, intrapersonal, logical–mathematical, spatial, body kinaesthetic, linguistic and musical intelligences.

Consider a simplified model in which intelligence could be described using three main themes: intellect (retention, recollection and application of facts), physicality (mastery of the physical body) and emotion (identification, recognition and mastery of emotional responses) (see Figure 4.2). Most people have varying levels or abilities in relation to these areas, and some aspects of the multiple-intelligences theory fit easily: spatial and body kinaesthesia are closely aligned with physical skills, as logical–mathematical and linguistic skills might be with intellect, and interpersonal and intrapersonal skills with the emotions. Musical skills cross all sectors.

It is not enough to be able to recall facts without being able to apply them. People with dogmatic views that are at variance with established facts may have a high emotional quotient: fundamentalism thrives on appeals to emotion (Yilmaz & Morieson, 2021). Emotion tempered with intellect fosters empathy, especially if non-verbal communication matches the spoken word.

A person with intellect and good physical skills but lacking empathy might have the capacity to design a highly efficient system, but without due concern or awareness of end-user acceptability and the capacity to engage with stakeholders, the initiative is likely to fail.

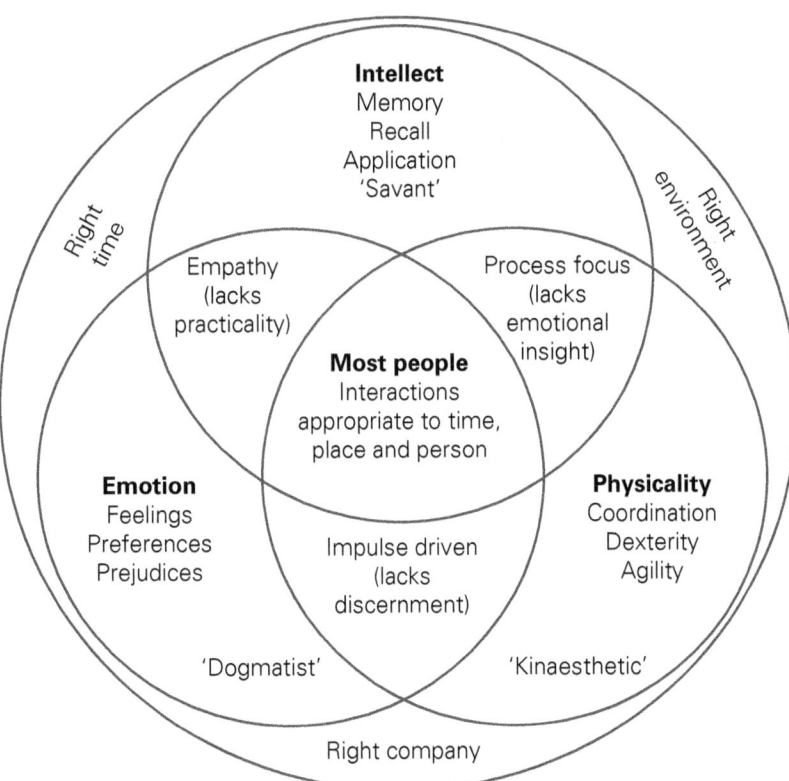

Figure 4.2 The interplay between selected 'intelligences' and how preferences and innate personal strengths may shape how a person interacts with others and is perceived by them. These are not fixed but are often determined by the context or environment, the company or interpersonal communication, and the space–time occurrence. Leadership requires appropriate use of memory, empathy and non-verbal communication

Emotional intelligence is as important as physical or intellectual intelligence (Sternberg, 2012). Just as people need to tailor the words they use to best suit the person with whom they are seeking to communicate, tone and mode of delivery should also seek to anticipate the recipient's feelings so as to communicate effectively and efficiently. An added complexity is the issue of context; for example, a particular conversation or action might be thoroughly appropriate in the company of friends at a social gathering and yet completely inappropriate or offensive in a professional or formal setting such as a staff meeting, even when the same people are involved.

Critical thinking

How might one exercise the choice suggested by self-management? For people in the health professions, **critical thinking** is an essential skill. The most practical example in the healthcare system is the accurate gathering of a patient's changing signs and symptoms. A non-critical thinking approach would be to simply record observations and fail to understand their significance, or to treat each of the signs and symptoms independently, with the inherent danger of overlooking underlying conditions or the interplay between them.

Critical thinking: The systematic evaluation or formulation of beliefs or statements, by rational standards, that forms the basis of problem-solving, decision-making and emotional intelligence (Vaughn & MacDonald, 2010, p. 119)

A related concept is that of critical thinkers, as described by Toplak, West & Stanovich (2014, p. 1039), as people who 'decouple their prior opinions from the evaluation of evidence and arguments and ... consider evidence in opposition to their own view'. A critical thinker never accepts things at face value and always seeks further information and validation. A critical-thinking approach involves considering all the factors, identifying and exploring possibilities, weighing up probabilities, arriving at a considered conclusion and being prepared to alter one's viewpoint upon further investigation. More information on critical thinking can be found in Chapter 18.

Motivation

So far, this chapter has explored the concepts related to intelligence, the gathering and processing of information and what someone may do as a result. It is timely to think about *why* one might choose to do certain things. Perhaps the best-known model of human motivation is Abraham Maslow's (1943) hierarchy of needs (see Figure 4.3), which states that motivation is driven by needs. Maslow stressed that the hierarchy is not linear and that there is fluidity between the levels of need. The most basic needs are those related to biology, such as air, food and water; without these, a person could not survive. The next level of need relates to safety, so that potential harms associated with the natural environment (shelter from extremes of cold and heat, animal predation, avoidable disease) and with societal factors (violence arising from lawlessness, social inequity) are either avoided or minimised. Maslow (1943) suggests that after this, the next emergent need is for love – he stresses that 'love is not synonymous

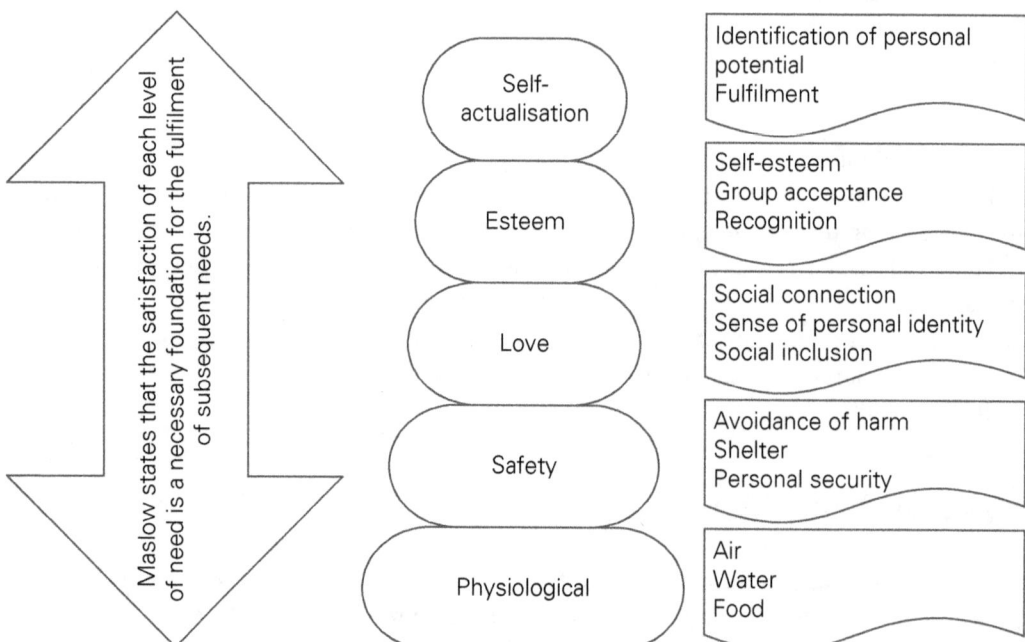

Figure 4.3 Maslow's hierarchy of human needs

Source: Adapted from Maslow (1943).

with sex', as it is also a physiological need – and that love must be reciprocated. Esteem, the next level, relates to the capacity of people to enjoy not only a good opinion of themselves but also the regard of their peers. At the apex is the need for self-actualisation, which relates to the identification of personal potential and personal achievement. Maslow states that self-actualisation is dependent upon satisfying prior needs, and that there is likely to be variance in the perception of different individuals: some needs may be conscious, while others are unconscious.

Maslow (1943) acknowledges that needs influence behaviours and that goals therefore become 'the [centring] principle in motivation theory' (p. 391), suggesting that needs generate aspirations, which are measured by, and have meaning for, the individual. The conclusion that may be drawn from this is that there are environmental factors required to achieve self-actualisation. It is unreasonable to expect a person to achieve optimal self-management in a workplace in which there are, for example, physical hazards, discord, disunity, or poor or ill-defined work practices. Individual self-management is not a solution for poor organisational design or a failure of general supervision or management. Although ubiquitous, Maslow's theory is not without criticism. Scholars have noted the need for greater empirical evidence, claiming that the model is specific to Westernised cultures and that not everyone can achieve self-actualisation (Cooke, Mills & Kelley, 2005; Navy, 2020; Wahba & Bridwell, 1976).

Notwithstanding, Frederick Herzberg (1923–2000) used Maslow's theories to develop his *Motivation–Hygiene Theory* (1964), which states that there are two major factors affecting job satisfaction and dissatisfaction. 'Motivation' refers to challenging and meaningful work that is possible to be achieved, with appropriate recognition, levels of autonomy and responsibility for decision-making. 'Hygiene', or environmental factors, refers to demotivating factors, which may include dissatisfaction with job status, remuneration, security of employment and/or poor management practices. The implication is that once a worker has a comfortable income (i.e. not having to live from one paycheque to the next), financial incentives may not necessarily increase their motivation, but being paid too little *will* reduce performance.

Social learning

Learning from academic or evidentiary sources is valuable and necessary, but the 'theory–practice gap' is often discussed – that someone may have good conceptual understanding but may fail to implement their knowledge in a practical manner. Social learning theory suggests that learning occurs not solely by memorisation of facts and figures but also by an individual modelling their behaviours on those of people they admire for their skills and expertise; that is, learning by observing and doing (Bandura, 1971; Baum, 1998; Boyce, 2011; Brauer & Tittle, 2012; Markham & Markham, 1995).

Bandura (1971) acknowledges the four key components of learning – attention, retention, reproduction and reinforcement – but says that the defining difference is that *most* learning, social or otherwise, occurs by observing others, and that positive or persuasive reinforcement occurs when the model exhibits 'status, prestige and power' (p. 18). It follows that those with status, prestige and power are more likely to influence others.

Aspirations and goals

Aspiration: Something one would like to achieve

Most people have a general idea of what they want to achieve in life. Some approach their **aspirations** with single-mindedness and determination, at the expense of other factors in their life. They have clearly defined plans with attainable goals and can describe exactly what they want to achieve and, perhaps more importantly, how they are going to pursue it and how they will know they have achieved it, because the goal is *measurable.*

Goal: An endpoint or reward

Then there are those who have a clear idea of what they would like to achieve but may not have access to the resources or information needed to develop a pathway towards achieving their **goals**. They may become discouraged and despondent because the pathway towards the goal is complex, and/or the intermediary steps have not been broken down into portions that the aspirant can progressively achieve. Alternatively, it may be that unexpected obstacles or barriers appear, or the person fails on their first attempt and is discouraged. At the other extreme, there are those who have little desire other than to meet immediate needs. Pathway choices to achieve an aspirational goal may depend on the options open to the individual: a process described by Sandorf, Campbell & Chorus (2022) as *satisficing,* whereby an individual makes choices based on the possibilities and associated implications.

Goal Setting Theory, proposed by Edwin Locke (1975), states that people are motivated to work towards goals, and this in turn will influence performance. Goals focus attention, energise and incentivise personal achievement, and encourage persistence. A person who sets personal goals is likely to develop an understanding of the strategies and tasks needed to achieve them, and it follows that increasingly difficult goals will lead to higher performance (Locke & Latham, 2002).

Locke and Latham (2019) maintain that goal setting is foundational to the possibility for success. Those who aspire establish progressive or incremental goals on a pathway, sometimes called objectives, which help them to identify whether they are on the right track. For example, sportspeople refer to achieving 'personal bests' as they strive to match or emulate the achievements of others, leading to progressive achievements on the pathways to their goals. Each incremental achievement is celebrated, and each celebration strengthens resolve to carry on in a positive feedback loop. Often, the necessary pathway may not be clear, or unexpected obstacles and setbacks may arise. Sometimes this can be catastrophic – or can have the *appearance* of being catastrophic – but experience teaches us that if we step back, often an alternative pathway becomes apparent.

Goals and objectives are most useful when they are capable of being measured. Doran (1981), possibly basing his work upon the earlier ideas of Raia (1965), uses the acronym SMART to identify goals that are Specific, Measurable, Achievable, Realistic and Time-related. SMART goals can be used by individuals and organisations (see Table 4.1) to effect change; they are discussed again in Chapter 31.

SMART goals need not be overly complex – for example: 'In seven days I will have completed the first draft of my 2000-word assignment'. This goal is specific, measurable (the deliverable being the draft), achievable and reasonable (people setting their own goals are unlikely to have unrealistic expectations), and it is time-related (it will be achieved within seven days).

The benefit of measurable goals is that they provide an opportunity for both reflection and a sense of achievement. The more one achieves, the more likely one is to continue progress. The more one does, the better one performs and feels. Positive feedback loops can explain

Table 4.1 Comparison of SMART goals in organisational and individual contexts

Organisational context	Individual context
Specific (capable of being exactly described)	Specific (capable of being exactly described)
Manageable (not too small but sufficient to build upon and develop existing skills)	Measurable (able to be measured against an external scale)
Assignable (within range of developing skills or competence of the team and able to be delegated)	Achievable (within range of developing skills or competence of the individual)
Realistic (likely to occur with the available resources open to the team)	Reasonable (within or slightly beyond the range of existing skills)
Time-related (predictable in terms of date of outcome)	Time-related (predictable in terms of date of outcome)

Source: Based on Raia (1965).

how and why some people thrive in certain jobs and others languish or harbour resentment, or give up. Those who receive positive feedback are often motivated to continue to do better and feel comfortable taking calculated risks to expand their knowledge and capacities.

Aids for self-management

Prioritisation

People often have competing demands for their attention, but successful people learn to prioritise tasks to achieve their goals. A decision-making model has been attributed to Dwight D. Eisenhower, who planned Operation Overlord, the D-Day landings of the Second World War, and later became president of the United States. Eisenhower is attributed with a simple decision-making framework to determine importance and urgency that thereby permitted him to prioritise his time (see Table 4.2). A model such as this helps identify what is needful. Using the examples in the table, we would hope that one would attend to whatever crisis was happening before pursuing a leisure activity (Ciarniené & Vienazindiené, 2014).

Table 4.2 The 'Eisenhower' matrix

	URGENT	NOT URGENT
IMPORTANT	DO IT YOURSELF Things that require your immediate attention (e.g. responding to an acute medical emergency)	DELAY IT Something you must achieve by a certain time and/or date (e.g. devoting time to meet a deadline)
NOT IMPORTANT	DELEGATE IT Things that must get done but may be delegated to someone *trusted* on your behalf (e.g. administrative tasks)	DEFER IT Most other things until there is time to engage in the activity *if desired* (e.g. engaging in social media)

Source: Based on Ciarniené & Vienazindiené (2014).

Reflective practice

Reflective practice is a process of actively thinking about one's experiences, behaviours and decisions in order to learn and improve. It is a process whereby one reviews a past event and the outcome, assessing what went well and what could have been done differently if the outcome was suboptimal. Insights gained from this practice have the potential to enhance future performance. Continuing professional development programs and professional competency frameworks, such as those of the 'ACHSM Master Competency Framework' (2022, p. 6), define reflective practice as a process whereby feedback is sought regarding strengths and limitations.

Mentors

Self-management need not be a solitary exercise. Social learning theory predicts that people will identify colleagues with more experience upon whom they may model behaviours, and some of whom may take an interest in their development (Kram, 1983). Mentors may provide advice, or sometimes unwelcome or confronting truths, which upon reflection are usually valuable. They will not (and should not) complete work for mentees, but rather help them understand how they are faring, be a source of external reflection and offer advice. The ideal mentoring relationship is professional and nurturing. The reward to the mentor is their mentee's success and the satisfaction from helping another person: mentoring is altruistic.

Summary

- Integration into the workforce is a gradual process, and the acquisition of skills and learning is facilitated by self-management.
- The transition from a predominantly clinical role to one of clinical leadership, or even a management role, can often feel like one is starting all over again.
- Intelligence is not simply a matter of good memory; it also includes understanding of emotions and reflection on personal characteristics and actions.
- Developing shorter, intermediate or incremental objectives is helpful in achieving detailed and challenging goals.
- People are more likely to be influenced by those they consider having prestige and power.
- Identifying people one encounters through one's career whose skills and knowledge are worthy of admiration and emulation may lead to wanting to work with them in a mentoring relationship.
- The decision to self-manage is an active, ongoing process that one can only make for oneself.
- Self-management is an important tool, if not the most important tool, to achieving lifelong learning.
- If individuals cannot appear to manage themselves, how can they be recognised as being capable of leading others?

Reflective questions

1. To what extent do you agree that Maslow's (1943) hierarchy of needs is true when he suggests that a person must be loved (that is, have positive social connections) in order to develop self-esteem?
2. Do you think it takes 2–3 years to achieve proficiency, as Benner (1982) suggests? If not, why not? What could be done to expedite development?
3. Have you given up on a particular goal because it was just too hard? If you had been given assistance in developing smaller steps and incremental goals, would it have made a difference? If so, how?
4. 'Economic affluence is directly proportional to future options: those who are miserable and affluent have more options open to them than those who are miserable and poor.' Is this a statement with which you disagree, or is it simply a disagreeable statement? Is there a difference?
5. Has there ever been a time when something happened that from your perspective seemed like the world was about to end, but when you look back on it now, you can see it was a blessing in disguise? What changed your perspective? Did this experience help you cope with later adversity?

Self-analysis questions

Where are you currently on Benner's (1982) spectrum of novice to expert? Does this spectrum only apply to nursing, or can it have wider applications? Are you where you expected to be at this stage in your career? What things could accelerate your development? Do you actively look for ways to improve your skills, or do you expect them to develop over time?

References

Arntz, M., Gregory, T. & Zierahn, U. (2016). *The risk of automation for jobs in OECD countries.* https://doi.org/10.1787/5jlz9h56dvq7-en

Australasian College of Health Services Management (ACHSM). (2022). Master Competency Framework. ACHSM.

Bandura, A. (1971). *Social learning theory.* General Learning.

Baum, F. (1998). *The new public health: An Australian perspective.* Melbourne: Oxford University.

Benner, P. (1982). From novice to expert. *American Journal of Nursing, 82*(3), 402–407.

Boyce, T. E. (2011). Applying social learning theory. *Training Journal,* (July), 31–4.

Brauer, J. R. & Tittle, C. R. (2012). Social learning theory and human reinforcement. *Sociological Spectrum, 32*(2), 1571–77. https://doi.org/10.1080/02732173.2012.646160

Breevaart, K., Bakker, A. B. & Demerouti, E. (2014). Daily self-management and employee work engagement. *Journal of Vocational Behavior, 84,* 31–8. https://doi.org/10.1016/j.jvb.2013.11.002

Ciarnienė, R. & Vienazindienė, M. (2014). The conceptual model of time management. *Mediterranean Journal of Social Sciences, 5*(13), 424–8.

Cooke, B., Mills, A. J. & Kelley, E. S. (2005). Situating Maslow in Cold War America – A recontextualization of management theory. *Group & Organization Management, 30*(2), 129–152. https://doi.org/10.1177/1059601104273062

Dachner, A. M., Ellingson, J. E., Noe, R. A. & Saxton, B. M. (2021). The future of employee development. *Human resource management review, 31*(2), 100732. https://doi.org/10.1016/j.hrmr.2019.100732

Doran, G. T. (1981). There's a S.M.A.R.T. way to write management's goals and objectives. *Management Review*, *70*(11), 35.

Gardner, H. & Hatch, T. (1989). Multiple intelligences go to school: Educational implications of the theory of multiple intelligences. *Educational Researcher*, *18*(8), 4–10. https://doi.org/10.2307/1176460

Gottfredson, L. S. (2003). Dissecting practical intelligence theory: Its claims and evidence. *Intelligence*, *31*, 343–397.

Hassi, A. & Storti, G. (2023). Wise leadership: Construction and validation of a scale. *Modern Management Review*, *28*(1), 47–69. https://doi.org/10.7862/rz.2023.mmr.03

Herzberg, F. (1964). The motivation-hygiene concept and problems of manpower. *Personnel Administration*, 27(1), 3–7.

Hirschi, A. & Koen, J. (2021). Contemporary career orientations and career self-management: A review and integration. *Journal of Vocational Behavior*, *126*, 103505. https://doi.org/10.1016/j.jvb.2020.103505

Houghton, J. D. & Neck, C. P. (2002). The revised self-leadership questionnaire. *Journal of Managerial Psychology*, *17*(8), 672–691. https://doi.org/10.1108/02683940210450484

Kram, K. E. (1983). Phases of the mentor relationship. *Academy of Management Journal* [pre-1986], *26*(4), 608.

Lawrence, P. S. (2023). *The wise leader: A practical guide for thinking differently about leadership*. Taylor & Francis Group.

Locke, E. A. (1975). Personnel attitudes and motivation. *Annual Review of Psychology*, *26*(1), 457–480. https://doi.org/10.1146/annurev.ps.26.020175.002325

Locke, E. A. & Latham, G. P. (2019). The development of goal setting theory: A half century retrospective. *Motivation science*, *5*(2), 93–105. https://doi.org/10.1037/mot0000127

——— (2002). Building a practically useful theory of goal setting and task motivation: A 35-year odyssey. *American Psychologist*, *57*(9), 705–717.

Luthans, F. & Davis, T. R. V. (1979). Behavioral self-management: The missing link in managerial effectiveness. *Organizational Dynamics*, *8*(1), 42–60. https://doi.org/10.1016/0090-2616(79)90003-2

Manz, C. C. (1992). Self-leading work teams: Moving beyond self-management myths. *Human Relations*, *45*(11), 1119–1140. https://doi.org/10.1177/001872679204501101

Manz, C. C. & Sims, H. P. (1980). Self-management as a substitute for leadership: A social learning theory perspective. *Academy of Management Review*, *5*(3), 361–367.

Manz, C. C. & Snyder, C. A. (1983). How resourceful entrepreneurs meet business challenges … and survive. *Management Review*, *72*(10), 68.

Markham, S. E. & Markham, I. S. (1995). Self-management and self-leadership reexamined: A levels-of-analysis perspective. *Leadership Quarterly*, *6*(3), 343–359. https://doi.org/10.1016/1048-9843(95)90013-6

Maslow, A. H. (1943). A theory of human motivation. *Psychological Review*, *50*(4), 370–396. https://doi.org/10.1037/H0054346

Navy, S. L. (2020). Theory of human motivation—Abraham Maslow. *Science education in theory and practice: An introductory guide to learning theory*, pp. 17–28, Springer International. https://doi.org/10.1007/978-3-030-43620-9_2

Raia, A. P. (1965). Goal setting and self-control: An empirical study. *Journal of Management Studies*, *2*(1), 34–53. https://doi.org/10.1111/j.1467-6486.1965.tb00564.x

Sandorf, E. D., Campbell, D. & Chorus, C. (2022). A simple satisficing model. *PLoS One*, *17*(10), e0275339. https://doi.org/10.1371/journal.pone.0275339

Saxena, P. (2015). Johari Window: An effective model for improving interpersonal communication and managerial effectiveness. *SIT Journal of Management*, *5*(2), 134–146.

Sternberg, R. J. (2012). Intelligence. *Wiley Interdisciplinary Reviews: Cognitive Science*, *3*(5), 501–511. https://doi.org/10.1002/wcs.1193

Tigner, R. B. & Tigner, S. S. (2000). Triarchic theories of intelligence: Aristotle and Sternberg. *History of Psychology*, *3*(2), 168–176.

Toplak, M. E., West, R. F. & Stanovich, K. E. (2014). Rational thinking and cognitive sophistication: Development, cognitive abilities, and thinking dispositions. *Developmental Psychology*, *50*(4), 1037–48. https://doi.org/10.1037/a0034910

Vaughn, L. & MacDonald, C. (2010). *The power of critical thinking* (2nd Canadian ed.). Oxford University Press.

Wahba, M. A. & Bridwell, L. G. (1976). Maslow reconsidered: A review of research on the need hierarchy theory. *Organizational behavior and human performance*, *15*(2), 212–240.

Yilmaz, I. & Morieson, N. (2021). A systematic literature review of populism, religion and emotions. *Religions*, *12*(4), 272.

5 Emotional intelligence and self-awareness

Leila Karimi and Jiri Rada

Learning objectives

How do I:

- gain insights into diverse models of emotional intelligence, including their components and intersections?
- acquire practical strategies to enhance my emotional intelligence, covering key aspects such as self-awareness, self-regulation, empathy and effective relationship-building communication skills?
- recognise the distinction between intelligence quotient and emotional intelligence, while acknowledging their synergistic effects on overall success?
- gain an appreciation for how EI significantly shapes behaviour, influences decision-making processes and influences interpersonal interactions within various spheres of life?
- apply EI principles to effectively navigate and enhance workplace dynamics, which encompass leadership, conflict resolution and team collaboration?

Introduction

The construct of **emotional intelligence (EI)**, also interchangeably referred to as EQ, has engendered considerable scholarly attention within the field of psychology over the past three decades. Despite its significant appeal in business, education and popular literature, EI remains a theme of scientific controversy and investigation. This scrutiny arises from discernible disparities between popular and scholarly interpretations of EI, which are further complicated by the methodological challenge of devising reliable measurement instruments.

This continuing scholarly exploration serves to bridge the dichotomy between passion and reason, thereby enriching our comprehension of human behaviour and cognition.

Definitions and new developments

The origins of the exploration of human intelligence can be traced to the late 19th century, when Sir Francis Galton, a prominent figure in the nascent field, initiated inquiries into this intricate trait. Often synonymous with assessments of intelligence quotient (IQ) and cognitive aptitude, the conceptualisation of intelligence has evolved beyond conventional metrics. Notably, psychologist E. L. Thorndike introduced the concept of social intelligence in the 1920s, delineating it as the acumen required for comprehending, navigating and managing interpersonal dynamics and complex social contexts (Thorndike, 1920). Building upon this foundation, Howard Gardner, a pioneering developmental psychologist, proposed the theory of multiple intelligences, contending that human cognition encompasses diverse forms of intelligence beyond the confines of traditional IQ assessments and emphasising the inherent variability in individual cognitive proficiencies (Gardner, 1987, 2011).

A consensus among scholars has emerged regarding the paramount significance of social intelligence in shaping quality of life at the individual level and the functioning of society. While conventional IQ assessments persist as valuable predictors of academic and occupational achievement, the role of social intelligence in fostering adaptive social behaviours, nurturing interpersonal relationships and facilitating emotional regulation is increasingly recognised as pivotal in determining overall wellbeing and life satisfaction.

The field of EI is relatively new. It was introduced in 1990 by Salovey and Mayer (1990) as the subset of social intelligence. In their model, emotions are understood as feeling states that convey relational information, which encompasses physiological responses and cognitions, while intelligence is the skill of reasoning accurately about this information.

These definitions provide a glimpse into the diverse conceptualisations of EI, ranging from abilities and skills to personality traits. They reflect the multi-dimensional nature of EI and its significance in various domains of human functioning.

Digital emotional intelligence (DEI) is an emerging concept that combines EI with digital competence. Audrin and Audrin (2023) define DEI as the ability to navigate digital environments while effectively managing emotions and relationships. The concept encompasses both EI and digital competence. DEI equips individuals to thrive emotionally in the digitalised world, emphasising the fusion of emotional awareness and digital literacy. It acknowledges that understanding emotions in a digital world requires a unique set of skills.

EI: Mayer and Salovey (2007) refined their earlier definition of EI, emphasising it as 'the ability to perceive accurately, appraise and express emotion; the ability to access and/or generate feelings when they facilitate thought; the ability to understand emotion and emotional knowledge; and the ability to regulate emotions to promote emotional and intellectual growth' (p. 10).

An emerging frontier in the landscape of technological innovation is the concept of emotion artificial intelligence (Emotion AI). Recent strides in artificial intelligence (AI) and the pervasive influence of digital transformation have catalysed a notable shift in the dynamics of human interaction with technology. As AI permeates various facets of organisational operations, a primary hurdle encountered by enterprises is the seamless integration of AI with EI. As posited by Kaur and Sharma (2021), Emotion AI serves as a conduit that bridges the divide between technological interfaces and human emotions, thereby fostering an environment of enhanced empathy and operational efficacy within digital workspaces.

Characteristics of emotional intelligence

EI encompasses a diverse array of attributes that empower individuals to discern, comprehend and regulate their emotions, both internally and externally. Drawing from seminal contributions by leading experts in the field of EI (Bar-On, 1997; Goleman, 1995; Mayer, Caruso & Salovey, 2016; Mayer, Salovey & Caruso, 2004; Petrides & Furnham, 2009; Salovey & Mayer, 1990), the following key characteristics are associated with EI:

1. Self-awareness: Recognising and understanding one's emotions and motivations.
2. Self-regulation: Managing emotions and behaviours effectively.
3. Empathy: Understanding and responding to others' emotions.
4. Social skills: Excelling in relationships and communication.
5. Motivation: Pursuing goals with persistence and resilience.
6. Emotional awareness: Perceiving emotions accurately.
7. Emotional regulation: Managing emotions adeptly.
8. Empathetic communication: Expressing understanding in interactions.
9. Conflict resolution: Navigating disagreements constructively.
10. Resilience: Bouncing back from challenges.

These traits form the foundation of EI, backed by extensive research in the disciplines of psychology, neuroscience and organisational behaviour.

Gender differences

The existing research on gender differences in EI reveals mixed findings but has only explored differences related to biological sex. While some studies show minimal disparities in overall EI scores between males and females, others highlight significant differences in specific EI components.

Petrides and Furnham (2000) propose divergent forms of EI for men and women, with women showing enhanced interpersonal skills and men demonstrating stronger self-awareness and independence. A systematic review examining various measures of EI reveals that certain instruments tend to yield higher EI scores among women when compared to men (Bru-Luna, Martí-Vilar, Merino-Soto & Cervera-Santiago, 2021). The review suggests that these disparities may be attributed to distinct modes of emotional processing within the brain or potential differences in emotional perception, as well as the influence of contextual factors.

Additional studies report varying degrees of gender disparities in EI. Naghavi and Redzuan (2011) suggest that females tend to display higher EI levels due to societal expectations promoting emotional expressiveness in girls. Conversely, Bosson, Vandello and Buckner (2018) caution that gender stereotypes may influence emotional expression, masking true gender differences in EI.

Cultural and contextual factors significantly shape gender differences in EI. Zeidner, Matthews and Roberts (2012) highlight the effects of societal norms on emotional expression and regulation. Moreover, discrepancies in research findings may stem from variations in measurement methodologies, with certain measures exhibiting greater sensitivity to gender-related nuances (Piefke, Weiss, Markowitsch & Fink, 2005). Gender differences in EI may also be influenced by neuroanatomy or brain structures rather than social determinants.

It is crucial to acknowledge that while gender differences may exist in EI and leadership styles, individual variances within each gender also significantly contribute to leadership effectiveness. Furthermore, societal and cultural factors play a pivotal role in shaping how EI is manifested and valued across different contexts. Recognising these nuances is essential in promoting diversity, equity and inclusivity in organisational leadership.

Improving emotional intelligence

Plato's assertion that all learning is rooted in emotion underscores the profound influence of EI on various aspects of life. Preliminary research demonstrates that individuals with high EI tend to experience greater happiness, career success, entrepreneurial prowess, leadership acumen and overall wellbeing than those with lower EI (Chamorro-Premuzic, 2016, 2013). Furthermore, evidence suggests that while our baseline level of EI may exhibit stability, it remains adaptable, implying that intentional practice and learning efforts can lead to its augmentation (Fariselli, Ghini & Freedman, 2008).

The effectiveness of EI enhancement initiatives hinges on several critical factors. Firstly, the quality of the training or coaching program is paramount. Interventions targetting interpersonal skills have shown significant efficacy, with benefits extending beyond professional spheres to enhanced personal happiness, health and relationships (Chamorro-Premuzic, 2013). Secondly, individuals seeking to augment their EI must actively seek and integrate specific feedback. This feedback facilitates self-awareness, enabling individuals to identify their strengths and weaknesses, and to analyse their behaviours. Additionally, selecting appropriate techniques for EI enhancement is essential, with cognitive behavioural therapy emerging as a promising avenue for favourable outcomes (Chamorro-Premuzic, 2013).

Individual differences and contextual factors must be considered in tailoring EI interventions. While some individuals may respond favourably to training, others may not, depending on factors such as enthusiasm, personality traits and willingness to embrace change (Bar-On, Maree & Elias, 2007). Moreover, recent empirical findings underscore the efficacy of EI interventions in fostering emotional skills. A comprehensive systematic review by Kotsou and colleagues (2019) reveals a significant improvement among groups receiving EI interventions when compared to control groups. Collectively, these findings underscore the potential effects of targeted EI training initiatives in facilitating personal growth and success across various domains of life.

Models of emotional intelligence

Three primary models dominate the discourse on EI: the Ability model, the Trait model and the Mixed models. Each offers distinct perspectives on the nature of EI and its implications for individual functioning.

Ability model

Proposed by Peter Salovey and John Mayer, this model emphasises EI as a set of practical competencies, focusing on an individual's ability to perceive, understand and manage emotions. Ability emotional intelligence (AEI) emphasises the cognitive aspect of EI, viewing it as a collection of practical skills. Based on this definition, AEI is usually measured through performance in tasks (Olderbak, Semmer & Doebler, 2019).

The AEI model (also called the four-branch model) describes four abilities that collectively illustrate the scope of EI (Mayer, Salovey, Caruso & Sitarenios, 2003; Papadogiannis, Logan & Sitarenios, 2009):

1. Emotion perception: Accurately recognising and interpreting emotions in oneself and others.
2. Facilitation of thought using emotions: Leveraging emotions to enhance cognitive processes, decision-making and problem-solving.
3. Emotion understanding: Grasping the underlying causes and implications of emotions.
4. Emotion management: Effectively regulating and expressing emotions in various situations.

According to this model, emotions serve as constructive sources of information. Each person has a unique way of perceiving, understanding and responding to emotions. The four abilities are arranged sequentially from areas specific to the emotions (perceiving emotions), to understanding emotions and, finally, to the areas more suited to personality (managing emotions). The capacity to accurately perceive non-verbal emotions in others is essential in advancing understanding of emotions.

In summary, the AEI model highlights that EI is not just about feeling emotions: it is about skilfully navigating them to enhance our thinking, relationships and overall effectiveness.

Trait model

This model, developed by Petrides (2009), focuses on the individual's self-perceptions of their emotional abilities, rather than treating EI as a cognitive ability (Petrides & Furnham, 2009).

The trait model centres on how individuals perceive their emotional abilities. It suggests that people perceive their emotional abilities differently; some feel in control of their emotions, while others find them surprising. Petrides believes that our perceptions are relatively stable and have a direct effect on our mood, achievements and behaviours. Trait emotional intelligence (TEI) encompasses a constellation of emotional self-perceptions situated at lower levels of personality hierarchies (Petrides, Pita & Kokkinaki, 2007). Traits include adaptability, empathy, expression of emotion, perception and self-esteem. Self-reported questionnaires are commonly used to assess TEI. TEI integrates affective aspects of personality and acknowledges that EI is intertwined with broader personality traits (Petrides et al., 2016).

Mixed models

Bar-On's Mixed model, developed in 1997, views EI as a blend of abilities, personality traits, competencies and skills. It emphasises an individual's capacity to cope with environmental demands and pressures. The model consists of five main domains:

1. Intrapersonal EI: Self-awareness and self-expression, recognising one's own emotions, strengths, limitations and constructive expression of feelings.
2. Interpersonal EI: Focuses on relationships and social interactions, including empathy, building relationships and social responsibility.
3. Adaptability: Coping with change, uncertainty and new situations, requiring flexibility, problem-solving and resilience.
4. Stress management: Coping with emotions during stress, including impulse control and emotional resilience, and maintaining focus under pressure.
5. General mood: Overall emotional wellbeing and life outlook, influenced by factors including optimism, happiness and life satisfaction, enhancing resilience and adaptability.

Goleman's mixed model of EI is a comprehensive framework essential for effective leadership and personal development (Goleman, 1995).

Structured around five key components, the model highlights fundamental aspects that are crucial in fostering EI:

1. Self-awareness: Recognising and understanding one's own emotions, strengths, weaknesses, values and goals.
2. Self-regulation: Managing and controlling emotions, impulses and reactions, even in challenging situations.
3. Motivation: Having the drive to achieve goals, and resilience and persistence in the face of setbacks.
4. Empathy: Understanding and appreciating the emotions of others and fostering strong interpersonal connections.
5. Social skills: Abilities related to interpersonal interactions, communication, conflict resolution, collaboration, leadership and influence.

Understanding EI models is crucial for the advancement of research and personal development that combine cognitive capabilities and self-perceptions of emotional traits. Further research will enhance our comprehension of human behaviour and cognition.

ENHANCING PATIENT CARE THROUGH EMOTIONAL INTELLIGENCE

Background

Susan, an experienced physician in a bustling hospital emergency department, grapples with consistently low patient-satisfaction scores. Despite her extensive medical expertise,

ENHANCING PATIENT CARE THROUGH EMOTIONAL INTELLIGENCE Continued

she recognises the pivotal role of EI in fostering positive patient experiences. Determined to address this issue, Susan resolves to refine her EI skills to enhance patient-care standards.

Key issues

1. Persistently low patient-satisfaction scores within the emergency department
2. Barriers in communication and empathy, which hinder patient interactions
3. Elevated stress levels among healthcare staff, which impede quality patient care

Approach

Susan embarks on a program to fortify her EI competencies, aiming to tackle these challenges head-on. She engages in workshops, seeks feedback from peers and patients, and implements targetted strategies to bolster her EI prowess.

Actions

1. **Self-awareness:** Susan initiates introspective exercises to identify her emotional triggers and biases. By recognising how her emotions influence interactions, particularly during busy shifts, she lays the groundwork for self-improvement.
2. **Self-regulation:** Through deliberate practice, Susan refines techniques for managing her emotions, particularly in high-pressure scenarios. She cultivates a calm and composed demeanour to help ensure empathetic and composed communication, even in emergencies.
3. **Empathy:** Susan prioritises understanding of her patients' emotions, perspectives and worries. Employing active listening and validation techniques, she fosters genuine empathy, which resonates with patients through her words and actions.
4. **Social skills:** Susan dedicates efforts to bolstering her communication and interpersonal aptitude. By refining active listening and fostering collaboration, she nurtures a supportive environment, thereby strengthening relationships with patients and colleagues alike.

Results

1. **Elevated patient satisfaction:** Susan's refined EI translates into improved patient experiences, evidenced by rising satisfaction scores. Patients feel acknowledged, validated and cared for, and this leads to more positive encounters overall.
2. **Enhanced patient–provider rapport:** Susan's heightened empathy and communication skills deepen her connections with patients. This fosters a conducive environment for open dialogue and active patient involvement in care decisions, ultimately yielding improved health outcomes.

> 3. Mitigated staff stress levels: Susan's EI-centred approach not only benefits patients but also alleviates stress among colleagues. By exemplifying effective communication, empathy and teamwork, she fosters a harmonious and supportive workplace culture.
>
> ### Conclusion
>
> Susan's commitment to enhancing EI heralds a transformative shift in patient-care dynamics within the emergency department. Through introspection and targeted skills development, she elevates communication, augments patient satisfaction and cultivates a culture of empathy among healthcare staff. This case underscores the indispensable role of EI in healthcare delivery and patient wellbeing.

Leadership and emotional intelligence

In today's evolving workplace, effective leadership extends beyond technical expertise and strategic thinking; it requires EI to navigate interpersonal dynamics. Studies show that managers spend more than 20 per cent of their time dealing with conflicts, which underscores the indispensability of conflict management skills in leadership (Lopes, Grewal, Kadis, Gall & Salovey, 2006). High EI equips leaders to resolve conflicts adeptly by empathising with others' viewpoints, defusing tensions and fostering collaborative solutions (Jordan & Troth, 2002).

Contrary to earlier conceptions that portray leadership as an inherent trait of exceptional individuals, contemporary scholarship highlights the role of EI in shaping leadership effectiveness. Leaders who are proficient in perceiving and managing emotions are better equipped to interpret emotional cues from subordinates and peers, ultimately enhancing organisational outcomes. Evidence suggests that leaders scoring high on EI assessments exhibit superior performance when compared to those relying solely on traditional measures such as personality traits and cognitive abilities (Rosete & Ciarrochi, 2005).

Research underscores EI as a pivotal leadership competency that can be cultivated and leveraged to enhance leadership effectiveness. The alignment between EI and leadership highlights its significance in human resource management practices (Saha et al., 2023). These theoretical foundations, complemented by practical insights, emphasise the imperative for organisations to invest in EI development and leadership effectiveness (Saha et al., 2023). A comprehensive analysis of existing literature reaffirms EI's crucial role in effective leadership within contemporary organisations, as leaders with high EI not only enhance organisational behaviours and outcomes but also positively influence team performance and members' attitudes toward work (Coronado-Maldonado & Benítez-Márquez, 2023).

Healthcare and emotional intelligence

EI is increasingly acknowledged as a fundamental aspect of healthcare delivery, exerting profound influence on patient-centred care, organisational effectiveness and professional wellbeing. Extensive research underscores EI's role in enhancing physician–patient relationships, thereby nurturing empathy, refining teamwork, communication and stress management, and bolstering leadership capabilities (Soriano-Vázquez, Cajachagua Castro & Morales-García, 2023; Warren, 2013). Particularly among nursing professionals, studies demonstrate a strong correlation between EI and job satisfaction, performance and resilience amidst occupational stressors (Birks & Watt, 2007; Codier, 2012; Karimi, Cheng, Bartram, Leggat & Sarkeshik, 2015; Karimi, Leggat, Donohue, Farrell & Couper, 2014).

Numerous nursing studies confirm the significant correlation between nurses' EI and their performance levels. For instance, Karimi and colleagues (2014) found that emotional labour and EI significantly influenced the wellbeing and perceived job stress among a group of Australian community nurses. Given the shortage of nurses globally, effective EI training may serve as a cornerstone for retaining nurses in their roles while alleviating job stress and burnout. Additionally, EI appears to correlate with both physical and emotional wellness in nurses, with their EI skills aligning with professionalism and expert practice standards (Codier, 2012).

Evidence suggests that healthcare leaders possessing high EI demonstrate the confidence to fortify their organisations and navigate through challenges, such as budget constraints and staff reductions. EI equips leaders with the necessary insights and skills to manage conflicts with patients, families and fellow staff, fostering a supportive team environment (Butler, 2021). Moreover, there is a pressing need to train all healthcare and medical personnel in addressing emotional issues, as every disease and health condition encompasses an emotional component. Goleman (1995) contends that by addressing individuals' emotional states alongside their illnesses, medical efficacy will see a significant increase.

Summary

- Emotional intelligence (EI) is the ability to recognise, understand and manage one's own emotions and those of others.
- EI includes emotional awareness, effective communication and empathy, and the ability to handle social interactions with skill and sensitivity.
- Key components of EI are self-awareness, self-regulation, social awareness and relationship management.
- Developing EI can enhance interpersonal relationships, improve decision-making and promote overall wellbeing.
- EI is increasingly viewed as essential for success in both personal and professional domains, complementing cognitive intelligence (IQ).
- Different types of EI are being explored, with continuing efforts to create reliable tools for measuring them.
- Research in neuroscience, cultural influences on EI and leadership ethics are deepening our understanding of the importance of EI.
- This growing perspective challenges the belief that intelligence is fixed at birth, and it opens the door to a more inclusive view of human potential.

Reflective questions

1. How do I perceive my emotional behaviour in different contexts?
2. What influences my self-perception regarding emotional behaviour?
3. Do I think others perceive my emotional behaviour similarly to how I perceive it?
4. Who can provide valuable insights into how others perceive my emotional behaviour?
5. How does my general demeanor affect my communication style and decision-making?

Self-analysis question

Drawing upon the insights garnered from this chapter and supplemented by personal research, how would you enhance your EI, integrate it into your daily routines and ensure its efficacy? In your response, explore actionable strategies and techniques, such as honing active listening skills, scrutinising your responses to interpersonal interactions and management of stress, evaluating the effects of your actions on others and conducting a comprehensive analysis of your strengths and weaknesses in EI.

References

Audrin, C. & Audrin, B. (2023). More than just emotional intelligence online: Introducing 'digital emotional intelligence'. *Frontiers in Psychology*, *14*, 1154355.

Bar-On, R. (1997). *The Emotional Intelligence Inventory (EQ-i): Technical manual*. Multi-Health Systems.

Bar-On, R., Maree, J. G. & Elias, M. J. (2007). *Educating people to be emotionally intelligent*. Bloomsbury.

Birks, Y. F. & Watt, I. S. (2007). Emotional intelligence and patient-centred care. *Journal of the Royal Society of Medicine*, *100*(8), 368–374. https://doi.org/10.1177/014107680710000813

Bosson, J. K., Vandello, J. A. & Buckner, C. E. (2018). *The psychology of sex and gender*. Sage.

Bru-Luna, L. M., Martí-Vilar, M., Merino-Soto, C. & Cervera-Santiago, J. L. (2021). Emotional intelligence measures: A systematic review. *Healthcare (Basel)*, *9*(12). https://doi.org/10.3390/healthcare9121696

Butler, J. (2021). Emotional intelligence in nursing leadership. *Australian Nursing and Midwifery Journal*, *27*(5), 18–21.

Chamorro-Premuzic, T. (2016). *Personality and individual differences*. John Wiley & Sons.

——— (2013, May 30). Can you really improve your emotional intelligence? *Harvard Business Review*. https://hbr.org/2013/05/can-you-really-improve-your-em

Codier, E. (2012). Emotional intelligence: Why walking the talk transforms nursing care. *American Nurse Today*, *7*(4), 3–7.

Coronado-Maldonado, I. & Benítez-Márquez, M. D. (2023). Emotional intelligence, leadership, and work teams: A hybrid literature review. *Heliyon*, *9*(10), e20356. https://doi.org/10.1016/j.heliyon.2023.e20356

Fariselli, L., Ghini, M, & Freedman, J. (2008). Age and emotional intelligence: Six seconds. The Emotional Intelligence Network [White paper research on emotional intelligence]. Retrieved from: https://prodimages.6seconds.org/media/WP_EQ_and_Age.pdf

Gardner, H. (1987). The theory of multiple intelligences. *Annals of dyslexia*, 19–35.

Gardner, H. E. (2011). *Frames of mind: The theory of multiple intelligences*. Basic Books.

Goleman, D. (1998). *Working with emotional intelligence*. Bantam Books.

——— (1995). *Emotional intelligence: Why it can matter more than IQ*. Bantam Books.

Goleman, D. & Boyatzis, R. (2008). Social intelligence and the biology of leadership. *Harvard business review, 86*(9), 74–81.

Jordan, P. J. & Troth, A. C. (2002). Emotional intelligence and conflict resolution: Implications for human resource development. *Advances in Developing Human Resources, 4*(1), 62–79.

Karimi, L., Cheng, C., Bartram, T., Leggat, S. G. & Sarkeshik, S. (2015). The effects of emotional intelligence and stress-related presenteeism on nurses' well-being. *Asia Pacific Journal of Human Resources, 53*(3), 296–310.

Karimi, L., Leggat, S. G., Donohue, L., Farrell, G. & Couper, G. E. (2014). Emotional rescue: The role of emotional intelligence and emotional labour on well-being and job-stress among community nurses. *Journal of advanced nursing, 70*(1), 176–186.

Kaur, S. & Sharma, R. (2021). Emotion AI: Integrating emotional intelligence with artificial intelligence in the digital workplace. In P. K. Singh, Z. Polkowski, S. Tanwar, S. K. Pandey, G. Matei & D. Pirvu (eds), *Innovations in information and communication technologies (IICT-2020)*. Cham.

Kotsou, I., Mikolajczak, M., Heeren, A., Grégoire, J. & Leys, C. (2019). Improving emotional intelligence: A systematic review of existing work and future challenges. *Emotion review, 11*(2), 151–165.

Lopes, P. N., Grewal, D., Kadis, J., Gall, M. & Salovey, P. (2006). Evidence that emotional intelligence is related to job performance and affect and attitudes at work. *Psicothema,* 132–138.

Martínez-Marín, M. D., Martínez, C. & Paterna, C. (2021). Gendered self-concept and gender as predictors of emotional intelligence: a comparison through of age. *Current Psychology, 40*(9), 4205–4218. https://doi.org/10.1007/s12144-020-00904-z

Mayer, J. D., Caruso, D. R. & Salovey, P. (2016). The ability model of emotional intelligence: Principles and updates. *Emotion Review, 8*(4), 290–300.

Mayer, J. D. & Salovey, P. (2007). *Mayer-Salovey-Caruso emotional intelligence test*. Multi-Health Systems Incorporated Toronto.

Mayer, J. D., Salovey, P. & Caruso, D. R. (2004). Emotional intelligence: Theory, findings, and implications. *Psychological Inquiry, 15*(3), 197–215.

Mayer, J. D., Salovey, P., Caruso, D. R. & Sitarenios, G. (2003). Measuring emotional intelligence with the MSCEIT V2.0. *Emotion, 3*(1), 97.

Naghavi, F. & Redzuan, M. (2011). The relationship between gender and emotional intelligence. *World Applied Sciences Journal, 15*(4), 555–561.

Olderbak, S., Semmler, M. & Doebler, P. (2019). Four-branch model of ability emotional intelligence with fluid and crystallized intelligence: A meta-analysis of relations. *Emotion review, 11*(2), 166–183.

Papadogiannis, P. K., Logan, D. & Sitarenios, G. (2009). An ability model of emotional intelligence: A rationale, description, and application of the Mayer Salovey Caruso Emotional Intelligence Test (MSCEIT). In J. D. A. Parker, D. H. Saklofske & C. Stough (eds), *Assessing emotional intelligence: Theory, research, and applications* (pp. 43–65). Springer. https://doi.org/10.1007/978-0-387-88370-0_3

Petrides, K. V. (2009). Psychometric properties of the trait emotional intelligence questionnaire (TEIQue). In *Assessing emotional intelligence: Theory, research, and applications* (pp. 85–101). Springer US.

Petrides, K. & Furnham, A. (2009). Trait emotional intelligence questionnaire (TEIQue). *Technical Manual*. London Psychometric Laboratory.

Petrides, K. V. & Furnham, A. (2001). Trait emotional intelligence: Psychometric investigation with reference to established trait taxonomies. *European Journal of Personality, 15*(6), 425–448.

——— (2000). Gender differences in measured and self-estimated trait emotional intelligence. *Sex Roles, 42,* 449–461.

Petrides, K. V., Mikolajczak, M., Mavroveli, S., Sanchez-Ruiz, M.-J., Furnham, A. & Pérez-González, J.-C. (2016). Developments in trait emotional intelligence research. *Emotion review, 8*(4), 335–341.

Petrides, K. V., Pita, R. & Kokkinaki, F. (2007). The location of trait emotional intelligence in personality factor space. *British Journal of Psychology, 98*(2), 273–289.

Piefke, M., Weiss, P. H., Markowitsch, H. J. & Fink, G. R. (2005). Gender differences in the functional neuroanatomy of emotional episodic autobiographical memory. *Human Brain Mapping, 24*(4), 313–324. https://doi.org/10.1002/hbm.20092

Rosete, D. & Ciarrochi, J. (2005). Emotional intelligence and its relationship to workplace performance outcomes of leadership effectiveness. *Leadership & Organization Development Journal, 26*(5), 388–399.

Saha, S., Das, R., Lim, W. M., Kumar, S., Malik, A. & Chillakuri, B. (2023). Emotional intelligence and leadership: Insights for leading by feeling in the future of work. *International Journal of Manpower, 44*(4), 671–701. https://doi.org/10.1108/IJM-12-2021-0690

Salovey, P. & Mayer, J. D. (1990). Emotional intelligence. *Imagination, Cognition and Personality, 9*(3), 185–211.

Soriano-Vázquez, I., Cajachagua Castro, M. & Morales-García, W. C. (2023). Emotional intelligence as a predictor of job satisfaction: The mediating role of conflict management in nurses. *Front Public Health, 11*, 1249020. https://doi.org/10.3389/fpubh.2023.1249020

Thorndike, E. (1920). Intelligence and its uses. *Harper's Magazine*, 140, 227–235.

Warren, B. (2013). Healthcare emotional intelligence: Its role in patient outcomes and organizational success. *Becker's Hospital Review*. Retrieved from: https://www.beckershospitalreview.com/honspital-management-administration-/healthcare-emotional-intelligence-its-role-in-patient-outcomes-and-organizational-success.html

Zeidner, M., Matthews, G. & Roberts, R. D. (2012). *What we know about emotional intelligence: How it affects learning, work, relationships, and our mental health*. MIT Press.

6 Exploring values

Eleanor Milligan and Jennifer Jones

Learning objectives

How do I:

- identify my personal values?
- learn how my personal values developed over time?
- understand and apply the importance and role of values in healthcare leadership?
- ensure an organisational culture that is based on appropriate values?
- develop my skills in values-based leadership strategies in my organisation?

Introduction

Mahatma Gandhi is attributed as saying, 'Your beliefs become your thoughts, your thoughts become your words, your words become your actions, your actions become your habits, your habits become your values, your values become your destiny' (Ganguly, 2019, p. S145). Values permeate every aspect of our lives, shaping individual actions and giving meaning, direction and scope to our work environments and organisational cultures. Defining positive behaviours and identifying unprofessional, disrespectful or negative behaviours shape and define every aspect of our work and personal lives. Values also have an emotional component: when we act in accordance with our values, we experience positive emotions; conversely, when we act against our values or are placed in situations that compromise our values, we experience emotional dissonance. It is this emotional component that drives us to seek values alignment in our personal and professional lives.

In healthcare, values-based leadership is particularly important. Patients seek our care often at the most vulnerable times in their lives. In their vulnerability, they must trust us to provide competent and compassionate care. They may have little choice but to trust that the healthcare system and those who work within it will act in their best interests. This power imbalance compels those who work within, manage and lead healthcare organisations to be trustworthy (Milligan, 2023). The significant financial resources, paid for by the community at large through taxation, further reinforce the social obligation on healthcare organisations to be trustworthy and act in alignment with community values. The values of care, trust and reciprocity, therefore, define effective healthcare, as caring for vulnerable others makes the provision of health services a moral, value-laden practice.

In this chapter, we explore where values come from, why they are important, how they can be used to form the basis of ethically sound leadership in promoting an organisation's ethical climate and culture, and how values-based leadership can build and maintain a trustworthy healthcare sector.

Definitions

Given the inextricable link between **values** and behaviour, the values we hold in our hearts inevitably become visible in our outward actions. The same is true for organisations: the values that shape the culture of an organisation are on display in the practices, norms, policies and codes that are endorsed within it. In his seminal work on organisational culture, *Culture's consequences: Comparing values, behaviors, institutions and organizations across nations*, Geert Hofstede (2001) proposes that our practices (heroes, symbols, rituals) are the outwardly visible representation of our hidden, or invisible, values.

Values: 'Underlying attitudes and beliefs that determine individual behaviour' (Viinamäki, 2012, p. 29)

As a leader, it is important to reflect upon questions like the following:

Who does your organisation hold as its heroes?
Does your organisation reward competitiveness while espousing collaboration?
What symbols represent your organisation, and what do they say about your
  organisation's values?
What rituals does your organisation adhere to?
Do the values evident in these behaviours align with the organisation's espoused values?

Values system: The ordering of values on the basis of their importance to individuals or organisations

Organisational values and **values systems** provide employees with norms that guide decision-making and behaviour in the workplace (Edwards & Cable, 2009). It is therefore important to give them careful attention.

In large and complex organisations, shared common values – or values congruence – are recognised as an important factor in forming a coherent and successful organisation in ways that benefit individual staff and the organisation itself (Howell, Kirk-Brown & Cooper, 2012). Buchko (2007) further explains that:

> Values are the glue that binds people together in organisations. When a group of people share a set of beliefs about the goals that need to be achieved and the means to be used to attain those goals, there is a basis for organisation. In fact without some common beliefs or values, organisations could not exist; people need a common set of beliefs to come together and create social organisations. (p. 37)

In the complex context of healthcare, it is almost inevitable that those in senior leadership roles will face challenges to their personal and professional values. Indeed, Graber and Kilpatrick (2008) argue that 'challenges and crises are in a sense necessary to not only test, but to evoke, the leader's values' (p. 186). In this environment, 'ethics and values may offer a more predictable, stable and sustainable base for leadership ... and provide a certain "warranty" on integrity and future prospects in organisations' (Viinamäki, 2012, p. 28). Knowing their personal and professional values can empower and equip leaders to make principle-based decisions in a way that models ethical leadership to their staff, builds trust and promotes confidence.

Personal values

Phenomenological philosophers such as Maurice Merleau-Ponty, Charles Taylor and Paul Ricoeur argue that the formation of a person's ethical framework and values system is a complex, multifaceted and highly individualised process. Each of us, from the day we are born, experience the world on multiple different levels, each bringing knowledge, social expectations and norms that mould our moral development and values framework (Isaacs, 2003, 2010).

The experiences that shape our values arise from how these values are embedded in the areas discussed here. From the examples given, we can gain an appreciation of the complex factors that make up each person's individual ethical framework and values system. Through appreciation and knowledge of our personal values, we can gain insight into our own and others' motivations and begin to challenge unreflective or habitual responses to various situations, including navigating values conflicts in the workplace (Clark, 2008).

The natural world

The natural world affects us physically, spatially and biologically. With respect to health, for example, our expectations and values concerning varied abilities, disabilities or physical incapacities are influenced by our own lived reality. How we view these factors in others is prejudiced by our assumptions, which are based on personal experience.

The social world

The social world is the area of multiple relationships, cultures, politics, economies, nations and communities of all shapes, moral understandings and identities. With respect to health, for example, if we have been embedded in a cultural norm of 'free' healthcare, this may shape our values and expectations when it comes to decision-making about access to high-cost care for our patients. In a culture of presumed plenty, we may feel justified in dismissing the financial considerations of health resourcing, as our expectation is that no-one will, or should, miss out.

Temporal space

The area of temporal space requires consideration of the ways in which our cultural norms relate to our historical context and how our historical temporality influences our perception of the present and imagining of the future. With respect to healthcare, for example, we may value growth in scientific knowledge and expect that this body of knowledge will continue to be pursued. We may also expect that technological advances will be fully implemented for the benefit of our patients.

Language

Language mediates our relationships with others. It supports understanding, shapes our identities and enables us to express our future growth and desires. With respect to health, the choice of language can alter and define clinical relationships. We may, for example, choose to call those who seek our care 'patients', or we may call them 'consumers'. The language we adopt defines the terms of the relationship. We may interact with a consumer who is purchasing a product or service. The use of a different term, such as 'patient', may frame the interaction as one in which a moral duty of care exists beyond the transactional nature of supplying goods or services. Hence, language shapes the moral tenor, assumptions and expectations of healthcare interactions, positively and negatively.

Spiritual horizons

For some people, spirituality gives direction and meaning to life. Many aspects of care evoke spiritual values that affect patients, staff and organisations. Issues concerning withdrawal of life-sustaining measures at the end of life, or a patient's request for termination of a pregnancy, may highlight challenges to the spiritual values of those involved (Isaacs, 2010).

Professional values

Once we enter a profession, another layer of shared socialisation and norms is added to our existing values framework (Hofstede, 2001). Similarly, when individuals become socialised in a particular organisation, yet another layer of shared experience and values is added. Like personal values, professional and organisational values are culminations of multiple layers of compounding and competing experience.

An essential first step in understanding and thoughtfully applying values-based leadership is to define one's own core values. A helpful tool for this is the VIA Character Strengths and Values Test (https://www.personality-quizzes.com/via-character-strengths). While it does not provide a definitive list, it is a starting point for recognising how values shape behaviour. It also enables users to reflect upon the origins of their values and can help foster appreciation of one's own motivations and the motivations of others' behaviours. As an example, imagine that one of your strong personal values is gratitude. Your leadership style will be one in which you consciously show appreciation to your colleagues, and you are likely to flourish in an environment in which you feel appreciated and noticed for your contribution. However, if you find yourself in a work environment where you feel undervalued, you are likely to interpret this as a negative workplace culture and to experience significant distress. In interactions with patients, those you perceive as 'ungrateful' may spark emotional reactions of resentment, or counter-transference. Understanding the source of these emotions as based on one of your values – that is, gratitude – and recognising the causes can help you to manage their consequences. For example, to minimise the effects of counter-transference on patient care, strategies such as implementing team-based care or having regular supervision or debriefing with colleagues can be helpful.

As a further example, imagine that one of your strong values is truthfulness. You will likely flourish in organisations that have a culture of transparency and openness, and your leadership style will model honesty and promote this in others. Moral distress may arise if you perceive that information is being withheld or an adverse event is not disclosed on the grounds of avoiding harm to a patient. In recognising your distress as based on one of your values – that is, honesty – you can frame discussions directly in language that identifies the ethical source of your concern.

Knowledge of your own values and those of your colleagues is therefore helpful, not only in enabling you to manage your own emotional reactions but also in understanding team dynamics and building values congruence within your organisation and with your colleagues.

Leadership and values

Leaders are tasked with ensuring the efficient and financially responsible management of their organisations. However, they are equally responsible for ensuring that appropriate ethical standards are promoted, modelled and upheld. Edgar Schein (2010) notes, 'leadership begins the culture creation process and … must also manage and sometimes change culture'. Similarly, Blanchard & O'Connor (1997, p. 3) claim that 'no longer is values-based organisational behaviour an interesting philosophical choice – it is a requisite for survival' (p. 3).

Since staff members take their cues from the actions of those in leadership positions, the ways in which values are modelled by managers and leaders are crucial. Leaders communicate organisational values to all employees; they model values in action, empower others to make principled decisions and promote trust. Individual leaders therefore have significant influence over the ethical culture of the organisation (Buchko, 2007). Positive role-modelling promotes confidence in leaders and improves values congruence for staff, which in turn promotes loyalty and optimism (De Hoog & den Hartog, 2008). The improved 'affective commitment' (Howell et al., 2012, p. 732) to an organisation because of improved trust and values congruence has also been correlated to the improved retention of staff (Buckley et al., 2001; Olson, 1995; Schluter, Winch, Holzhauser & Henderson, 2008).

This has significant implications for organisational stability, which is especially important in healthcare organisations, in which workforce instability can have negative effects on patient care (Schluter et al., 2008).

At the organisational level, the ability to articulate shared values is an important strategy in managing complex organisations, since values are the foundation of shared principles of decision-making. Promoting shared values creates a vehicle through which the diverse views and expectations of individuals within an organisation can be focused towards a commonly agreed, overarching goal. Authentic alignment to a set of organisational values, or core values, is consistently recognised as a characteristic of successful organisations (Viinamäki, 2012).

Ethical climate and culture

When the ethical climate, organisational culture and the values of employees align in a healthcare organisation, there are significant benefits, including improved organisational stability, stronger emotional commitment and trust from staff, and improved quality of care, confidence and trust for the public (Olson, 1995; Schluter et al., 2008).

Ethical climate

One of the most important enablers of ethical behaviour is being situated in a climate that supports ethical decision-making. The **ethical climate** is shaped by the prevailing organisational practices, procedures and codes that have ethical content or determine ethical action. In their seminal work, Victor and Cullen (1988) claim that ethical climates centre around three dimensions: egoism, benevolence and principles. Further research has confirmed that benevolent and principled climates are more likely to reduce unethical conduct. Ego-based climates, on the other hand, are more likely to create unethical behaviour (Kish-Gephart, Harrison & Triveno, 2010; Wimbush & Shepard, 1994). Hence, a leader's ability to promote a climate of acting on principle through values-based leadership, giving attention to the good of the whole, can reduce unethical workplace behaviour (Kish-Gephart et al., 2010).

Ethical climate: 'A group of prescriptive climates reflecting the organisational procedures, policies and practices with moral consequences' (Martin & Cullen, 2006, p. 177)

For further exploration of ethical climate in an organisation, the Ethical Climate Questionnaire (Victor & Cullen, 1987, 1988; Cullen, Victor & Bronson, 1993) is a validated tool and useful resource.

Organisational culture

Organisational culture is described as the shared values, meanings, beliefs, assumptions, rituals, myths, language and metaphors that describe an organisation. It predicts how people behave and determines the behaviours that are rewarded or punished. It also demonstrates the values at play within the organisation.

Organisational culture: The shared values, meanings, beliefs, assumptions, rituals, myths, language and metaphors that describe an organisation

It follows that through ethical climate and organisational culture, organisations and their leaders can proactively create ethical environments that can either promote or undermine ethical choices (Kish-Gephart et al., 2010). Furthermore, employees look to leaders to display authenticity, to match their espoused values with their enacted values.

Values-based leadership

Despite the hierarchical nature of health service structures, all staff at every level of the organisation can influence care, culture and patient outcomes by exhibiting **values-based leadership** within their own sphere of influence. Values-based leadership provides a framework

Values-based leadership: Leadership based on foundational moral principles (Viinamäki, 2012)

for making the inherent moral aspects of healthcare explicit, inviting and challenging everyone in healthcare, in particular leaders, to model ethical behaviour, to make decisions based on ethical principles, to provide clear leadership, to strengthen the ethical climate and culture, and to improve alignment of organisational and personal values, thereby reducing moral distress for staff and promoting alignment.

The defining feature of values-based leadership is communicating the values of the organisation and consistently acting in accordance with them. Leaders who lead from an authentic values foundation are more effective than those who do not, as they provide credible and legitimate role models and effectively set standards of behaviour by rewarding ethical conduct. They also have the standing to identify and effectively respond to unethical conduct. The four elements discussed following are crucial in ensuring the success of values-based leadership.

Values recognition

To act from a values base, a person must first recognise the situation as having an ethical, or values, dimension. Failure to do so results in the adoption of another decision-making schema, such as economic rationality or egocentric self-interest. Practical steps for healthcare leaders to promote recognition of values include knowing their personal and professional values and increasing employee knowledge of values and ethics through education – for example, using public forums such as grand rounds, in which the values aspects of the organisation's work are openly discussed and modelled. Such forums can be used to explore ethically challenging situations – for example, unlikeable patients, withdrawal of life-sustaining measures and resource allocation. An organisation's willingness to openly discuss ethically laden issues demonstrates authenticity and transparency, promoting a culture of openness and honesty.

A further practical step is working with internal stakeholders to create a shared sense of values and to link these to organisational values and principled decision-making. For example, if an organisational value is honesty, an open disclosure policy might outline an organisational pathway for principled decision-making with respect to sharing information concerning adverse events with all those affected, even when this is uncomfortable.

Values awareness

Leaders model values awareness when they demonstrate concern for the collective good of the whole group and for the impact of the means and ends of the decision-making process; consider the long-term and short-term consequences of the decision; and commit to seeking the views and input of multiple stakeholders who will be affected by the decision.

Practical steps for healthcare leaders in promoting values awareness include clarifying the extent to which the organisation promotes the values its leaders aspire to implement. For example, if an organisation's values include justice, its leaders might consider pathways to promoting access for socially and financially disadvantaged patients. Healthcare leaders can also facilitate discussions that communicate the enduring values of the organisation. For example, during staff meetings, decision-making should be linked to organisational values. If one of the organisation's values is community, then a proactive invitation to external stakeholders to participate in decision-making within the organisation will demonstrate living that value. Other practical steps involve committing to ensure that organisational values are embedded into the ethical codes, procedures and practices adopted by the organisation; ensuring that organisational values are visible to employees – for example, through a tagline on all email correspondence or the design of a logo that has meaning related to the values; making organisational values visible to the community through a public website and communications; and monitoring feedback and evaluation systems, and acting upon what they say about the enactment of organisational values.

> ## RESOURCE ALLOCATION
>
> A 59-year-old man, Joe, presents to the emergency department of a hospital, breathless and blue in the face. On examination he appears confused and weak. His history reveals a diagnosis of an advanced form of renal cancer two years previously, which has been treated aggressively at his request. Discussion further reveals that Joe has refused palliative care despite his poor prognosis, and his condition has continued to deteriorate.
>
> Despite the reality that he is nearing the end of his life, Joe's wife is advocating for 'all possible treatments', citing Joe's wishes and the family's future financial security: the amount of Joe's superannuation payment will decrease significantly if he is not alive on his 60th birthday, now six days away. Following the accidental death of their son and daughter-in-law 3 years ago, Joe and his wife are now also the legal guardians of their 12-year-old grandson.
>
> As Joe's condition deteriorates further, a decision needs to be made in relation to the allocation of resources to care for him. He requires more care than can be provided on a regular ward, and now staff must consider whether it is a justifiable use of resources to care for him in the intensive care unit, at a cost of around $4500 per day (Hicks et al., 2019), when there is no prospect of improvement. Staff are further aware that delaying Joe's death, which could be possible if he is cared for in the intensive care unit, will have significant financial benefit for his wife and grandchild.
>
> In considering Joe's case, it is evident that there are multiple competing demands. For instance, if equitable healthcare for all is a major value, the use of a finite resource to delay Joe's inevitable and imminent death will be a primary concern as it may deny this resource to other patients with better prognoses. If, however, patient autonomy, the right to self-determination, is a core value, consideration of Joe's wishes will be the primary consideration. These competing and compelling demands, in the broader context of 'caring' – which incorporates the amelioration of suffering (physical, mental, emotional or spiritual) – make evident the multilayered nature of the ethical challenge. Legal advice is sought, and all clinical options being considered are legally appropriate.
>
> In making sense of the situation and in seeking a best-practice outcome, practitioners are guided and supported by the personal, professional and organisational values, which have arisen from multiple layers of compounding and competing experience.
>
> What would you do in this situation? What outcome would you advocate for? What values are informing your decision? What values stance might others adopt that differs from yours? How would you navigate a disagreement? Whatever decision is made, some staff members will be distressed by the outcome. As a leader, how will you bring your team back together and provide space for moral reflection?

Values practice

Since ethical problems are often characterised by uncertainty and ambiguity, leaders must have the skills to make principled decisions and to demonstrate the practical application of values. Steps that demonstrate competence include:

- communicating and reinforcing values through strategic avenues within the organisation
- rewarding behaviour that aligns with organisational values
- seeking consensus when values clash
- providing feedback to strengthen capacity and understanding
- providing organisational structures at all levels where values can be shared, debated and agreed.

Values commitment

Commitment to values-based leadership requires the ongoing communication of values, establishment of reward systems that reinforce organisational values and authentic modelling of organisational values by those in leadership positions. If any of these steps is weak or missing, the success of values-based leadership implementation will be compromised and may ultimately fail (Graber & Kilpatrick, 2008; Olson, 1995; Viinamäki, 2012).

Summary

- Values are underlying attitudes and beliefs that shape our behaviour.
- Values arise from multiple sources and are related to our individual experiences with respect to the natural world, our social norms, the time and historical context of our experiences, the language we are exposed to and choose, and the spiritual dimensions that give meaning to these experiences.
- Organisational values evolve in response to internal and external factors that shape the purpose, role and expectations held by the organisation and its stakeholders.
- Important values inherent in effective leadership are authenticity, integrity, trustworthiness and social responsibility.
- The organisational and individual benefits of values in healthcare leadership include improved confidence, commitment, trust, loyalty and retention, and reduced likelihood of unethical behaviour.
- The promotion of values through strong ethical climates and organisational cultures can create healthy ethical environments to promote sound ethical choices.

Reflective questions

1. What are your core values?
2. Think of a time when your individual values were at odds with the values of a colleague or with the organisational values of your workplace. How did this make you feel? What steps, if any, did you take to resolve the tension?

3. Faced with a situation today in which your individual values are at odds with the values of a colleague or with the organisational values of your workplace, what new understanding could you bring in resolving the situation?
4. Think about a time when you felt most effective in your professional or personal life. What made this time memorable? What values were foremost at this time?
5. Do you believe values-based leadership would benefit your organisation? What are the barriers and enablers to values-based leadership in your organisation?

Self-analysis questions

After listing your values, consider how your values are evident in your personal and professional behaviours. Are there any inconsistencies in your list? Do you feel this list has evolved and changed as you have grown in your personal and professional life? How can you use your awareness of your values to understand your motivations and the motivations and behaviours of others?

References

Blanchard, K. & O'Connor, M. (1997). (With J. Ballard.) *Managing by values*. Berrett-Koehler.

Buchko, A. (2007). The effect of leadership on values-based management. *Leadership & Organization Development Journal*, *28*(1), 36–50. https://doi.org/10.1108/01437730710718236

Buckley, R. M., Beu, D. S., Frink, D. D., Howard, J. L., Berkson, H., Mobbs, T. A. & Ferris, G. R. (2001). Ethical issues in human resources systems. *Human Resource Management Review*, *11*, 11–29. https://doi.org/10.1016/S1053-4822(00)00038-3

Clark, L. (2008). Clinical leadership: Values, beliefs and vision. *Nursing Management*, *15*(7), 30–35. https://doi.org/10.7748/nm2008.11.15.7.30.c6807

Cullen, J. B., Victor, B. & Bronson, J. W. (1993). The ethical climate questionnaire: An assessment of its development and validity. *Psychological Reports*, *73*, 667–674. https://doi.org/10.2466/pr0.1993.73.2.667

De Hoog, A. H. B. & den Hartog, D. N. (2008). Ethical and despotic leadership, relationships with leader's social responsibility, top management team effectiveness and subordinates' optimism: A multi-method study. *Leadership Quarterly*, *19*, 297–311. https://doi.org/10.1016/j.leaqua.2008.03.002

Edwards, J. R. & Cable, D. M. (2009). The value of value congruence. *Journal of Applied Psychology*, *94*(3), 654–677. https://doi.org/10.1037/a0014891

Ganguly, K. K. (2019). Life of M. K. Gandhi: A message to youth of modern India. *The Indian Journal of Medical Research*, *149*(Suppl), S145–S151. https://doi.org/10.4103/0971-5916.251672

Graber, D. & Kilpatrick, A. (2008). Establishing values-based leadership and value systems in healthcare organizations. *Journal of Health and Human Services Administration*, *31*(2), 179–197.

Hicks, P., Huckson, S., Fenney, E., Leggat, I., Pilcher, D. & Litton, E. (2019). The financial cost of intensive care in Australia: A multicentre registry study. *Medical Journal of Australia*, *217*(7), 324–325.

Hofstede, G. (2001). *Culture's consequences: Comparing values, behaviors, institutions and organizations across nations*. Sage.

Howell, A., Kirk-Brown, A. & Cooper, B. K. (2012). Does congruence between espoused and enacted organizational values predict affective commitment in Australian organizations? *International Journal of Human Resource Management*, *23*(4), 731–747. https://doi.org/10.1080/09585192.2011.561251

Isaacs, P. (2010). Ontology, narrative and ethical engagement. In E. Milligan & E. Woodley (eds), *Confessions: Confounding narrative and ethics* (pp. 121–42). Cambridge Scholars.

——— (2003). *Doing ethics: An action based approach.* Paper presented at the Peninsula Behavioural Health Conference, Gatlinburg, TN.

Kish-Gephart, J., Harrison, D. & Triveno, L. K. (2010). Bad apples, bad cases and bad barrels: Meta-analytic evidence about sources of unethical decisions at work. *Journal of Applied Psychology, 95*(1), 1–31. https://doi.org/10.1037/a0017103

Martin, K. D. & Cullen, J. B. (2006). Continuities and extensions of ethical climate theory: A meta-analytic review. *Journal of Business Ethics, 69,* 175–194. https://doi.org/10.1007/s10551-006-9084-7

Milligan E. (2023). Ethics in healthcare leadership – Knowing, doing, being and becoming. In S. Lloyd et al. (eds), *Leading in health and social care.* https://oercollective.caul.edu.au/leading-in-health-and-social-care/

Olson, L. (1995). Ethical climate in health care organizations. *International Nursing Review, 42*(3), 85–90.

Schein, E. H. (2010). *Organizational culture and leadership* (4th ed.). Jossey-Bass.

Schluter, J., Winch, S., Holzhauser, K. & Henderson, A. (2008). Nurses' moral sensitivity and hospital ethical climate: A literature review. *Nursing Ethics, 15*(3), 304–321. https://doi.org/10.1177/0969733007088357

Victor, B. & Cullen, J. B. (1988). The organisational basis of ethical work climates. *Administrative Science Quarterly, 33*(1), 101–25. https://doi.org/10.2307/2392857

——— (1987). A theory and measure of ethical climate in organizations. In W. C. Frederick (ed.), *Research in corporate social performance and policy* (pp. 51–71). JAI.

Viinamäki, O. (2012). Why leaders fail in introducing values-based leadership? An elaboration of feasible steps, challenges, and suggestions for practitioners. *International Journal of Business and Management, 7*(9), 28–39. https://doi.org/10.5539/ijbm.v7n9p28

Wimbush, J. C. & Shepard, J. M. (1994). Toward an understanding of ethical climate: Its relationship to ethical behaviour and supervisory influence. *Journal of Business Ethics, 13*(8), 637–647. https://doi.org/10.1007/BF00871811

Ambiguity and leadership

Mark Avery

7

Learning objectives

How do I:

- develop a clear understanding of how ambiguity in organisational settings affects management and leadership?
- reduce ambiguity?
- enhance the ability to confidently recognise, diagnose and effectively address ambiguity within healthcare organisations?
- acquire skills and knowledge in useful approaches to managing positions, directions and outcomes related to ambiguous circumstances and problems?

Introduction

The complexities inherent in healthcare organisations highlight the multifaceted nature of their operations. Regardless of role, scale, procedural intricacies or governance structures, these organisations need to deal with the complexities of both internal dynamics and external landscapes. The diversity of stakeholders involved adds layers of challenge to effectively managing clinical and social processes, optimising outcomes, allocating resources equitably, developing and retaining a skilled workforce, making informed decisions and upholding ethical standards.

Navigating this complex framework demands more than managerial capacity; it necessitates a blend of skills, strategies and personal competencies tailored to the nuances of healthcare leadership. Leaders must adeptly steer their organisations while also cultivating the resources and capabilities to inspire and guide individuals, teams and entire workforces toward shared goals amidst this landscape.

Definitions

Ambiguity is defined as lack of certainty or dependability of meaning in communication, action or knowledge. It describes a situation in which information could be interpreted, construed or understood in more than one way. It is a natural aspect of the operations of healthcare facilities and the environments in which they engage with many stakeholders. Leading and managing health organisations requires awareness, understanding and focused action to ensure that ambiguous situations are managed for impact and usefulness to the health facility.

Ambiguity: Lack of certainty or dependability of meaning in communication, action or knowledge

Uncertainty: Limited or no understanding of knowledge or information regarding a given state or situation

Clarity: Intelligible and comprehensible thoughts, actions and purposes

Vagueness: Imprecision in communication or language regarding a situation

Three important elements align with **ambiguity**: uncertainty, clarity and vagueness. The purpose of a strong understanding of the roles of these elements in dealing with ambiguous situations in organisations relates to the leader's strength of understanding and comprehension of information and knowledge.

Firstly, **uncertainty** has been associated with human conceptions and understandings that may not be objective. For example, health managers may be uncertain about whether the services provided to consumers are valued or seen as high quality. These are situations that can be addressed by obtaining facts from consumers (directly or indirectly), but given the large and varied number of consumers in healthcare, there can be ambiguity in understanding their views on service needs and quality of care. Secondly, **clarity** is important in leadership, as it is the mechanism by which to ensure that staff or followers in an organisation understand requirements, directions, interpretations and purposes. The opposite of clarity is ambiguity. Health managers aim for clarity in direction and communication. Finally, **vagueness** – where communication and language about facts in a matter or situation are not certain or firm in imparting understanding – is also relevant. A healthcare leader might aim to use feedback from consumers as part of the organisation's quality review process. A vague approach here might result in consumer feedback that is not useful.

Healthcare

In health organisations and in leading them, two aspects of ambiguity are important: organisational ambiguity and role ambiguity.

Organisation ambiguity

Organisation, or bureaucratic, ambiguity concerns the development and values of the organisation. Best (2012) highlights the central role that ambiguity plays in the complex organisation. Organisations are formed for many reasons, and it is in the architecture and operation of their structures that ambiguity can be both identified and valued.

Health organisations operate in uncertain, risky and constantly changing service and environmental contexts (Page, Irving, Amalberti & Vincent, 2024). The managers must actively work to manage uncertainty by addressing and mitigating unpredictable environments through key activities. These include planning, developing systems and processes, and setting strategic and operational directions. Standardisation is essential in supporting efficiency and effectiveness, which are achieved by developing policies and procedures for the organisation as a whole, as well as for specific, localised applications. Additionally, organisations need to measure and quantify their processes, goals and outcomes to support planning, operations and achievements.

Standardisation and development of policies and procedures support effective management in these contexts and enable clear communication and agreement with staff members. Quantification supports both operational clinical and non-clinical activities and establishes the basis for process and outcome evaluation. Leaders in health organisations can capitalise on the management of ambiguity through a bureaucratic organisational framework of systems and planning, policies and procedures, and qualification of performance. Casting of situations and paradigms onto these frameworks enables the leader to reduce complexity and ambiguity, and therefore to focus on interpretation and action.

Role ambiguity

Problems associated with ill-defined or ill-formed roles and lack of understanding about roles have a negative effect on organisational performance and can cause stress and lowered job satisfaction for individuals (Maden-Eyiusta, 2021). Key requirements associated with **role ambiguity** in an organisation or among workers include the existence of comprehensive role delineation, management of new or changing roles and general or wide communications regarding roles. In relation to healthcare, a study of nurses reports that role conflict and ambiguity can be associated with stress in professional roles (Zhang, Liu & Lang, 2024).

Role ambiguity: Lack of clarity about expected actions and behaviours associated with roles or positions in an organisation

When discussing ambiguity in health organisations, it is useful to consider ambiguity in the role of leadership. Leadership is a complex role with complex actions. At times and in some contexts, leadership is difficult to define and evaluate. Leadership behaviours, characteristics and styles can make assessing the effectiveness of leadership and its influence on the performance of an organisation difficult. Ziegert and Dust (2021) examine the concepts of leadership, the effectiveness of leaders and the attribution of leadership. This brings into focus the need for leaders to connect impact and effectiveness to the key organisational issues, including dealing with ambiguity.

The healthcare organisation and the key responsibility of service provision and delivery are often planned and structured in the context of internal and external ambiguity. Complex healthcare organisations (as opposed to complexity in the organisation) provide both an operational and an environmental setting for ambiguity, but they also provide structures, processes and problem-solving constructs that can be used to address the issues of ambiguity.

AMBIGUITY RELATED TO EMERGENCY DEPARTMENT SERVICE PLANNING

MetroVista General Hospital, a public hospital located in an outer-metropolitan area, serves a diverse community through its 24/7 Emergency Department (ED). Despite meticulous planning and resource management, the ED grapples with unpredictable challenges stemming from the inherent nature of emergency services and external economic and environmental factors. The complexity of forecasting patient access is influenced by strategic management, leadership and the decision-making processes tailored to navigate the ED's uncertainties.

Effective leadership in the ED, particularly regarding service availability and access, requires a comprehensive approach that encompasses data-driven decision-making, scenario planning and robust staff support. Anticipating the demand for ED services entails a deep understanding of patient care needs and proactive engagement with external conditions.

At MetroVista, the ED's planning to respond with emergency services is complicated by several factors, including:

- seasonal fluctuations and specific community health trends affecting patient volumes
- challenges in staffing, particularly in recruiting and retaining qualified personnel while also addressing staff resilience and burnout
- constraints on resources that strain service-delivery capabilities
- economic shifts and insurance cover changes affecting patients' ability to afford care privately
- availability of access to healthcare providers outside normal service hours
- enhancing community education on the ED's role to be able to effectively manage expectations.

MetroVista's management recognises the importance of comprehensive service-demand planning, considering both operational and external factors to deal with ambiguity and strengthen the ED's operational strategy. This strategic clarity is essential for ensuring the ED's capacity to deliver timely and effective care to its community.

Management and ambiguity

Ambiguity affects key areas of planning, development and decision-making, and requires a comprehensive approach. In most complex organisations, the management of ambiguity is not handled alone or in a simple, straightforward way. Two key areas in which ambiguity interrelates are in organisations' change management programs and processes, and in strategies and processes of evaluation. Both are discussed following.

Change management approaches

Managing change and leading in ambiguity are closely linked as both require adaptability, resilience and a clear vision. In change management, leaders guide organisations through transitions, helping teams navigate in ambiguous settings and contexts. Leading in ambiguity involves making decisions with incomplete information, nurturing a culture of trust and maintaining direction despite unknowns. Leaders operating in ambiguous environments empower others, encouraging flexible responses and continuous learning. These application areas are essential for managing change successfully and building organisational resilience in uncertain times.

Healthcare managers use change-management approaches with varying degrees of sophistication. The nature and complexity of the reform and development agenda that organisations face and develop influence the different types of changes and transformation approaches. Related here is the issue of ambiguity, which can be affected by timeframes (planning over medium and longer terms), the clarity of the growth and development agenda and the capacity of the organisation in the development of the change process and in all forms of its resourcing.

Changes in an organisation evolve at different rates, and variations in the organisation's activity levels, tolerance and resourcing affect these rates. The ability to describe and instil key aspects of organisational development is an important factor in the change management process. Whether processes enable review and understanding of internal and external environments will affect the content, quality and rates of change. Nadler and Tushman (1995) identify four key types of changes in organisations:

1. **Tuning** is the seeking of better ways of performing or defending, and these are generally initiated internally.
2. **Adaption** concerns responses to external pressures that are mainly influential on incremental and adaptive shifts in behaviour and operations.
3. **Re-orientation** affects the redefinition of the organisation or its system and engenders knowledge and support in nature.
4. **Re-creation** involves reactive change to transform the organisation or its system.

The alignment and influence of ambiguity relate to the complexity and needs of the change processes outlined. For example, change that in nature is tuning for an organisation (where incremental and other less-complicated ways of working are at hand) requires less sophistication and information to support reform. This is compared with re-orientation and re-creation, which compel more novel and unique information about, and opportunities for, new ways of working that may not be readily recognisable to organisations.

The change-management process needs to address these key levels of response, as the environment is dynamic, driven by research, technology, consumer demand, ageing populations and health economics. Associated with this is a matrix of change drivers: environmental factors, risk and safety dynamics, and significant and finite resourcing.

Several studies (Bass et al., 2020, Harvey & Kudesia, 2023) identify important skills and competencies that enhance leaders' capacity and effectiveness in managing problems of ambiguity and change-management processes:

- **Problem-finding** involves the identification of the right problem through judgement, intuition and logic, and then recognition of the opportunities available.
- **Map-building** is the ability to generate one or more conceptualisation approaches to a situation by relating organisational and personal values and identities to situational demands.
- **Janusian thinking** (from the Greek god Janus, who faces two directions at once) involves constructively joining contradictory beliefs through mapping a direction that compensates for poorly structured issues with creative thinking.
- **Controlling and not controlling** is application of judgement: knowing which factors can be influenced and when.
- **Humour** diffuses stress and encourages creativity, reassuring and fusing tense and hostile situations.
- **Charisma** is the provision of enthusiasm, commitment and confidence to the problem-solving situation. (McCaskey, 1988)

These skills and competencies align with research undertaken by Hodgson and White (2003) in terms of effective skills for leadership and strategy in handling ambiguity and the feelings of uncertainty. To overcome fear of failure, the high levels of uncertainty experienced by leaders and managers in modern organisations should be addressed, and the need for them to experiment and take risks, along with associated reconditioning in their organisations and their agendas, stressed.

Leaders who are effective in the management of ambiguity in organisations are good at helping others to find energy and fun through the introduction of experimentation in new approaches to confronting situations. Simple and clear questions and communication are features of dynamic and responsive organisations. This relates not only to problem identification and generation of alternatives but also to the process and effectiveness of implementation. Achieving balanced focus is necessary; it should not be too narrow and blinded to the possibilities but should be able to hold and retain clear understanding of a few key tasks. Mastery of inner sense involves combining skills in management of rational and factual activity with use and confidence of instinct, experience and intuition.

Evaluating health services

The effectiveness of goals, objectives and tasks in health organisations needs evaluation, to appraise the outcomes of leadership of change, development and problem-solving, and to progressively and iteratively consider the strengths and weaknesses of the efforts made. An evaluation logic model is useful in informing the evaluation of problem-solving in the context of ambiguous situations and in focusing targets of knowledge and information. Use of an evaluation logic model gives context, structure and mechanisms in grounding thinking and review, thereby reducing ambiguity.

There are several forms and approaches in such models, but one that is useful comes originally from a system evaluation developed in the 1970s by Carol Weiss (1998; see Figure 7.1). The model highlights three core components that are useful in evaluation of programs and structures in health organisations. The first relates to inputs, processes and outputs in health organisations' clinical and non-clinical operations. Focus gives clarity to issues associated with resourcing, systems and approaches to organisation of direct and indirect care, and differentiation of outputs from those processes.

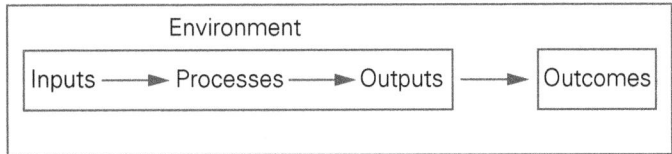

Figure 7.1 Evaluation logic model

Source: Adapted from W. K. Kellogg Foundation (2004).

The second component relates to outcomes of care and services. Outcomes are the results that may or may not have been intended from the service, activity or care provided. Ambiguity regarding resources and processes affects the success of outcomes.

Finally, healthcare organisations operate in complicated and sophisticated environments (e.g. ownership, stakeholder, regulatory, economic and research and development environments). Environments are multifaceted; therefore, a high degree of complexity is found within them.

Leadership and ambiguity

Communication

Eisenberg (1984) highlights important subtleties in interpretation and flexibility associated with leadership of ambiguity, particularly as it relates to communication in organisations. While leaders often strive for clarity and open communication in organisations, Eisenberg cautions against an over-emphasis on such clarity. A degree of ambiguity in development and communication of strategy supports development of an environment for change. Where ambiguity exists, there is opportunity to encourage multiple viewpoints or opinions, to create debate and discernment. Opportunities to foster agreement on abstract issues without limiting interpretation provide for contribution and goal focus in thinking and problem-solving. Many organisations articulate goals and objectives with a degree of ambiguity in them to enable the freedom to alter plans and operations over time.

Managing ambiguity

In large healthcare systems, particularly with development agendas related to networking and aggregation of impact, sometimes simplistic assumptions of problems or standardisation may be limiting. Best (2012) discusses the unexpected nature of complex political, economic and scientific environments and makes a case for a degree of discretion and judgement in ambiguous situations. The power and expertise of the managers in an organisation can help solve complex situations by working within the ambiguity. Therefore, ambiguity may be an effective management strategy to bring about complex change.

Leadership and ambiguity

Key qualities and activities that leaders can bring to health organisations to sensitively manage ambiguity include personal characteristics and processes that support discernment, and development of strategic planning and decision-making processes.

Priorities and effectiveness

Leaders contribute through evolving and articulating mind maps of strategies to handle ambiguous situations and problems. Key leadership behaviours include direction-setting, role-acting and role-modelling, while important discernment and action processes include situational awareness, communication, knowledge, agility, trust, framing, needful interrelating, adjusting and ongoing management of ambiguity itself (Baran & Scott, 2010).

Tolerance of ambiguity

Healthcare situations and the environment of uncertainty need to be appropriately and proportionately supported as they work in ambiguous situations and contexts. Tolerance of Ambiguity (TOA) gauges individuals' experience in navigating uncertain environments in which they work (de Vries, 2023 Elembilassery, Jain & Aggarwal, 2024). To support leaders and managers in response to TOA, clear communication strategies are critical. Expectations and working context guidelines and protocols reduce uncertainty, and focused training enhances skills in critical thinking and decision-making. Enabling and fostering open dialogue ensures that staff, at all levels in this context, can seek clarification. For individuals, this can mean assigning mentors or coaches to provide guidance and support when faced with ambiguous situations. Self-awareness and stress management techniques can encourage staff to build resilience. Fostering a supportive environment can empower them to navigate ambiguity with confidence.

Information and direction articulation

Health organisations collect significant amounts of data. In scoping direction and leading for resolution in messy and complex problems, healthcare leaders need to align opportunities for situational and decision-making analysis with useful and focused information.

Framing

Framing: Careful choice of the language used to describe an issue, so as to adopt a more positive or negative appearance

Framing involves the deliberate use of conscious and less conscious skills within a sense of perception, so as to present an issue in a way that enables individuals and teams to understand what might be taking place beyond the limits of their knowledge. It provides insight into the meaning and significance of the situation in order to make sense of it.

Framing is a valuable strategy for leaders involved in the discernment and development of change and problem-solving in organisations. Considerable work on the usefulness and techniques of framing has been developed by Bolman and Deal (2008), who set out four key frames for perspective in organisations:

1. **Structural frames** focus on the organisation and its structure.
2. **Human resource frames** give perspectives on the people and relationships in the organisation.
3. **Political frames** consider power and the tensions of competition in the organisation.
4. **Symbolic frames** look at meaning in the organisation through examination of its rituals, stories and culture.

Sensemaking

Sensemaking is a useful illustrative mechanism for understanding and articulating complexity in situations and activities, and it can generate emerging maps, or pictures, that can be built upon with information, option development and strategic decision-making to produce engaging agendas for action. There are three core activities in sensemaking: exploring the wider system, creating a map of the current system and acting to change the system to learn more about it (Ancona, 2012).

Sensemaking: A method of giving meaning to situations and activities

Summary

- Healthcare organisations operate in complex internal and external environments, and their situations foster ambiguous situations in structures, processes, roles and directions.
- Awareness, identification, management and minimisation of, and engagement with, ambiguity are critical parts of effective leadership in healthcare organisations.
- Framing, articulating and communicating about ambiguous situations within health organisations are important for strategic direction-setting and decision-making processes.
- Healthcare leaders are responsible for bringing individual traits, characteristics and skills to the management of ambiguity to match the nature and complexity of ambiguous situations to the processes and methods designed to manage them.

Reflective questions

1. Discuss the relationship between uncertainty, clarity and ambiguity.
2. Identify ambiguous situations that might have a negative effect on healthcare organisations.
3. Identify situations in which working with ambiguity can provide positive or useful opportunities for healthcare organisations.
4. What issues or situations might bring ambiguity into the role and function of a health professional's job? What problems can arise for individuals and organisations from role ambiguity?
5. What would be effective ways of supporting managers and staff working in situations of sustained ambiguity?

Self-analysis questions

Consider an ambiguous situation in a healthcare organisation. List two or three contributions that a healthcare leader could make to bring clarity and resolution to the situation. Then list two or three identification and conceptualisation approaches that could be used to bring context, structure and meaning to the situation. What experience and skills would you personally need to take on a leadership or management role in the situation?

References

Ancona, D. (2012). Sensemaking: Framing and action in the unknown. In S. Snook, S. Nohria & R. Khurana (eds), *The handbook for teaching leadership* (pp. 3–19). Sage.

Baran, B. E. & Scott, C. W. (2010). Organizing ambiguity: A grounded theory of leadership and sensemaking within dangerous contexts. *Military Psychology, 22*(Suppl. 1), S42–S69. https://doi.org/10.1080/08995601003644262

Bass, A. E., Maric, S., Milosevic, I., Uhl-Bien, M., Groves, K. S., Kim, D., Lord, J., Silvera, G., Clark, J., Feyerherm, A. E., Hollingsworth, J., Owen-Smith, J., Twyman, M. D. & Vogus, T. J. (2020). Future of leadership in healthcare: Enabling complexity dynamics across levels. *Management Faculty Publications*.

Best, J. (2012). Bureaucratic ambiguity. *Economy and Society, 41*, 84–106. https://doi.org/10.1080/03085147.2011.63733

Bolman, L. G. & Deal, T. E. (2008). *Artistry, choice and leadership* (4th ed.). Jossey-Bass.

de Vries, H. (2023). Tolerance of ambiguity. In *The Palgrave encyclopedia of the possible* (pp. 1654–1669). Springer International Publishing.

Eisenberg, E. M. (1984). Ambiguity as strategy in organizational communication. *Communication Monographs, 51*, 227–242. https://doi.org/10.1080/03637758409390197

Elembilassery, V., Jain, N. K. & Aggarwal, D. (2024). What influences individuals' tolerance for ambiguity? Exploring the role of social comparison orientation, tendency to maximize and feel regret. *Personality and Individual Differences, 217*, 112436.

Harvey, J. F. & Kudesia, R. S. (2023). Experimentation in the face of ambiguity: How mindful leaders develop emotional capabilities for change in teams. *Journal of Organizational Behavior, 44*(4), 573–589.

Hodgson, P. V. & White, R. P. (2003). Leadership, learning, ambiguity, and uncertainty and their significance to dynamic organizations. In R. S. Peterson & E. A. Mannix (eds), *Leading and managing people in the dynamic organization* (pp. 185–199). Lawrence Erlbaum.

Leatt, P. & Porter, J. (2003). Where are the healthcare leaders: The need for investment in leadership development. *HealthcarePapers, 4*(1), 14–31. https://doi.org/10.12927/hcpap.2003.16891

Maden-Eyiusta, C. (2021). Role conflict, role ambiguity and proactive behaviours: Does flexible role orientation moderate the mediating impact of engagement? *The International Journal of Human resource Management, 32*(13), 2829–2855. https://doi.org/10.1080/09585192.2019.1616590

McCaskey, M. B. (1988). The challenge of managing ambiguity and change. In L. R. Pondy, R. J. Boland & H. Thomas (eds), *Managing ambiguity and change* (pp. 1–30). Wiley.

Nadler, D. A. & Tushman, M. L. (1995). Types of organization change: From incremental improvement to discontinuous transformation. In D. A. Nadler, R. B. Shaw & A. E. Walten (eds), *Discontinuous change: Leading organization transformation* (pp. 15–34). Jossey-Bass.

Page, B., Irving, D., Amalberti, R. & Vincent, C. (2024). Health services under pressure: A scoping review and development of a taxonomy of adaptive strategies. *BMJ Quality & Safety, 33*(11), 738–747.

Weiss, C. H. (1998). *Evaluation: Methods for studying programs and policies* (2nd ed.). Prentice Hall.

W. K. Kellogg Foundation. (2004). *Logic Model Development Guide*. Retrieved from: https://www.naccho.org/uploads/downloadable-resources/Programs/Public-Health-Infrastructure/KelloggLogicModelGuide_161122_162808.pdf

Zhang, H., Liu, F. & Lang, H. (2024). The relationship between role ambiguity and anxiety in intensive care unit nurses: The mediating role of emotional intelligence. *Intensive & Critical Care Nursing, 81*, 103597. https://doi.org/10.1016/j.iccn.2023.103597

Ziegert, J. C. & Dust, S. B. (2021). Integrating formal and shared leadership: The moderating influence of role ambiguity on innovation. *Journal of Business and Psychology, 36*(6), 969–984. https://doi.org/10.1007/s10869-020-09722-3

Leadership and critical reflective practice

8

Ahmad Saedisomeolia
With acknowledgement to Lorraine Venturato

Learning objectives

How do I:

- improve my ability to reflect on my own practice?
- benefit from a critical reflection approach?
- reflect for action, reflect in action and reflect on action?
- enhance my leadership abilities through reflective practice?
- choose an efficient reflective technique?

Introduction

Reflection is an action in which we step back and take another look (Grimm, 2016). It is not a new concept in the health sciences. Contemporary conceptions of reflective practice are underpinned by the classic works of John Dewey (1916, 1933), Carl Rogers (1969) and Donald Schön (1983, 1987). Nowadays, reflection is considered one of the core components of healthcare education and is evident in the governing codes and guidelines underpinning professional practice in many health disciplines in Australasia (Manton & Williams, 2021). References to reflection appear in the health disciplines' code of professional practice or codes of conduct. Effective and purposeful reflection is seen to be a core component of proficiency and continuing professional development. Despite this, students, practitioners and healthcare leaders often find reflection – and critical reflective practice – challenging.

This chapter explores the concepts of reflection and critical reflective practice. It offers advice on how to adopt a critically reflective attitude and foster reflective skills in leadership, and explores how leaders can benefit from critical reflection to support growth and change at the personal, team and organisational levels.

Definitions

Why should we reflect?

A popular example of reflection is when we look in a mirror. In this passive action, we can easily see our image reflected. Despite the passivity, a mirrored reflection invites us to do more than merely recognise our own image.

Firstly, gazing upon our reflected image invites a critical inspection and active engagement. When we look in a mirror, our gaze often carries the following implied questions: Is my face clean? Is my hair tidy or messy? Should I grow a moustache? That is, we actively engage in a cognitive process based on a question-and-answer dialogue with ourselves. Secondly, it is often these questions that direct us to the mirror in the first place: looking in the mirror does not occur by accident; it is an intentional activity. Finally, the mirror may also reflect our location, based on the background to our image.

When it comes to the professional level, reflection is an intentional and active process, which involves thinking and questioning, and helps us to find the broader context of our professional experiences. Indeed, the term reflection is often used interchangeably with 'thinking', but reflection is more than just thinking about our experiences (Rolfe, 2014; Thompson, Byerley & O'Bryan, 2024). **Reflection** is defined as an intentional, active cognitive process of interpreting, understanding and giving meaning to an experience by considering and critically assessing the content and process, and by critiquing our assumptions and/or practices (Mezirow, 1991). Schön (1983) identifies three broad elements of reflection, and these appear in most definitions of reflection today (Hathazi, 2021): reflection involves an active intellectual engagement, it entails the exploration of experiences or problems, and it results in a subsequent change in perspective or practices and/or generates new insights.

Reflection: An intentional cognitive process of thought and contemplation regarding an issue and its relationship to one's practice, beliefs, values or behaviour

Definitions of critical reflection and critical reflective practice extend this definition to the broader social, political and/or moral contexts in which such experiences occur (Morley & O'Bree, 2021). **Critical reflection** goes beyond reflection to include an awareness and challenge to the hidden assumptions of practitioners or leaders, as well as the broader social and political contexts. Critical reflection is often associated with the deconstruction of long-held beliefs or habitual practices. **Critical reflective practice** moves critical reflection beyond consideration of a specific problem or incident. As an everyday practice, critical reflection occurs on a continuing basis and features as the practitioner's and leader's way of practising or leading. It has been suggested that critical reflective practice generates knowledge for better care (Rolfe & Freshwater, 2020).

Critical reflection: Reflection that includes an awareness of, and challenge to, the hidden assumptions of practitioners and leaders, as well as the broader social and political contexts

Critical reflective practice: Critical reflection that occurs on a continuing basis and is seen as a way of practising or leading

Types of reflection

Classically, Schön (1992) identifies three types of reflection based on temporal considerations: reflection *for* action, reflection *in* action and reflection *on* action. Reflection *for* action, or anticipatory reflection, occurs before an action. Here, a leader may consider ways of dealing with a situation prior to doing anything about it. There is some debate and confusion regarding the two concepts of 'reflection *on* action' and 'reflection *in* action' (Thompson et al., 2024). In general, reflection *in* action is conceptualised as 'thinking on your feet', often occurring rapidly in the midst of an activity, while reflection *on* action entails looking back at actions, processes and outcomes after a certain activity or event.

Hatton and Smith (1995) propose a hierarchical framework as a way of distinguishing between types of reflection. They identify four levels of reflection in writing:

1. *descriptive information*, which describes events without reflection
2. *descriptive reflection*, which describes events and attempts to provide some justification or explanation, with evidence of alternative viewpoints
3. *dialogic reflection*, which involves distancing from the events to explore the experience, is analytical and/or integrates alternative perspectives and factors, and recognises inconsistencies while providing a rationale or critique
4. *critical reflection*, which situates events and actions within multiple perspectives, recognising the influence of numerous historical and sociopolitical contexts.

As a pioneer in reflective teaching, Pollard (2002, 2005) identifies seven characteristics of reflective teaching that fit equally well with characteristics of critical reflective practice. Reflective teaching:

1. Is concerned 'with aims and consequences, as well as means and technical efficiency' (Pollard, 2002, p. 12). This situates critical reflection in everyday practice as well as in the broader sociopolitical and moral contexts.
2. Is 'a cyclical (continuing a same pathway) or spiral (improving) process' in which practice is continuously monitored, evaluated and revised (Pollard, 2002, p. 12). Critical reflection is not a one-off event but a continuous and embedded way of practising – a critical reflective practice.

3. Requires a degree of competence in evidence-informed inquiry; thus, it is a key element of experiential learning in continuing professional development and evidence-based practice (Stewart, 2012), and it supports the higher-order thinking skills that constitute clinical reasoning (Akpur, 2020; Donaghy & Morss, 2000).
4. Requires 'open-mindedness, responsibility and whole-heartedness' (Pollard, 2002, p. 13; see also Dewey, 1933). Critical reflection encompasses inquisitiveness and openness to other ways of thinking and doing. This does not imply a naivety or blind acceptance; rather, it implies curiosity and lack of defensiveness in thinking and questioning.
5. Requires judgement. Critical reflection and critical reflective practice draw on experience, practice, evidence and context to evaluate and innovate.
6. Entails dialogue, which may be with colleagues (Pollard, 2002) or internally with oneself and is essential as it serves as a trigger for learning and thinking (Snyder, 2014).
7. Entails creative mediation: negotiating between opposing or conflicting ways of thinking or acting, and movement towards a resolution in terms of thought or action.

Perhaps an eighth defining characteristic of critical reflective practice lies in a focus on action and activity (Bradbury-Jones, Coleman, Davies, Ellison & Leigh, 2010), which differentiates it from only thinking about something (Rolfe, 2014). Its focus on activity and its continuous, or cyclical, nature make reflection a practice rather than a one-off or occasional event, often in response to a critical incident. Reflective practice is active and continuous – a way of being or, as Rolfe (2014) suggests, a way of doing.

Reflective practice is experiential in nature; that is, we get better at it the more we do it and the more experience we have to build on (Wainwright, Shepard, Harman & Stephens, 2010). Therefore, reflective practice is a key element in experiential learning (Spencer, 2024), contributing to the progression of clinicians and leaders from novice to expert (Stewart, 2012). It is also a key element in professional development and adult learning, and a central feature of professional practice.

Part of the strength of critical reflective practice lies in the premise that self-reflective and self-initiated learning involving both feelings and cognition are the longest-lasting and most pervasive types of learning. Independence, self-reliance, creativity and personal growth are all facilitated when self-criticism and self-evaluation are strong, and evaluation by others is of secondary importance.

Given its active, continuous and experiential learning components, critical reflective practice is also identified as an important method for integrating theory and practice (Binding, Morck & Moules, 2010; Plack, Dunfee, Rindflesch & Driscoll, 2008; Wainwright et al., 2010), and it can help us to understand and resolve contradictions in expectations and practice (Johns, 2006). Therefore, critical reflective practice facilitates the integration of new theories and practices with previous beliefs and practices (see Figure 8.1).

Critical reflective practice is also closely linked to critical thinking (Cendon, 2020), higher-order thinking (Akpur, 2020; Mezirow, 1991) and critical awareness (Rolfe & Freshwater, 2020). These skills facilitate examination of attitudes, values, beliefs and goals (self-awareness), appreciation of the perspectives of others, awareness of alternative positions and evaluation and sensemaking of one's own position (Plack et al., 2008), as well as consideration of broader policies, social and political circumstances, and moral obligations.

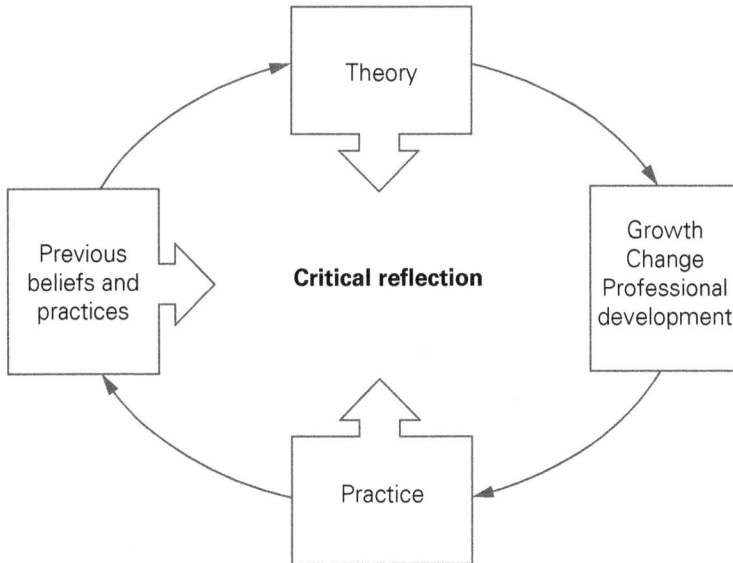

Figure 8.1 The cycle of critical reflective practice

Leadership and critical reflective practice

Critical reflective practice is an important aspect of professional practice and leadership in contemporary healthcare environments (Rowe, Moore & McKie, 2020). The rationale for its importance draws on the links between learning and self-awareness, and the ability to be innovative, to manage and to cope with change (Horton-Deutsch, Young & Nelson, 2010).

Benefits of critical reflective practice

Critically reflective leaders are self-aware and thoughtful, and they critically question and evaluate their leadership in a continuous and active cycle of development and learning. Reflective leaders have moral purpose and build relationships that can integrate theories and practices with their past experiences to lead through change at personal and organisational levels. The key benefits of critical reflective practice are further discussed in this section.

Self-awareness

Self-awareness is an essential element in leadership development and growth (Spencer, 2024) and in enhanced learning in practice (Bradbury-Jones et al., 2010). Self-awareness supports recognition of our strengths and limitations, assists us to deal with challenges and relationships with others, and to maintain a sense of openness (Bradbury-Jones et al., 2010; Enterkin, Robb & McLaren, 2013; Horton-Deutsch et al., 2010; Snyder, 2014; Spencer, 2024).

Transferable learning

Critical reflective practice can offer insights into our previous experiences that may help us to understand and make sense of future experiences and facilitate future learning processes (Rowe et al., 2020).

Understanding

Critical reflective practice can help leaders to clarify career goals and identify career development needs at the personal and team levels (Enterkin et al., 2013). Opportunities for career development are central to staff empowerment, which is intrinsic to retention and change (Snyder, 2014).

Exploration

Critical reflective practice is also associated with a wider, contextualised viewpoint. Social and organisational contexts must factor into reflective leaders' strategic thinking in developing supportive networks and engaging in change activities at the organisational or political level (Pool-Funai & Summers, 2023; Enterkin et al., 2013).

Adaptability

Understanding and working with change are parts of daily practice in contemporary healthcare settings for both leaders and clinicians. Adaptability requires self-awareness and a broad understanding of the context in which change occurs (Horton-Deutsch et al., 2010). Critical reflective practice is transformative, and 'reflective leaders model an adaptive capacity, manage conflict, and … [enable others] to embrace the future and share in the creation of it' (Pool-Funai & Summers, 2023; Horton-Deutsch, 2013, p. 4).

Innovation

Critical reflection can expand thinking about further developments and new ways of thinking and acting, and can develop and drive innovation (Rowe et al., 2020).

CRITICAL REFLECTIVE PRACTICE AND CAREER-PLANNING

I was invited to speak to a group of first-year nursing students about my career and career-planning in general. My initial thought was that there had not been a lot of planning involved! On reflection, I recognised that there were pivotal moments and considered choices underpinned by careful and critical reflection.

In my speech, I described my growing realisation that the career I thought I wanted before studying to be a nurse was, in fact, not the one presenting itself to me. When I entered nursing, I thought I wanted a career in intensive care or emergency, or maybe to travel to exotic lands doing medical aid work. With each practicum, I grew increasingly aware of situations that ignited a response in me – ways of working that were most satisfying.

For example, during a much sought-after practicum in a busy emergency department, I realised that having patients in and out so quickly was not satisfying. I recognised over future practicums that I liked working in areas where I got to know patients' names, preferences, family. It did not matter if it was an oncology, rehabilitation, palliative care or long-term care facility; there were significant connections to be made, and the therapeutic relationship was central.

> I also realised that I enjoyed working with people who were dealing with 'big' issues. I had a million questions and I enjoyed seeking answers in a systematic way. Thinking like this led me to a career I could never have foreseen, but one that fits me well. My advice to the students that day was to remain open to possibilities, to think about what they most connected with and to reflect on their experiences; that's how you build a career.

The relationship between reflection and leadership

Like reflection, leadership is a complex concept and is frequently discussed in terms of leadership styles, such as transformative, authoritarian or democratic. Critical reflective leadership may be embedded in different styles of leadership, though it may be more evident and compatible with leadership styles such as transformative or congruent leadership (Anselmann & Mulder, 2020; Latimer, 2011).

Warwick and Swaffield (2006) note that reflection contributes to 'good' leadership in much the same way that it contributes to 'good' practice. They highlight the value of reflection in leadership in relation to facilitating clear aims, goals and directions that are underpinned by values; being able to build relationships, collaborations and engagement in dialogue; and being able to understand and facilitate change through a process of monitoring, evaluating, reflecting and revising. The link between 'good' leadership and reflection lies in the capacity for self-awareness and self-regulation, as well as in enhancing relationships and empowering others (Enterkin et al., 2013; Spencer, 2024), thereby improving emotional intelligence and, ultimately, communication, teamwork, goal-setting and attainment, and effective change management.

Strategies for developing critical reflection

Numerous strategies for developing reflective skills are available to clinicians and healthcare leaders.

Reflective writing

Reflective writing is one of the main strategies identified and is often considered essential in integrating concepts, context and experience (Artioli et al., 2021; Binding et al., 2010). Reflective writing may take many forms, including diaries, journals and, increasingly, personal blogs (Anselmann & Mulder, 2020; Latimer, 2011). It is one of three reflective activities identified by Stewart (2012), along with reflective thinking and reflective practice. However, reflective thinking and writing may both support reflective practice. Reflective writing is most often seen in educational settings and is one way in which reflective thinking and practice are taught and assessed in health professional training programs.

Supervision and mentorship

Clinical supervision and mentorship are also important strategies for developing critical reflective practice. Latimer (2011) and, more recently, Koh, McNulty & Toh-Heng (2022) believe that clinical supervision is particularly useful in this regard when timely clarification and advice are required, when the student is learning and may benefit from expert guidance and mentorship, and when there is a significant emotional toll; in the latter case, a mentor or supervisor may provide the emotional distance required for critical reflection.

Learning circles and group reflection

Learning circles and group reflection are other ways to support and develop critical reflective practice (Rowe et al., 2020; Enterkin et al., 2013; Snyder, 2014; Walker, Henderson, Cooke & Creedy, 2011; Walker, Cooke, Henderson & Creedy, 2013). Group reflection methods support shared learning and peer support and can minimise isolation (Enterkin et al., 2013), while learning circles can promote individual and organisational growth and change (Walker et al., 2013). Learning circles may also be useful in work-integrated environments in which negotiation, communication and relationship-building are key elements. Group reflection can assist in identifying and exploring problems and issues in the workplace, can generate new insights and can assist in developing action plans (Walker et al., 2011). It is also useful in uncovering the voice of the other and supporting listening and empathy in novice reflective practitioners.

Critical questioning

Critically reflective students, clinicians and leaders ask tough questions. Critical questioning involves identifying and resolving problems and issues through a process of question and answer (Snyder, 2014). What is the issue? Why do certain problems exist? Why did this occur? How can this be resolved? Who benefits? Whose voices are heard and not heard? Bradbury-Jones and colleagues (2010) suggest that questions should also include subjective questions on thoughts and feelings: How did I feel? Why did I feel like that? What was I thinking? What were the consequences of my feelings and thinking? What would I do next time?

Such questions can be useful prompts for novice practitioners and new leaders as they learn to integrate critical reflection into their everyday practices, establishing it as a part of the inner dialogue necessary to developing new roles.

Creativity and arts-based approaches

Creativity and arts-based approaches, which provide 'a hope to foster meaningful learning, based on the reactions to artistic assignments or learning contents by learners' (Rieger, Chernomas, McMillan & Morin, 2020), are also useful in developing critical reflective practice. They include arts-based learning, research and knowledge translation (practice change), while creative thinking is closely aligned with change and innovation (Latimer, 2011). Creativity and creative thinking challenge the status quo and generate new possibilities for practice and leadership. Whether arts-based learning supports critical reflection has been reviewed recently (Timpani, Sweet & Sivertsen, 2021). Such an approach is particularly useful when experience is limited, as it can expose novice practitioners and leaders to previously unencountered situations.

A cautionary note

While reflection is widely espoused in healthcare as an important underpinning strategy for learning and change, it is not without its critics (Rolfe & Freshwater, 2020; Rolfe, 2014).

One of the questions about the nature of reflection is whether it can be taught or is a predisposition. Farrell (2020) and others (Stewart, 2012; Wainwright et al., 2010) argue that reflection and reflective writing skills can be taught, while Rolfe (2014) contends, following Dewey's (1916) and Schön's (1987) argument, that reflection as experiential learning is essentially unteachable. This argument is largely based on the differences between teaching and learning, and in particular teaching about learning. Rolfe's (2014) argument is that while reflective practice is unteachable, it can be learned through experience and practice. Despite this, many studies recommend intentional instruction and explicit, purposeful development of reflective capabilities as part of professional preparation for practice in health disciplines, and when it is followed up in the workplace (see e.g. Wainwright et al., 2010).

Secondly, some authors point out that critical reflective practice needs time (Wainwright et al., 2010). Sufficient time to reflect, to listen and to have the space to question is often lacking in today's busy and complex healthcare environments.

A third critique argues that reflection is often difficult and may not come easily. The focus on reflective writing in education may challenge those who reflect best through oral traditions and storytelling and who struggle to write, losing key elements when confronted with the need to construct reflections in writing. Despite this criticism, writing can force us to be clearer in reflection, and being able to think and communicate clearly in writing is a part of professional life (Farrell, 2020). Reflective writing offers potential to develop not just reflective ability but also writing skills – an important skill combination in healthcare environments that is initially linked with our thoughts and gradually develops.

Critically reflective leaders establish critical reflection as a daily way of doing; it is who they are as leaders. Critically reflective practice is an important skill and attribute of successful and sustainable healthcare leadership in the 21st century.

Summary

- Reflection is a way of thinking and doing that for practitioners and leaders combines theory and practice to facilitate learning and development.
- Critical reflective practice is a core element of professional practice in healthcare.
- Critical reflective practice is associated with critical thinking and experiential learning.
- There are different models and ways of thinking about reflection, including reflection for action, reflection in action and reflection on action.
- Critically reflective leaders are self-aware and thoughtful, questioning all aspects of their practice.
- Strategies promoting critical reflection in leadership include reflective writing, clinical supervision or mentorship, learning circles and group reflection, critical questioning techniques and creativity and arts-based approaches.

Reflective questions

1. What is reflection?
2. How does critical reflection differ from reflection?
3. What is meant by the term 'critical reflective practice'?
4. How do principles of critical reflective practice apply to leadership in healthcare?
5. Why is critical reflective practice important to the work of professionals?

Self-analysis questions

Regarding your current practice or leadership style, what are your strengths and challenges in relation to critical reflective practice? How might you apply some of the critical reflection strategies identified in this chapter to develop your leadership potential?

References

Akpur, U. (2020). Critical, reflective, creative thinking and their reflections on academic achievement. *Thinking Skills and Creativity, 37*, 100683. https://doi.org/org/10.1016/j.tsc.2020.100683

Anselmann, V. & Mulder, R. H. (2020). Transformational leadership, knowledge sharing and reflection, and work teams' performance: A structural equation modelling analysis. *Journal of Nursing Management, 28*(7), 1627–1634. https://doi.org//10.1111/jonm.13118

Artioli, G., Deiana, L., De Vincenzo, F., Raucci, M., Amaducci, G., Bassi, M. C. … & Ghirotto, L. (2021). Health professionals and students' experiences of reflective writing in learning: A qualitative meta-synthesis. *BMC Medical Education, 21*(1), 1–14. https://doi.org/org/10.1186/s12909-021-02831-4

Binding, L., Morck, A. C. & Moules, N. J. (2010). Learning to see the other: A vehicle of reflection. *Nurse Education Today, 30*(6), 591–594. https://doi.org/10.1016/j.nedt.2009.12.014

Bradbury-Jones, C., Coleman, D., Davies, H., Ellison, K. & Leigh, C. (2010). Raised emotions: A critique of the Peshkin approach to reflection. *Nurse Education Today, 30*, 568–572. https://doi.org/10.1016/j.nedt.2009.12.002

Cendon, E. (2020). From reflective practice to critical thinking: The reflective practitioner in higher education. In W. Nuniger & J. M. Châtelet (eds), *Handbook of research on operational quality assurance in higher education for life-long learning* (pp. 189–211). IGI Global. https://doi.org/10.4018/978-1-7998-1238-8.ch008

Dewey, J. (1933). *How we think: A restatement of the relation of reflective thinking to the educative process.* DC Heath.

——— (1916). *Democracy and education: An introduction to the philosophy of education.* MacMillan.

Donaghy, M. & Morss, K. (2000). Guided reflection: A framework to facilitate and assess reflective practice within the discipline of physiotherapy. *Physiotherapy Theory and Practice, 16*, 3–14.

Enterkin, J., Robb, E. & McLaren, S. (2013). Clinical leadership for high quality care: Developing future ward leaders. *Journal of Nursing Management, 21*, 206–216. https://doi.org/10.1111/j.1365-2834.2012.01408.x

Farrell, T. S. (2020). Professional development through reflective practice for English-medium instruction (EMI) teachers. *International Journal of Bilingual Education and Bilingualism, 23*(3), 277–286. https://doi.org/org/10.1080/13670050.2019.1612840

Grimm, S. R. (2016). The value of reflection. In M. A. Vargas (ed.), *Performance epistemology: Foundations and applications* (pp. 183–195). Oxford University Press.

Hathazi, A. (2021). The implementation of reflection-based approaches in the education and rehabilitation of children with disabilities. *Proceedings 11th International Scientific Conference Special Education* and *Rehabilitation Today*, Belgrade, 29–30 October, pp. 23–26.

Hatton, N. & Smith, D. (1995). Reflection in teacher education: Towards definition and implementation. *Teaching and Teacher Education*, *11*(1), 33–49. https://doi.org/10.1016/0742-051X(94)00012-U

Horton-Deutsch, S. (2013). Thinking it through: The path to reflective leadership. *American Nurse Today*, *8*(2). Retrieved from: http://www.americannursetoday.com

Horton-Deutsch, S., Young, P. K. & Nelson, K. A. (2010). Becoming a nurse faculty leader: Facing challenges through reflecting, persevering and relating in new ways. *Journal of Nursing Management*, *18*, 487–493. https://doi.org/10.1111/j.1365-2834.2010.01075.x

Johns, C. (2006). *Engaging reflection in practice: A narrative approach*. Blackwell.

Koh, D., McNulty, G. & Toh-Heng, H. L. (2022). Reflective practice through clinical supervision: Implications for professional and organisational sustainability. *British Journal of Guidance & Counselling*, *50*(6), 879–896. https://doi.org/org/10.1080/03069885.2021.1978056

Latimer, S. (2011). Reflection. In D. Stanley (ed.), *Clinical leadership: Innovation into action* (pp. 265–276). Palgrave Macmillan.

Manton, D. & Williams, M. (2021). Strengthening Indigenous Australian perspectives in allied health education: A critical reflection. *International Journal of Indigenous Health*, *16*(1), 223–242. https://doi.org/10.32799/ijih.v16i1.33218

Mezirow, J. (1991). *Transformative dimensions of adult learning*. Jossey-Bass.

Morley, C. & O'Bree, C. (2021). Critical reflection: An imperative skill for social work practice in neoliberal organisations? *Social sciences*, *10*(3), 97. https://doi.org/org/10.3390/socsci10030097

Plack, M. M., Dunfee, H., Rindflesch, A. & Driscoll, M. (2008). Virtual action learning sets: A model for facilitating reflection in the clinical setting. *Journal of Physical Therapy Education*, *22*(3), 33–42.

Pollard, A. (2005). (With J. Collins, M. Maddock, N. Simco, S. Swaffield, J. Warin & P. Warwick). *Reflective teaching* (2nd ed.). Continuum.

——— (2002). (With J. Collins, M. Maddock, N. Simco, S. Swaffield, J. Warin & P. Warwick). *Reflective teaching: Effective and evidence-informed professional practice*. Continuum.

Pool-Funai, A. & Summers, T. (2023). *The reflective administrator: A leader-centered focus*. Taylor & Francis.

Rieger, K. L., Chernomas, W. M., McMillan, D. E. & Morin, F. L. (2020). Navigating creativity within arts-based pedagogy: Implications of a constructivist grounded theory study. *Nurse Education Today*, *91*, 104465. https://doi.org/10.1016/j.nedt.2020.104465

Rogers, C. (1969). *Freedom to learn: A view of what education might become*. Charles Merill.

Rolfe, G. (2014). Rethinking reflective education: What would Dewey have done? *Nurse Education Today*, *34*(8), 1179–1183. https://doi.org/10.1016/j.nedt.2014.03.006

Rolfe, G. & Freshwater, D. (2020). *Critical reflection in practice: generating knowledge for care*. Bloomsbury Publishing.

Rowe, L., Moore, N. & McKie, P. (2020). The reflective practitioner: the challenges of supporting public sector senior leaders as they engage in reflective practice. *Higher Education, Skills and Work-Based Learning*, *10*(5), 783–798. https://doi.org/10.1108/HESWBL-03-2020-0038

Schön, D. A. (1992). The theory of inquiry: Dewey's legacy to education. *Curriculum Inquiry*, *2*(2), 119–139.

——— (1987). *Educating the reflective practitioner: Towards a new design for teaching and learning in the professions*. Jossey-Bass.

——— (1983). *The reflective practitioner: How professionals think in action*. Basic Books.

Snyder, M. (2014). Emancipatory knowing: Empowering nursing students towards reflection and action. *Journal of Nursing Education*, *53*(2), 65–69. https://doi.org/10.3928/01484834-20140107-01

Spencer, R. (2024). Reflection, self-awareness, and cultural competency as a foundational pedagogy for clinical legal education. In *Contemporary Challenges in Clinical Legal Education* (pp. 76–86). Routledge.

Stewart, J. (2012). Reflecting on reflecting: Increasing health and social care students' engagement and enthusiasm for reflection. *Reflective Practice: International and Multidisciplinary Perspectives, 13*(5), 719–733. https://doi.org/10.1080/14623943.2012.670627

Thompson, P. W., Byerley, C. & O'Bryan, A. (2024). Figurative and operative imagery: Essential aspects of reflection in the development of schemes and meanings. In *Piaget's Genetic Epistemology for Mathematics Education Research* (pp. 129–168). Springer International Publishing. https://doi.org/10.1007/978-3-031-47386-9_5

Timpani, S., Sweet, L. & Sivertsen, N. (2021). Storytelling: One arts-based learning strategy to reflect on clinical placement. An integrative review. *Nurse Education in Practice, 52,* 103005. https://doi.org/10.1016/j.nepr.2021.103005

Wainwright, S. F., Shepard, K. F., Harman, L. B. & Stephens, J. (2010). Novice and experienced physical therapists clinicians: A comparison of how reflection is used to inform the clinical decision-making process. *Physical Therapy, 90*(1), 75–88. https://doi.org/10.2522/ptj.20090077

Walker, R., Cooke, M., Henderson, A. & Creedy, D. (2013). Using a critical reflection process to create an effective learning community in the workplace. *Nurse Education Today, 33*(5), 504–511. https://doi.org/10.1016/j.nedt.2012.03.001

Walker, R., Henderson, A., Cooke, M. & Creedy, D. (2011). Impact of a learning circle intervention across academic and service contexts on developing a learning culture. *Nurse Education Today, 31*(4), 378–382. https://doi.org/10.1016/j.nedt.2010.07.010

Warwick, P. & Swaffield, S. (2006). Articulating and connecting frameworks of reflective practice and leadership: Perspectives from 'fast track' trainee teachers. *Reflective Practice: International and Multidisciplinary Perspectives, 7*(2), 247–263. https://doi.org/10.1080/14623940600688704

Empathic leadership

Sandra G. Leggat

9

Learning objectives

How do I:

- support staff to provide compassionate care?
- understand and incorporate empathy and spirituality in my leadership style?

Introduction

Compassionate care: The action taken to deal with the emotional resonance in another's concerns, distress, pain or suffering (Lown, McIntosh, Gaines, McGuinn & Hatem, 2016)

Lack of compassion among health service staff has been identified as a concern around the world. High-profile scandals and inquiries in the United Kingdom have suggested that health systems and services 'are struggling to provide safe, timely, and **compassionate care**' (de Zulueta 2016, p. 1). In the United States, only half of patients and staff surveyed believed the health system provides compassionate care (Lown, Rosen & Marttila, 2011). Similarly, a recent study in Australia identified a gap between the intentions of organisational leadership to provide consistently high-quality care and the ability of staff to do so at point of care (Leggat & Balding, 2017). Healthcare managers are looking for proven ways to support staff to recognise and provide compassionate care.

Healthcare raises profound questions about the meaning and purpose of life, and concerns about loss, death and issues of life after death, for patients and their families and for staff (Vance, 2001). This has led to the suggestion that healthcare should ensure empathy for the spiritual needs of patients and family members in the care provided (Kashi Komala & Ganesh, 2006; Holmes, 2018). There is substantial evidence of a positive association between spirituality and health outcomes (Koenig, McCullough & Larson, 2001), further supporting the need to ensure spiritual needs are addressed in care processes.

Similarly, there is evidence that spirituality can enhance both organisational and staff outcomes in healthcare and in other industries. There is growing research supporting a positive relationship between workplace spirituality and work attitudes (Shankar Pawar, 2009), employee wellbeing (McKee, Driscoll, Kelloway & Kelley, 2011) and organisational outcomes (Mitroff & Denton, 1999), as well as a relationship between individual spirituality and workplace spirituality (Duchon & Plowman, 2005, Shankar Pawar, 2009).

Organisational culture: The shared meanings of organisational values, attitudes and beliefs that influence patterns of behaviours (Denison, 1990)

Spiritual leadership: Comprises attitudes and behaviours that help individuals experience intrinsic motivation through finding life's meaningfulness and membership (Fry, 2003)

Empathic leadership: Enhances a leader's capacity to perceive internal and external stakeholders' concerns and feelings in leading others (Natale & Libertella, 2019)

Reinforcing the suggested link between spirituality and compassion, Craigie (1998) stresses that the culture within healthcare organisations should reinforce the duty of everyone in the organisation to provide compassionate care and to respect spiritual values. 'Practical compassion is also the quintessential outcome of both spiritual traditions and effective spiritual care' (Sinclair et al., 2016, p. 18). **Organisational culture**, broadly defined as the shared meanings of organisational values, attitudes and beliefs that influence patterns of behaviours (Denison, 1990), although elusive, is influenced by organisational leaders. The formal (managers) and informal leaders influence staff practices through the systems and processes they implement and oversee (Glickman, Baggett, Krubert, Peterson & Schulman, 2007). Staff perceptions of their leaders' attitudes strongly influence their own attitudes, as well as the norms of staff working groups (Fogarty & Shaw, 2010).

Organisational leadership has been studied extensively, with a recent focus on exploring the effects of empathic and **spiritual leadership** styles on valued organisational outcomes (Klaus & Fernando, 2016), especially during times of crisis (Guntuku, Boini, Mary & Kummeta, 2021). Empathic leaders have been found to be effective because when leaders feel compassion for staff they are motivated to address issues, and emotional connection has been shown to improve performance (Brescoll, 2016). If compassionate care is enhanced by the spirituality of health professionals, healthcare managers and leaders have a role to play in facilitating this spirituality through **empathic leadership**. This leads to the aim of this chapter: to explore management and leadership practices that support staff to provide high-quality, compassionate healthcare.

The loss of compassionate care

While acknowledged as an important aspect of care, compassion is not well understood in the literature. The Oxford English Dictionary's definition of compassion is simply 'to suffer with'. Various disciplines have discussed what this means in practice. The business literature outlines three components, comprising noticing, feeling and acting (Kanov et al., 2004). Similarly, in psychology, compassion is described as sensemaking that includes noticing that someone is suffering, feeling emphatic concern and acting on this concern (Dutton, Workman & Hardin, 2014). Empathic concern is described as feeling sympathy towards others and is altruistically motivated (Batson, 1987). The nursing literature suggests seven dimensions of compassion, comprising: attentiveness, active listening, naming suffering, involvement, helping, being present and understanding suffering (van der Cingel, 2014). In a detailed review, Strauss and colleagues (2016, p. 19) propose a comprehensive definition of compassion as 'a cognitive, affective and behavioural process with five elements'. The elements comprise:

1) recognising suffering;
2) understanding the universality of suffering in human experience;
3) feeling empathy for the person suffering and connecting with the distress (emotional resonance);
4) tolerating uncomfortable feelings in response to the suffering person (e.g. distress, anger, fear) so remaining open to and accepting of the person suffering; and
5) motivation to act to alleviate suffering.

These definitions suggest that compassion has aspects of both recognition and action, encompassing empathy, pity and kindness.

While much of the literature focuses on compassion as an issue with, and concern for, individual care providers, Crawford and colleagues (2014) stress the need to consider the organisational context as an important facilitator or barrier to the provision of compassionate care. These authors suggest that compliance-focused health systems have contributed to the reduction in delivery of compassionate care. Tick-box procedures that are associated with compliance-based risk-reduction quality systems result in staff distancing themselves from patient compassion. For example, Leggat and Balding (2018) report that staff working in hospitals with compliance-focused quality systems described quality of care as bureaucratic tasks likened to audits and attending meetings, and did not relate quality with the care they provided all day, every day.

Five factors were found to interfere with the provision of compassionate care:

1. Burnout or overload of the staff members (Fernando & Consedine, 2014). The stress experienced when the needs for care exceed the resources the caregiver has to offer decreases their capacity to provide compassionate care (Vitaliano, Zhang & Scanlan, 2003).
2. Cynicism among staff; that is, the belief that nothing makes a difference (Benson & Magraith, 2005).
3. External distractions in the role, including bureaucratic requirements (de Zulueta, 2016; Fernando & Consedine, 2014). For example, bureaucratic processes and goals seen by nursing staff as largely irrelevant to the care tasks at hand reduce relationship-based compassionate care among nurses (Maben, Latter & Clark, 2006).

4. Patients and families who are difficult to deal with (Fernando & Consedine, 2014).
5. Complex clinical situations (Fernando & Consedine, 2014).

Although the literature has suggested that these five factors can reduce the compassion shown by health professionals, there are no studies to date that have measured their effects on compassionate care, as there are no validated tools to measure compassionate care. A review found a self-administered compassionate care scale, patient-reported compassion scales and an organisational compassionate care scale, but indicates than none provides a comprehensive measure of compassionate care with psychometric validation (Sinclair, Russell, Hack, Kondejewski & Sawatzky, 2017). Although not supported by empirical research as yet, it is proposed that certain types of health professional–client interactions can increase resources for compassion, as opposed to the long-held belief that these interactions tend to be draining for health professionals (Lilius, 2012).

Workspace spirituality theory

There has been increasing interest in spirituality in the workplace, with Fox, Webster and Casper (2018) finding that spirituality provides a 'backdrop for how individuals think about, feel, and perceive themselves and their work environment' (p. 206). Spirituality theory is based on the notion that a person's intangible spirit gives the body life in all human beings. McKee and colleagues (2011) suggest that workplace spirituality comprises three elements: meaningful work, sense of community and values alignment. Additionally, the survey responses of 131 senior human resource managers stress that spirituality (but not necessarily religion) is one of the most important determinants of organisational performance (Mitroff & Denton, 1999). Not surprisingly, spiritual leadership, as one of the value-based leadership theories, shares many elements with servant leadership, relationship-oriented and leader–follower leadership theories (Frisdiantara & Sahertian, 2012).

While there is need for further research, there is sufficient evidence for healthcare managers and leaders to consider how they might incorporate spirituality into their practice,

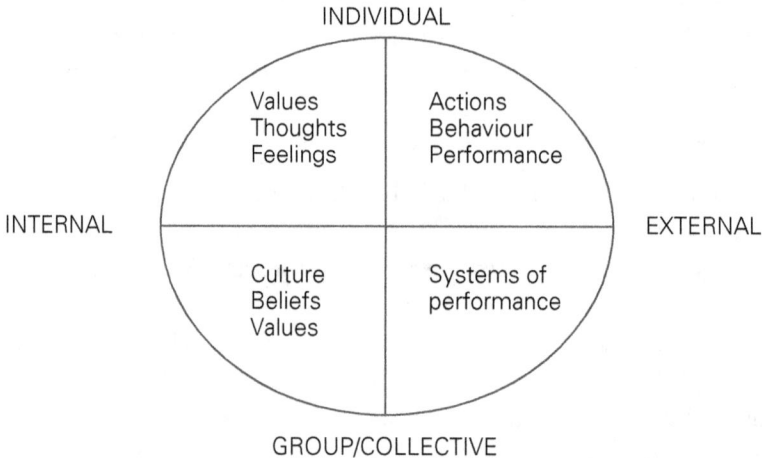

Figure 9.1 Individual and collective spirituality

Source: Adapted from Wilber (1996).

both to foster their own empathy and to assist staff to provide compassionate care. Wilbur's (1996) four-quadrant model suggests focusing on empathy for individuals, as well as the internal organisational culture, beliefs and values and the external systems of performance (Figure 9.1). In support of these relationships, person–organisation fit predicts that the greater the consistency among the individual values, thoughts and feelings and the organisation's culture, beliefs and values, the greater the job satisfaction and organisational commitment of employees (Kristof-Brown, Zimmerman & Johnson, 2005).

Fostering organisational culture through spiritual beliefs and values

IMPROVING HOSPITAL PERFORMANCE

In 2005, Judith Dwyer and I published an article 'Improving hospital performance: Culture change is not the answer' (Leggat & Dwyer, 2005) lamenting that health-system inquiries in the early 2000s suggested that performance issues in hospitals and health systems were the result of poor organisational culture. These systemic issues remained, with the previously described lack of compassion and continuing acceptance by 'the medical community, and indeed the public at large ... of a fatal [hospital] accident rate estimated at three times that of road accidents and a significant multiple of the rates in aviation and the oil and gas industries' (Hudson, 2003 p.11). If cultural change was a feasible solution, two decades seems sufficient time to have made the necessary changes. Different solutions are required.

Based on our increasing understanding of how to create compassion, empathic and spiritual leadership that encourages staff to live the vision, beliefs and values of the organisation in their day-to-day jobs presents a more viable strategy than organisational culture change (Frost et al., 2006). Large-scale organisational cultural-change programs are rarely successful (Smith, 2003), while management actions that reinforce achievement of the mission and vision through organisational values have greater potential for success. It has long been understood that compassion is incorporated by staff into workplace roles when those staff members see it as consistent with the organisation's norms and values (Katz & Kahn, 1978). In fact, it has been suggested that, under the right conditions, complex adaptive systems such as hospitals and other healthcare organisations will self-organise for compassion (Madden, Duchon, Madden & Plowman, 2012). However, when management imposes bureaucratic systems and processes that are inconsistent with the beliefs and values of health professionals and their perceptions of the organisation, compassionate care is lost (Maben et al., 2006). Recent research in Victorian hospitals has found that health professional staff actively craft their jobs, responding to the messages conveyed by their managers (Leggat & Balding 2019). For example, when managers focus communication on access to care, a key government priority for public healthcare systems, the staff modify their jobs to ensure access, often at the expense of compassion.

Empathic and spiritual leadership for compassion also encompasses regular feedback and emotional support, and encourages opportunities for reflection on actions, behaviour and performance (Frost et al., 2006). Madden and colleagues (2012) hypothesise that 'motivated, empathetic agents inside an organisation characterised by diversity among agents, role interdependence and high levels of social interaction are likely to self-organise [for compassion] around the pain trigger' (p. 698). This may be the case in organisational life in many industries, but pain triggers are found in healthcare in every minute of every day and every work shift. As a result, even though healthcare staff are diverse and have high levels of role interaction and social interaction, they can become immune to the need for compassion. It therefore becomes the manager's responsibility to assist their staff to recover their passion for compassion through regular feedback, emotional support and encouraging reflection. There is evidence of a negative correlation between individuals who participate in feedback and their reports of fatigue (Fritz, Lam & Spreitzer, 2011), such that 'reflection will prevent the pitfalls of compassion, such as projection, pity or self-sacrifice' (van der Cingel 2014, p. 1256). Researchers suggest that, through feedback and reflection, health professionals and their leaders can use the evidence from management research to understand and build upon the interactions that restore compassion and recognise when support is needed for interactions that deplete compassion (Fritz et al., 2011; Lilius, 2012).

In summary, organisational culture can be influenced by specific actions of managers and leaders. As Fry (2003) suggests, the first step is to create and communicate a vision that calls staff to meaningful action. That is, to have an organisational purpose that intrinsically motivates. Then, by consistently responding with empathy, leaders and followers must develop genuine care, concern and appreciation for both self and others. Consistent actions are required to inform and embed culture (Leggat & Dwyer, 2005). Fry (2003) stresses that this shared empathy enables a sense of membership and of being understood and appreciated – the organisational culture that has been found to promote compassionate care.

Using spirituality to improve the relevance of healthcare performance systems

Public healthcare systems of performance have become largely compliance-based despite the recognition that regulation and bureaucracy that are inconsistent with health-professional values impede the flow of compassion (de Zulueta, 2016). The over-emphasis on compliance has contributed to the reduction in compassionate care. Staff do not see the relevance of quality systems focused on achieving bureaucratic results that ignore the needs of their patients (Balding & Leggat, 2019). In addition, despite the benefits of management support for healthcare staff (McClelland & Vogus, 2014), the difficulties in providing emotional support for healthcare staff who face suffering every day have long been recognised (Menzies Lyth, 1988). This has become even more difficult in the age of performance-driven public-sector budget cuts and organisational constraints (Meyer, 2010). 'We cannot expect staff to give compassionate care if they do not feel respected and supported by the organisations in which they work. Current policy focuses too much on the needs of patients, occasionally on the needs of families and rarely on the needs of staff' (Meyer, 2010 p. 72). In addition, Burke (2006) argues that while we have always thought of leadership in terms of the social, psychological and the technological, we need to incorporate spirituality.

Health professionals already have the 'calling' that mediates the relationship between management spirituality, comprising vision, faith and altruistic love, and the positive organisational outcomes that have been reported in the literature (Fry, 2003). This suggests that leaders need to reinterpret the performance systems for their staff, so as to better align health-professional values and beliefs with patient, client and organisational values and beliefs.

Summary

- There is evidence that health care has increasingly become devoid of compassion.
- Research shows a positive relationship between empathic and spiritual leadership, and both health and organisational outcomes, and suggests that empathic leadership may be an effective strategy to support healthcare staff in the provision of compassionate care.

Reflective questions

1. What support will your team need from you to succeed this year?
2. What would your actions, and how you spend your time, reveal about you to the objective observer?
3. Do you believe that you can consistently demonstrate empathy for your team while still meeting your goals?
4. Are your actions and behaviours consistent with your values, thoughts and feelings?
5. What would you like to be known for?

Self-analysis question

If you came to work tomorrow and a miracle had happened ... the people you worked with were getting along and working well as a team, and everyone in the organisation was compassionate towards your patients and each other, what would be different? What could you document as the new ways of doing things?

References

Balding, C. & Leggat, S. G. (2019). *The impact of quality management as a hospital strategy: Findings from a mixed methods longitudinal study in Australian hospitals*. La Trobe University.

Batson, C. D. (1987). Prosocial motivation: Is it ever truly altruistic? *Advances in Experimental Social Psychology, 20*, 65–122.

Benson, J. & Magraith, K. (2005). Compassion fatigue and burnout: The role of Balint groups. *Australian Family Physician, 34*, 497–498.

Brescoll, V. L. (2016). Leading with their hearts? How gender stereotypes of emotion lead to biased evaluations of female leaders. *The Leadership Quarterly, 27*(3), 415–428.

Burke, R. (2006). Leadership and spirituality. *Foresight*, 8(6), 14–25.

Craigie, F. C. (1998). Weaving spirituality into organizational life: Suggestions for processes and programs. *Health Progress, 32*, 25–28.

Crawford, P., Brown, B., Kvangarsnes, M. & Gilbert, P. (2014). The design of compassionate care. *Journal of Clinical Nursing, 23*(23–24), 3589–3599.

de Zulueta, P. (2016). Developing compassionate leadership in health care: An integrative review. *Journal of Healthcare Leadership, 8*, 1–10.

Denison, D. (1990). *Corporate culture and organizational effectiveness*. John Wiley.

Duchon, D. & Plowman, D. A. (2005). Nurturing spirit at work: Impact on work unit performance. *Leadership Quarterly, 16*, 807–833.

Dutton, J. E., Workman, K. M. & Hardin, A. E. (2014). Compassion at work. *Annual Review of Organisational Psychology and Organisational Behaviour, 1*(1), 277–304.

Fernando, A. T. & Consedine, N. (2014). Development and initial psychometric properties of the barriers to physician compassion. *Postgraduate Medical Journal*, *90*, 388–395.

Fogarty, G. J. & Shaw, A. (2010). Safety climate and the theory of planned behavior: Towards the prediction of unsafe behavior. *Accident Analysis & Prevention*, *42*(5), 1455–1459.

Fox, C., Webster, B. D. & Casper, W. C. (2018). Spirituality, psychological capital and employee performance: An empirical examination. *Journal of Managerial Issues*, 2, 194–213.

Frisdiantara, C. & Sahertian, P. (2012). The spiritual leadership dimension in relation to other value-based leadership in organization. *International Journal of Humanities and Social Science*, *2*(15), 284–290.

Fritz, C., Lam, C. F. & Spreitzer, G. M. (2011). It's the little things that matter: An examination of knowledge workers' energy management. *Academy of Management Perspectives 25*(3), 2839.

Frost, P. J., Dutton, J. E., Maitlis, S., Lilius, J. M., Kanov, J. M. & Worline, M. C. (2006). Seeing organisations differently: Three lenses on compassion. In S. R. Clegg, C. Hardy, T. B. Lawrence & W. R. Nord (eds), *Handbook of organisational studies* (2nd edn, pp. 843–865). Sage.

Fry, L. W. (2003). Toward a theory of spiritual leadership. *The Leadership Quarterly*, *14*(6), 693–727.

Glickman, S. W., Baggett, K. A., Krubert, C. G., Peterson, E. D. & Schulman, K. A. (2007). Promoting quality: The health-care organization from a management perspective. *International Journal for Quality in Health Care*, *19*(6), 341–348.

Guntuku, R. K., Boini, S., Mary, D. R. & Kummeta, R. S. (2021). Impact of empathetic leadership behaviour on organizational outcomes: Reference to global political leaders and companies during COVID times. *Turkish Online Journal of Qualitative Inquiry*, *12*(10).

Holmes, C. (2018). Stakeholder views on the role of spiritual care in Australian hospitals: An exploratory study. *Health Policy*, *122*(4), 389–395.

Hudson, P. (2003). Applying the lessons of high risk industries to health care. *BMJ Quality & Safety*, *12*(1), i7–i12.

Kanov, J. M., Matilis, S., Worline, M. C., Dutton, J. E., Frost, P. J. & Lilius, J. M. (2004). Compassion in organizational life. *American Behavioral Scientist*, *47*(6), 808–827.

Kashi Komala, R. R. & Ganesh, L. S. (2006). Spirituality in health care organisations. *Journal of the Indian Academy of Applied Psychology*, *32*(2), 119–126.

Katz, D. & Kahn, R. (1978). *The social psychology of organisations*. Wiley.

Klaus, L. & Fernando, M. (2016). Enacting spiritual leadership in business through ego-transcendence. *Leadership & Organization Development Journal*, *37*(1), 71–92.

Koenig, H. G., McCullough, M. E. & Larson, D. B. (2001). *Handbook of religion and health*. Oxford University Press.

Kristof-Brown, A. L., Zimmerman, R. D. & Johnson, E. C. (2005). Consequences of individuals' fit at work: A meta-analysis of person-job, person-organization, person group, and person-supervisor fit. *Personnel Psychology*, *58*(2), 281–342.

Leggat, S. G. & Balding, C. (2019). *Resilient health care: Necessary but not sufficient*. La Trobe University.

―――― (2018). Effective quality systems: implementation in Australian public hospitals. *International Journal of Health Care Quality Assurance*, *31*(8), 1044–1057.

―――― (2017). A qualitative study on the implementation of quality systems in Australian hospitals. *Health Services Management Research*, *30*(3), 179–186.

Leggat, S. G. & Dwyer, J. (2005). Improving hospital performance: Culture change is not the answer. *Healthcare Quarterly*, *8*(2), 60–66.

Lilius, J. M. (2012). Recovery at work: Understanding the restorative side of 'depleting' client interactions. *Academy of Management Review*, *37*(4), 569–588.

Lown, B. A., McIntosh, S., Gaines, M. E., McGuinn, K. & Hatem, D. S. (2016). Integrating compassionate, collaborative care (the 'Triple C') into health professional education to advance the triple aim of health care. *Academic Medicine*, *91*(3), 310–316.

Lown, B. A., Rosen, J. & Marttila, J. (2011). An agenda for improving compassionate care: A survey shows about half of patients say such care is missing. *Health Affairs*, *30*(9), 1172–1178.

Maben, J., Latter, S. & Clark, J. M. (2006). The theory-practice gap: Impact of professional bureaucratic work conflicts on newly qualified nurses. *Journal of Advanced Nursing*, *55*(4), 465–477.

Madden, L. T., Duchon, D., Madden, T. M. & Plowman, D. A. (2012). Emergent organizational capacity for compassion. *Academy of Management Review*, *37*(4), 689–708.

McClelland, L. E. & Vogus, T. J. (2014). Compassion practices and HCAPHS: Does rewarding and supporting workplace compassion influence patient perception? *Health Services Research*, *49*(5), 1670–1683.

McKee, M. C., Driscoll, C., Kelloway, E. K. & Kelley, E. (2011). Exploring linkages among transformational leadership, workplace spirituality and well-being in health care workers. *Journal of Management, Spirituality and Religion*, *8*(3), 233–255.

Menzies Lyth, I. (1988). The function of social systems as a defence against anxiety: A report on a study of the nursing service of a general hospital. *Containing anxiety in institutions. Selected essays. I. Menzies Lyth*. Free Association Books.

Meyer, J. (2010). Promoting dignity, respect and compassionate care. *Journal of Research in Nursing*, *15*(1), 69–73.

Mitroff, I. I. & Denton, E. A. (1999). *A spiritual audit of corporate America: A hard look at spirituality, religion, and values in the workplace*. Jossey-Bass.

Natale, S. M. & Libertella, A. F. (2019). *Empathic leadership. Encyclopedia of Business and Professional Ethics*. D. Poff & A. Michalos (eds). Springer.

Shankar Pawar, B. (2009). Individual spirituality, workplace spirituality and work attitudes: An empirical test of direct and interaction effects. *Leadership & Organization Development Journal*, *30*(8), 759–777.

Sinclair, S., Norris, J. M., McConnell, S. J., Chochinov, H. M., Hack, T. F., Hagen, N. A. … Bouchal, S. R. (2016). Compassion: A scoping review of the healthcare literature. *BMC Palliative Care*, *15*(1), 6–22.

Sinclair, S., Russell, L. B., Hack, T. F., Kondejewski, J. & Sawatzky, R. (2017). Measuring compassion in healthcare: A comprehensive and critical review. *The Patient-Patient-Centered Outcomes Research*, *10*(4), 389–405.

Smith, M. E. (2003). Changing an organisation's culture: Correlates of success and failure. *Leadership & Organization Development Journal*, *24*(5), 249–261.

Strauss, C., Taylor, B. L., Gu, J., Kuyken, W., Baer, R., Jones, F. & Cavanagh, K. (2016). What is compassion and how can we measure it? A review of definitions and measures. *Clinical Psychology Review*, *47*, 15–27.

van der Cingel, M. (2014). Compassion: The missing link in quality of care. *Nurse Education Today*, *34*(9), 1253–1257.

Vance, D. L. (2001). Nurses' attitudes towards spirituality and patient care. *Medsurg Nursing*, *10*, 264–268.

Vitaliano, P. P., Zhang, J. & Scanlan, J. M. (2003). Is caregiving hazardous to one's physical health? A meta-analysis. *Psychological Bulletin*, *129*, 946–972.

Wilber, K. (1996). *A brief history of everything*. Shambhala.

Part 3
Engages Others

10 Communication leadership

Mark Keough

Learning objectives

How do I:

- use the basic principles of communication theory to improve my communication?
- understand communication as a process in a health service context?
- identify the barriers to effective communication, particularly in health services?
- develop skills to improve the use of communication in team-based, health services settings?
- adapt to evolving communication practices, including electronic communication?

Introduction

Critical to successful engagement in any organisation is an understanding of the important elements affecting good communication. There are many dimensions to the study of communication in the 21st century, both generally and in health service settings. This chapter considers the foundational concepts, with references to help students discover more about communication in organisational, social and cultural settings.

Many believe that even the definition of communication is worth questioning. As a notion it is so discursive and diverse that any definition other than the simplest becomes so complex as to cease being useful (Newman, 1960).

Communication, knowledge and learning are inextricably linked. Not all our daily communication is merely functional. Increasingly, communication contains significant amounts of information, some of it important and some of it not so important. The information transmitted has become so great in volume that there is a need for better information science to absorb what is important for now, store what is important for later and discard or archive what is not important at all. This classification process requires considerable skill, and everyone is engaged in analysing large numbers of incoming communications daily, if not hourly or by the minute.

Definitions

Communication between people is so fundamental to life that it is somewhat surprising that it is only since the Second World War that it has been a significant domain of academic study. This interest was fuelled by the extensive advances in the technology of human communication that took place in the late 19th century and the 20th century, and it has been accelerated by the **globalising** effects of the internet and the worldwide web since the 1990s. The study of communication has become the cornerstone of any review of socialised human endeavour, including our use of media, organisational behaviour and human, family and interpersonal relations.

Until the 20th century, the focus of study was the art of communication rather than the process of communication. The art of communication can be observed through language, visual representation, drama and music. After the Second World War, the Bell Laboratories, a division of the Bell Telephone Company, proposed the first model of communication (Shannon & Weaver, 1949). Not surprisingly, it was the development of radio and telephone communications technologies that gave rise to the model. The basic model proved too simplistic for most people and thus was progressively developed, from a simple process to describe communication using telephony to a model applicable in the much broader realm of human social relations. In the early 1960s, based on the work of David Berlo (1960), the model was expanded and clarified to what is now widely accepted as the basic model of communication: that of source, message, channel and receiver.

Understanding of communication and its effects has grown rapidly in recent years, beginning with the modernist premise that preceded the growth in advertising communications in the 1960s. The idea that 'the medium is the message' was promoted by Marshall McLuhan (1964) and has been further developed into our contemporary understanding that communication

> **Communication:** A two-way exchange of information through writing, speaking or another medium
>
> **Globalisation:** The process through which an organisation or concept develops a presence or influence in more than one country

can be initiated by the inanimate. For example, the structure of an organisation, the architecture of a building, the clothing people wear (such uniforms and dress codes) are all media to convey a message. And the media may be the message. This is further complicated by evolving notions of identity and ideas about self. People's self-awareness, their preferences and personalities, even their mood: all form part of the source of messages.

Essential elements of communication

Sender

Sender: The person or system initiating a communication

The **sender** of human communication (usually, but not always, a person) retains the belief that the techniques they employ, their message and the information contained therein are always received in the detail and context with which they were intended. Messages rely heavily on language, and of course the language used must be understood. When sending a message, it is important to ensure that the language is simple, clear and to the point. Messages constructed carefully have the best chance of being understood. Think about a simple request like, 'I would like you to make a cup of coffee for me, please'. When messages are clear they contain a reference to the source ('I' and 'for me'), the subject ('you'), the object ('a cup of coffee') and an emotive adjunct to the phrase to support the desired behaviour ('please').

When messages are ambiguous, receivers may start to look for other meanings than that which was originally intended. For example, if the message is simply, 'I would like a cup of coffee', the receiver may assume it has nothing to do with them, because the subject ('you') is not identified. Of course, if the sender says, '*Fais-moi un café, s'il te plaît*', they are assuming the subject can speak French. Language and its careful construction, tone and use are often critical to communication.

To assist with comprehension when communicating with individuals or groups, it is recommended that plain language is used and aimed at a standard reading level (e.g. upper primary or lower secondary).

Emotion

When messages are loaded with emotion, such as anger or happiness, the meaning can also become unclear. In fact, an angry or happy message will most likely convey the emotion rather than the message itself: emotion can cloud a message to the point at which no part of the message is retained save for the emotional effect. How people send a message – the language, tone and medium – is critical to the message that will be received.

Distortion

Distortion: A change in the usual, original, natural or intended meaning, condition or shape

Ambiguity is only one of the possible distortions that result in a message being lost or a communication being ineffective. Message **distortion**, or noise, can have several causes. Sometimes it is accidental, but sometimes it is a deliberate and disruptive act by the receiver or a third-party stakeholder with an interest in skewing the message.

A distortion effect can occur in a workplace when a communication between one person and another, or one person and many other people, becomes skewed by external interference. If communication is to be clear, understood and acted upon, sources of distortion must be eliminated or minimised. A critical skill in communication leadership is establishing an intuitive alert mechanism for distortion.

Feedback

One way in which it is possible to test whether a message is getting through is by asking for **feedback** from the receiver. Feedback is essential if the sender is to achieve confirmation that the message is heard and understood. Without feedback, even in the most straightforward of personal communications, the sender may have no idea whether the message has been received, let alone understood.

Feedback: An indication of the reaction of the receiver

Non-verbal communication

A smile, a happy disposition, an open stance, or a warm handshake or greeting immediately indicates a positive disposition between a communication sender and receiver. Folded arms, clenched teeth, hands covering the face and an agitated disposition have the opposite effect. Non-verbal acts can communicate vividly and can undermine attempts to communicate with equal and stunning effect. More subtle clues lie in interpersonal behaviours, such as eye contact and shuffling in one's seat, or perhaps in the choice of clothing for a particular situation. Any of these factors can enhance or detract from the effectiveness of communication. Good communicators pay close attention to non-verbal cues; understanding them in their cultural, social and workplace contexts is critical to successful communication (Dwyer & Boyd, 2003).

> **HEALTH COMMUNICATION, THE SMARTPHONE AND ETHICS**
>
> Since the release of the smartphone in 2007, personal, asynchronous communication has become a 24/7 phenomenon. We 'wear' our smartphones, and we often have connected smartwatches, which enable social media tools, SMS texts and email communication to be available all the time. For some people this is a blessing, while for others it is a pervasive and intrusive pest. Some employers, in all industries, take advantage of this ubiquity, sending messages to employees when they are off duty with the expectation of a response.
>
> Amendments in 2024 to the *Fair Work Act 2009* (Cth) allow Australian workers the right to disconnect from work after working hours (Golding, 2023). Within the bounds of reasonableness, they are no longer compelled to respond to workplace communication sent when they are off duty. This can be problematic for human services industries, such as health services, where the care of a patient or client is of paramount concern. It is a worthy reflection to consider your right to switch off from work and truly rest and recover, as well as the primary care consideration in health settings. For example, a vital piece of information forgotten at the time of patient handover may need to be communicated.
>
> The amended legislation makes responding optional, but even reading a work communication out of one's working hours can be stressful. While most organisations are likely to develop employee-led policies on such matters, it is important that you form your own view of how to consider the ethics of the situation, and to care for yourself, patients and clients, especially in critical-care settings.

Receiver

Receiver: The person or system who perceives a communication

The perception of the **receiver** of a message or group of messages is completely dependent on their reading comprehension, and their skills in listening and analysing the message – that is, it depends on their situational awareness. If the receiver is not aware or listening, they will not receive the message. Given that they are not the initiator of the message, it is highly likely that the sender may need to first gain their attention. With a telephone call this is relatively simple: the sender dials a number, the phone rings and the receiver answers. Most cultural protocols include some identifying language and confirmation that the receiver is ready to listen.

When this is translated into a workplace situation it can be either simpler or more complicated. For example, we should assume that in the earlier example someone would not ask another person to make them a cup of coffee unless the subject could hear the request and there was some idea or evidence that they were listening or taking it in. In other situations, such as during a speech or while giving instructions to a group, it is difficult to guarantee that individuals in the receiving group are alert and listening. In more complex situations, the true message may be couched in such neutral or inoffensive language, in order not to offend members of an audience, that comprehension of the request becomes very difficult. If the receiver is not skilled, capable or ready to receive a message, the communication will be lost.

Healthcare and communication

Communication in health services settings can be broadly grouped into three streams: administrative (financial, human resources and organisational), clinical (medical and interprofessional) and client (patient and family). This chapter focuses on the second two; many good texts about organisations are available that describe the nature and importance of sound administrative communications, while special skills and structures are needed to lead clinical and client communications successfully.

Formal and informal communication

In health management settings, understanding when a communication should be formal or informal is critical. For new team leaders, it can be embarrassing to have written a formal memorandum-style email to a team member and colleague and afterwards discover that a personal conversation would have been more appropriate. An important part of managers' and leaders' skillsets is a consistent set of formal and informal protocols for communication.

Upward communications (reports, proposals, requests for approval) are often formal. Most managers respect, however, that subordinates may need to talk over an idea in an informal setting. Downward communications (procedures, requests, memorandums, meeting minutes) are also often formal, whereas peer, or sideways, communications are more likely to be informal, except when a structured communication is called for due to an administrative requirement or clinical situation.

Clinical communication

In any health-service context, strong communication skills can literally be a matter of life and death. The lore of human health experience is littered with examples and anecdotes of situations in which poor communication led to a terrible health outcome, escalating illness or even unnecessary loss of life (see e.g. the executive summary in the Mid Staffordshire NHS Foundation Trust Public Inquiry, 2013). A challenging issue in healthcare is the unintended 'silo' effect of having experts from many differently focused fields of healthcare advising on a single situation without first communicating with each other. This can, and has, led to many unfortunate outcomes in which information was conveyed without the correct context, and a tragic result occurred.

Structured communication

New developments derived from experiences of the United States military have led to a popular model for structured communication in clinical practice: the formalising of communication protocols for situations in which information and context must be conveyed with as much accuracy as possible. An example is the clinical handover of information from one daily rostered shift to the next, or from one health service location to the next. The Introduction, Situation, Background, Assessment and Recommendation (ISBAR) model is one such framework that is commonly in use in many health settings. Figure 10.1 shows the model and the core questions required to establish the critical clinical information. ISBAR is not only useful in clinical settings but can also be used to manage organisational communications in which the use of a formal protocol is likely to be well known and understood. Whenever communication is of a critical nature and distortion must be minimised, following this structured method will assist in ensuring clarity.

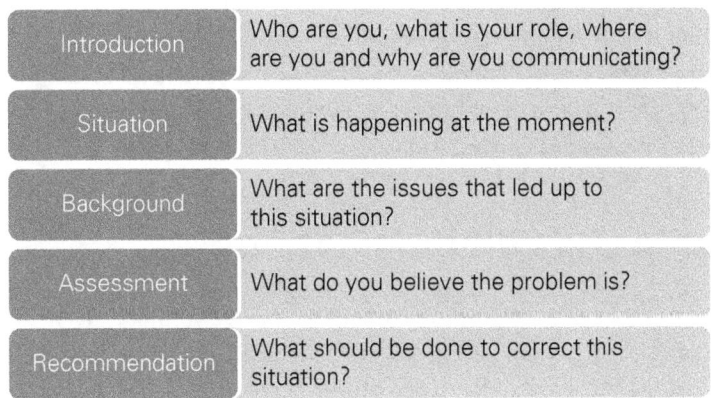

Figure 10.1 The ISBAR model

Source: Hunter New England Health (2009) and SA Health (2016).

Electronic communication

In any study of communication, we cannot ignore the effects of communications technologies and how they have changed society through communicative action (Habermas, 1987). Mobile communications technology, in particular, has 'taken on the full figure of the discursive action: it has inserted itself into the daily needs of the projective selves who carry and operate it' (Keough, 2011, p. 519).

While the principles of good communication and the attributes of poor communication apply universally, there are some important characteristics of electronic communication that are worthy of special note. Every time we communicate electronically, there are three important and common aspects that are often overlooked. Firstly, non-verbal markers are severely discounted. Online communication is mostly written and often brief. We mistakenly assume that the receiver can see the wink in our eye or the 'tongue in our cheek'. Secondly, many people falsely believe that electronic communication is more anonymous than interpersonal communication and therefore sometimes write a little too courageously, only to later regret the message's tone. Finally, we often believe that the only person reading an electronic communication is the person to whom it was directed.

All people in organisations rely heavily on emails to communicate, which makes writing an effective email a fundamental skill. An effective email will ensure that receivers understand the message quickly and will generate a faster and more effective response. Ineffective emails are often ignored.

When writing an email, especially when it is aimed at work colleagues, it is important to start with the key message, using the best comprehension level and tone, having taken time to understand the demographics of the intended audience. When the purpose of the email is clear from the start, it will be opened and read, so a descriptive subject header is a critical first component. Then, the most important information should be positioned at the top of the email, in the opening paragraph. There should be one piece of information in each paragraph. If an email message is longer than one screen, people are often tempted to print it out, so it is recommended that the most important aspect of the message is provided in one or two short paragraphs and then additional or supporting material is appended in a PDF or other attachment. Understanding the audience involves knowing the role and position of the receiver, whether they will understand the chosen terminology and whether a message being sent to more than one person should be the same for all recipients or tailored for different people. It is important to use plain language, avoiding jargon and complicated wording, to make sure the key message is understood.

Leadership and communication

Communicating within teams is both challenging and rewarding, given that we seek to establish successful and functional groups with a shared purpose. Team communications are critical when the outcome of a service can be achieved only by several people working together. These complex situations are common in all health services.

Active listening

Active listening is a key skill in health-service teams. It means listening with focus and intent. Some methods for putting active listening into action are discussed here.

Firstly, ask rather than tell, by using open questions that encourage others to express their views. Open questions invite the listener to provide information, such as, 'Jenny, I would like your opinion on this'. Closed questions are designed to narrow the focus of the answers and are often used to qualify information in a situation, leading to a yes or no answer. They are helpful in some situations – for example, 'Are you allergic to peanuts?' – but can stifle conversation and limit onward discovery.

It is also important to try to suspend judgement and consider matters from other people's perspectives without filtering what is heard through a narrow viewpoint. This is quite a skill, but it is always helpful to quietly ask yourself, 'If I were in their shoes, how would I feel about this?' in order to maintain a sense of accurate context for the information being received.

Ensuring genuine interest in understanding the other person is vital. Take time to actively check the listener's understanding by reflecting and paraphrasing their answer before responding. Listen for the true message the person is trying to convey. This can be enhanced by taking careful notice of tone, body language and situational context.

The results of active listening are usually more beneficial than those of a passive approach. Conversations become two-way, and the participants feel more engaged.

Difficult conversations

Holding regular conversations about difficult topics can help to avoid workplace tension and reduce the likelihood of a crisis and can lead to healthier and more productive relationships at work. Difficult conversations may take place one-to-one or during team sessions. When a difficult conversation becomes necessary, before starting it is important to think about the most suitable place and time for it to occur. Grabbing someone in the corridor on their way to lunch is not a good idea. In some cases, a witness may be required.

For a difficult conversation to be successful, the facts of the situation need to be checked and corroborated. It is important to ensure that the other person or audience understands the problem, the expectations and desired outcomes. During the conversation, it is best to keep to the main point without bringing up other issues. This helps to ensure that trust is kept intact, which is most important to a beneficial outcome. No matter what occurs with the receiving party, the initiator of the conversation must be respectful and keep their emotions in check.

When tackling difficult conversations, 'I' messages should be used when the issue is more complex or is ongoing. Such messages have four parts. Firstly, if the conversation is about the person's problem-causing behaviour, it should be described in an objective, non-blaming way. Secondly, the phrase 'the effects are' is used to help the person understand the consequences of the behaviour. Then, the manager describes how the behaviour makes them feel; a simple 'I feel' avoids a direct accusation. Finally, such phrases as 'I'd prefer' are used, rather than 'you should', to identify the preferred behaviour. For example, 'When you raised your voice in front of my peers, it was uncalled for in that setting, and I felt stupid. I'd rather you had pulled me aside to speak about this in private'.

It is useful when tackling difficult conversations to use plain language, so as to avoid feelings being misunderstood. For example, saying 'I'm angry' could mean a person is either furious or just irritated. It can be misread. If there is uncertainty in a situation, of course, it is important to say so.

Electronic communications

A challenge for health-service managers exists in the ways in which tools for electronic communication blur boundaries between our personal and professional lives. Social networking tools can engender the feeling of anonymity, often encouraging us to write our emotional responses to an issue or event with the feeling that we are in a safe 'social' situation among friends and family. However, social networking tools come with the permanence of writing, the forensic accuracy of a time and date stamp, and occasionally an escalation in audience numbers from local to global.

The responsibility of employees and managers to carefully and responsibly navigate this area is not helped when clear legislation, policies and procedures have lagged well behind social and organisational practices. Local organisational policies and procedures that are clear and unambiguous are essential in health-services settings.

Communication and learning

The communication revolution of the late 20th and early 21st centuries is truly remarkable and, for the most part, has initiated a great leap forwards for all humankind. Online webs of communication have dramatically influenced learning: imagine a world without search engines such as Google, Yahoo, Bing, ChatGPT search and Openverse, to name just a few. What can be known and authenticated from online information is astonishing; internet tools save lives, speed learning and make knowledge truly global. Provided there exists the privilege of access to these global learning networks, there is no excuse for ignorance or decisions based on significantly out-of-date information.

There are many ways to learn about the expanding domains of communication, but leaders in health-services settings may consider the work of Etienne Wenger (1998a, 1998b) in his definition of a **community of practice and interest**. This body of thinking offers managers and leaders a framework for understanding how organisations function, communicate and learn. It offers a useful way of understanding the role of mature communication in an organisation, supporting improvement in service quality, and client and employee satisfaction.

Community of practice and interest: A group of people who share a concern or passion for something they do and who learn how to do it better as they interact regularly (Wenger 1998a, 1998b)

All communication in this era is contributing to our learning about communication, and all communication networks create new societal benefits. Although, as Castells (2013) cautions, too much control over communication networks may lead to unintended and unfortunate consequences, such as stifling innovation and creativity. Through improved communication skills and technologies, the future of society and working relationships is surely in everyone's interest.

Communication and marginalised groups

In the Australian context, what might we consider a marginalised group? A marginalised group is one that experiences discrimination and exclusion through social, political and economic disadvantages. They are often pushed to the edge of the power structures within society and thereby experience disempowerment.

There is a wide range of groups that may be considered marginalised, including:

- cultural groups such as recent immigrants, many of whom experience English as a second or subsequent language
- First Nations peoples of Australia
- individuals and families experiencing housing and other personal financial crises
- victims of domestic violence or family violence
- victims of crime
- people living with physical or mental impairment.

Key principles for health communication with First Nations peoples

Effective health communication with First Nations peoples in Australia and Aotearoa New Zealand hinges on fostering trust, respect and cultural safety. These principles are vital for addressing health inequities and developing effective interventions.

Cultural awareness

Cultural appropriateness is paramount, recognising the unique values and worldviews of Indigenous peoples. This includes respecting their connection to land, language and tradition, and acknowledging the historical trauma of colonisation.

Culturally safe communication involves incorporating First Nations' languages and perspectives, thereby building trust between healthcare providers and Indigenous patients.

Health literacy should be a collaborative process, incorporating both Indigenous and biomedical knowledges. This fosters shared understanding and can help to ensure both patient and provider are aligned in their comprehension of health information. Health communication interventions are best when co-designed with Indigenous communities to ensure cultural relevance and resonance.

Co-design

Indigenous leadership and governance are essential in shaping health systems that address the specific needs of First Nations communities. Indigenous peoples must play a central role in developing policies, programs and services that affect them, emphasising local engagement and self-determination.

Education

Addressing systemic barriers, such as institutional racism, and improving Indigenous representation in the health workforce are critical. Healthcare providers should engage in cultural safety training and create an environment in which Indigenous patients feel respected and understood. By embedding these principles into health communication, we can strive for more equitable health outcomes for First Nations peoples in both Australia and Aotearoa New Zealand.

Key principles for health communication with people who have impaired physical or mental ability, and culturally and linguistically diverse communities

Principles for health communication with people from Culturally and Linguistically Diverse (CALD) groups and people with impaired ability must focus on addressing barriers that hinder their access to healthcare and ensure inclusive, equitable services.

Contextual, cultural and linguistic appropriateness

Healthcare information should be available in relevant languages and tailored to the cultural beliefs and practices of the respective CALD communities. This helps to bridge the gap between providers and patients, and can help to reduce misunderstandings arising from language and cultural differences.

Reducing healthcare inequalities

People with impaired ability and some people from CALD communities may experience barriers such as limited access to healthcare services, limited health literacy and institutional racism. Addressing these issues involves improving service-delivery models to meet community needs, with a focus on cultural safety and respect.

Collaborative approaches

Health policies and interventions must be co-designed with the relevant communities to ensure they are contextual and effective. This includes engaging community leaders in the planning and implementation of healthcare initiatives.

Data and policy refinement

National standards for collecting and reporting data on CALD populations need to reflect the diversity within these communities. Accurate data is crucial for understanding healthcare needs and designing effective health communication strategies.

Communication needs, as well as therapeutic approaches, will be different based on the social ecology of the group (or individuals) concerned. Making assumptions without proper consultation is likely to lead to poor outcomes.

It is important to consider the needs of marginalised people as individuals first. Some people's needs are unique and may be influenced by several factors that cause marginalisation. Only when appropriate consultation has occurred would it be prudent to seek to meet the needs of a marginalised group.

Summary

- Communication consists of a five-step process: source, sender, message, channel and receiver.
- Team-based communication is not helped by the common silos that exist in many professional and administrative settings in health services.
- Communication in health settings is helped by structures and protocols such as the ISBAR model, particularly in sensitive areas.
- Poor communication practices can lead to harmful outcomes in health services, including loss of life.
- Recent events and trends such as the COVID-19 pandemic and the increased use of communications technologies have changed expectations and practices significantly in health communications.
- Community centred approaches to health communication are essential for marginalised groups.

Reflective questions

1. Is communication an art or a process?
2. What types of distortions are common in health-services communication?

3. What technologies are present in health-services settings?
4. When is it better to communicate with patients and clients electronically and when must it be face-to-face? Explain why.
5. Why are non-verbal signals important in communication?

Self-analysis questions

Reflect on what makes a leader a good communicator, considering aspects of leadership that you think most affect communications – for example, self-assurance or confidence. Is it important to be organised with structured protocols or is flexibility and a listening ear more critical? The ability to listen and identify with a wide range of people is desirable, but is it critical in a health-service setting? Is being reflective considered more important than being timely and decisive? How has your experience of the COVID-19 pandemic and the role of communications technologies changed your practice?

Consider your leadership strengths and how they naturally support good communication. Then ask some trusted friends whether they agree with your analysis.

References

Berlo, D. K. (1960). *The process of communication: An introduction to theory and practice*. Holt, Rinehart & Winston.

Castells, M. (2013). *Communication power*. Oxford University Press.

Golding, G. (2023). The right to disconnect in Australia: Creating space for a new term implied by law. *UNSW Law Journal, 46*(2), 728–757. https://doi.org/10.53637/HJMQ5885

Habermas, J. (1987). *The theory of communicative action: Vol. 2. Lifeworld and system: A critique of functionalist reason*. Polity Press.

Hunter New England Health. (2009). ISBAR revisited: Identifying and solving barriers to effective clinical handover. [Project toolkit]. Retrieved from: https://www.safetyandquality.gov.au/sites/default/files/migrated/ISBAR-toolkit.pdf

Keough, M. (2011). *Toward learning utility: The evolution of online learning as a network utility in industry settings*. University of South Australia.

McLuhan, M. (1964). *Understanding media: The extensions of man*. Routledge & Kegan Paul.

Mid Staffordshire NHS Foundation Trust Public Inquiry. (2013). *Report of the Mid Staffordshire NHS Foundation Trust Public Inquiry: Executive summary* (Chaired by R. Francis QC). Retrieved from: https://www.gov.uk/government/uploads/system/uploads/attachment_data/file/279124/0947.pdf

Newman, J. B. (1960). A rationale for a definition of communication. *Journal of Communication, 10*(3), 115–124. https://doi.org/10.1111/j.1460-2466.1960.tb00530.x

SA Health (2023). *A standard mnemonic to improve clinical communication*. Retrieved from: https://www.sahealth.sa.gov.au/wps/wcm/connect/8a8b26804896068a9cb8fc7675638bd8/15111.3-+Clinical+Handover+Fact+Sheet+%28V1%29WebS.pdf?MOD=AJPERES&CACHEID=ROOTWORKSPACE-8a8b26804896068a9cb8fc7675638bd8-nwKWYoN

Shannon, C. E. & Weaver, W. (1949). *The mathematical theory of communication*. University of Illinois.

Wenger, E. (1998a). Communities of practice: Learning as a social system. *Systems Thinker, 9*(5), 2–3.

——— (1998b). *Communities of practice: Learning, meaning, and identity*. Cambridge University.

11 Leading interprofessional teams

Katrina Radford
and Janna Anneke Fitzgerald

Learning objectives

How do I:

- understand the place of interprofessional teams in healthcare organisations?
- analyse the enablers and barriers to leading interprofessional teams?
- enhance my teamwork skills by applying principles of successful leadership of interprofessional teams?
- work with the benefits and challenges associated with leading interprofessional teams?

Introduction

Leadership is an elusive concept. Key authors cannot agree on the characteristics of leaders, but all agree that leadership is about relationships and evolves over time. For example, Rost and Barker (2000) state that 'leadership is an influence relationship among leaders and followers who intend real changes and outcomes that reflect a shared purpose' (p. 3). Meanwhile, Landsdale (2002) suggests that 'effective leaders enable people to move in the same direction, toward the same destinations, at the same speed, but not because they have been forced to, but because they want to' (p. 56). This raises the question of how we get people to want to go in the same direction and at the same pace. In the health services, this is particularly challenging because of the multidisciplinary nature of the key stakeholders. It requires appropriate leadership of interprofessional teams.

There is widespread recognition that providing high-quality patient care includes working in interprofessional teams (Ingels, Zajac, Kilcullen, Bisbey & Salas, 2023). In addition, interprofessional teams produce greater patient satisfaction and outcomes, reduced healthcare costs and improved job satisfaction (Clarke & Hassmiller, 2013).

This chapter stresses the importance of leading interprofessional teams and presents some suggestions for how collaborative teams can work together effectively to achieve common goals. By the end of this chapter, you will better understand how to lead interprofessional teams by acknowledging the place of interprofessional teams in healthcare organisations today, as well as the benefits and challenges of such a collaborative approach to healthcare.

Definitions

Working with a variety of different professionals in a team enables the sharing of expertise and perspectives to meet the common goal of providing quality care to patients within a healthcare setting. This form of teamwork is commonly known as interprofessional

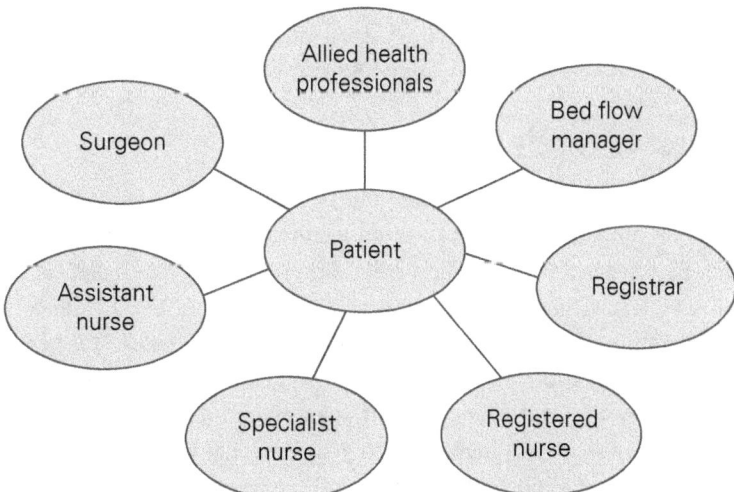

Figure 11.1 Example of an interprofessional team within an acute-care setting

Source: Adapted from Gopee & Galloway (2009).

collaborative practice and involves 'health professionals working collaboratively in integrated teams to draw on individual and collective skills and experiences across disciplines' (Clarke & Hassmiller, 2013, p. 334). An example of the types of professions that could make up an **interprofessional health team** is provided in Figure 11.1.

Interprofessional health team: A group of professionals from different disciplines working collaboratively in an integrated team to draw on individual and collective skills and experiences

Teams with professional boundaries

There are many terms used within healthcare settings to indicate the context within which health professionals work together.

Mumma and Nelson (2002) propose three different types of teams: multidisciplinary, interdisciplinary and transdisciplinary teams.

Multidisciplinary teams

Multidisciplinary team: A group of professionals from different disciplines working collaboratively and with clear disciplinary boundaries

Multidisciplinary teams have discipline-specific goals. There are clear boundaries between disciplines, and effective communication is essential for success and to ensure that crossover of workloads does not occur. This model involves each discipline working within the parameters of its profession to provide appropriate, patient-centred care.

Interdisciplinary teams

Interdisciplinary team: A group of professionals from different disciplines working closely together to achieve common outcomes through regular meetings, using a collaborative patient-care approach and not bound by discipline-specific boundaries

In contrast to multidisciplinary teams, **interdisciplinary teams** collaborate to identify patient goals and use an expanded problem-solving model that goes beyond discipline-specific boundaries in order to maximise patient outcomes. This model involves working together to achieve common outcomes and may mean holding regular patient-centred meetings with representatives from a variety of disciplines in order to maximise patient outcomes through a collaborative patient-care approach.

Transdisciplinary teams

Transdisciplinary team: A group of professionals from different disciplines working collaboratively across boundaries with flexibility between disciplines to minimise duplication

Transdisciplinary teams tend to work across boundaries between disciplines and have the flexibility to minimise duplication of effort. However, this model takes the most work to manage in terms of effective communication and teamwork.

Dyad leadership models

Dyad leadership models have recently come to be accepted as best practice across North American hospitals (Ingels et al., 2023). Dyad leadership models involve pairing a clinical leader and another leader with a complementary background – such as a non-clinical administrator – to lead a system, division or area (Sanford, 2015). Evidence suggests that this type of leadership enables better decision-making and greater ability to lead change initiatives (American Hospital Association, 2018; Biga, 2024). Moreover, dyad leadership models in a cardiology team have been shown as enabling increased communication across interdisciplinary teams as well as demonstrating 'operational efficiencies, strategic planning and execution, integration of clinical expertise with decision making processes' (Biga, 2024, p. 2128).

In the Australian setting, calls have been made to innovate leadership in the aged-care setting (Radford & Meissner, 2024). As such, a dyad leadership model has been trialled in a residential aged-care setting in Adelaide (Radford et al., 2024). That study reports that dyad leadership models improve patient, family and staff satisfaction with the care provided. In addition, the co-creation of a dyad leadership models is said to improve staff career opportunities, reduce stress and encourage operational integration across the whole of the organisation, thereby leading to stronger teamwork outcomes (Radford et al., 2024).

Teams with role-related boundaries

In addition to interprofessional teams that are delineated by professional boundaries, there are teams that are delineated by their roles – for example, clinical leaders, managers and practitioners (or clinicians). These roles can exist within and across professions, making leadership of this type of interprofessional team more challenging because the principal concerns of practitioners and those of managers are distinct, as evident in Table 11.1 (Edwards, Kornacki & Silversin, 2002; Edwards, Marshall, McLellan & Abbasi, 2003). Note that in the table 'clinician' refers to a clinical position not involving management (e.g. registered nurse). A manager refers to any position that involves managing a team within a healthcare environment.

Table 11.1 Principal concerns of clinicians and managers

Clinicians	Managers
Patient or client outcomes	Patient experience
Individual patients or clients	Population or organisation
Optimal care for each patient or client	Managing competing claims
Professional autonomy	Public accountability
Self-regulation	Systems
Evidenced-based practice	Fair allocation of resources
Personal responsibility	Delegation
Role clarity	Role ambiguity
Explicit knowledge	Tacit knowledge

Source: Adapted from Edwards et al. (2002); Edwards et al. (2003); Fitzgerald (2002).

There are deep differences in clinicians' and managers' backgrounds, as well as varying concerns, which give rise to 'unavoidable conflict between the reductionist approach to medicine and the messy political and complex world of policy' (Edwards et al., 2002, p. 837). For example, practitioners' work is rooted in the biological sciences, based on cause-and-effect relationships, and has a strong academic focus. Clinicians are responsible for their own patients and enact professional discretion in treatment decisions; they tend to think operationally, work to short timeframes and function in a professional culture. In contrast, managers draw from the economic, financial, social and behavioural sciences, which operate within the qualitative paradigm. Their focuses are groups and populations, and they tend to base their decisions on rational processes or legal policy. Managers think strategically, plan for distant time horizons and work well in teams. They function in task-and-role cultures (Parkin, 2009). Consequently, because of the differences in the paradigms in which they work, practitioners and managers may not always agree on core matters.

For example, a residential aged-care manager may be concerned with the site accreditation results and implementation of new monitoring or reporting requirements to fulfil their outcomes at the clinical level by the nurse manager. However, that nurse manager may already be overwhelmed with the volume of administration that takes them away from caring for residents, and they may not feel they can fit any more administration tasks into their daily activities without compromising care quality. As such, without open communication and respect for each other's perspectives, serious issues may arise, such as staff burnout and lack of reporting required for the next accreditation visit.

Thus, leaders must shift their mindsets from working in silos and power struggles to working in partnerships that build trust and respect within teams. This begins with understanding the view of the other party in negotiations and daily activities; to help with this, it is important to focus on building a culture of teamwork and open communication between leaders in the organisation. This may include cross-role buddying whereby one leader shadows the other for a day to help them understand the role boundary that exists and to provide deep insight into the other profession; this should aim to create and maintain trust in each other.

Building on the previous example, having strategic workload discussions as a team helps members understand each other's perspectives and enables a group decision to be made. In the previous example of the residential aged-care manager setting additional reporting requirements for the nurse manager, regularly bringing together the entire senior leadership team in a strategic conversation regarding current reporting arrangements will enable all perspectives to be taken and considered. This also allows the organisation to explore not only how much administration is being asked for and by whom but also to reflect and identify any duplication that can affect workload. This approach opens the door for a win–win scenario to occur, whereby the manager can add the reporting requirements they need, and the nurse manager does not need to compromise care quality as their administrative workload is being considered in decision-making.

Leadership of interprofessional teams

Effective leadership of interprofessional teams is critical to maximising productivity (Seaton, Jones, Johnston & Francis, 2024; Trivedi et al., 2013). Yet, leading these teams can be a difficult and challenging experience, especially as communication styles differ and leadership styles need to be flexible to support such diverse teams.

Successful team dynamics are achieved when members see their roles as important to the team and when there is open communication between team members, autonomy and equality of resources (Morrison, 2007). Further, a blending of professional cultures is necessary, which includes sharing skills and knowledge to improve the quality of patient care (Bridges, Davidson, Odegard, Maki & Tomkowiak, 2011). Thus, leaders must be conscious of the team dynamics involved and must influence the outcomes by creating opportunities for understanding, empathy and resource-sharing between professions in the broader team.

One way this can occur is through **integrated care**, which involves training and education, open communication and mutual respect (Interprofessional Education Collaborative Expert Panel, 2011). Clarke and Hassmiller (2013) propose four key competencies for successful interprofessional collaborative practice:

1. understanding and demonstrating values and ethics of interprofessional practice throughout the organisation and unit
2. espousing clear roles and responsibilities for each team member
3. providing clear interprofessional communication
4. encouraging effective teams and teamwork.

The following list contains important guidelines for leaders of interprofessional teams:

- Identify key stakeholders and know who matters most.
- When problem-solving, be sure to examine the diversity within the team to provide varying perspectives for members; this means decisions will be more widely accepted.
- Understand how team members respond to conflict and expectations.
- Work towards understanding and valuing the benefit of individuals' differences and appreciating all contributions.
- Avoid assumptions that all professional groups act and respond in the same ways.
- Recognise similarities between team members.
- Treat resistance as a form of communication.
- Seek out different experiences from the majority and from those who matter most.
- Pay close attention to verbal and non-verbal communication.
- Ask for clarification, to avoid making assumptions.
- Assist those in minoritised groups to be successful by including them in informal networking within the team culture.

Working within an interprofessional team is not easy and requires strong leadership to be successful. This is because working in a team calls for cooperation, understanding and the use of effective communication (Burzotta & Noble, 2011). Strong leadership of such a team requires the following values and traits to be established by the leader within the team before collaboration begins: responsibility, accountability, coordination, communication, cooperation, assertiveness, autonomy, and mutual trust and respect (Bridges et al., 2011; Burzotta & Noble, 2011; Clarke & Hassmiller, 2013).

Integrated care: A team approach involving training and education, open communication and mutual respect (Interprofessional Education Collaborative Expert Panel, 2011)

Management of interprofessional teams

Healthcare organisations are driven by the need for cost reductions and organisational efficiencies; this is known commonly as the business of health, and it responds to organisational targets such as cost reduction and performance measures driven by the economic and political climate. As a result, the business of health has had an increasing influence over the practice of health in recent years, and practitioners have expressed resentment towards health service managers because they perceive that economic and political imperatives, more than clinical need, drive the structural and operational changes implemented in healthcare organisations. From the practitioners' perspective, managers limit practitioners' autonomy and control over their clinical practice (Spurgeon, Clark & Ham, 2011). In contrast, managers may feel that change is warranted, based on the social, political, historical and economic needs of the environment within which they are operating. These two perspectives are continuing to merge as the competition for clinical talent continues following the COVID-19 pandemic, the emergence of dyad leadership models and increasing use of interprofessional teams to manage caseloads across healthcare environments. Thus, healthcare leaders must lead interprofessional teams effectively.

The successful management of collaborative teams involves addressing some key challenges, which include managing knowledge held by team members about other team members' disciplines, personal values and beliefs, **professional identity**, perceptions of occupational esteem and workload (Reese & Sontag, 2001).

> **Professional identity:** The way in which each profession categorises itself and differentiates itself from other professions (Schein, 1978).

Understanding the professional identity of team members is critical to the management of interprofessional teams, as it cannot be assumed that team members will respond to management in similar ways. Deconstructing professional identities is sometimes useful in seeking to understand interprofessional team difficulties. This can be achieved by categorising and analysing how each discipline views its professional autonomy, authority and sovereignty. Some idea of these views can be gained by discovering how team members see their roles and tasks (occupational or professional), how they define their roles (ambiguous or clear), what kind of knowledge they enact (tacit, intuitive or explicit, scientific) and the nature of their work (dirty or clean). In addition, the manner and aptness in which professionals are rewarded are also useful identity constructs (Fitzgerald, 2002).

Poor team dynamics can be a result of poor communication styles within the team, lack of time investment in team development and poor understanding of other professional roles and codes of conduct (Burzotta & Noble, 2011). Working interprofessionally can also mean problems are identified by different team members through different means and at different times. Fortunately, over the past 10 years there has been an increasing occurrence of interprofessional education in tertiary education, which paves the way for harmony in interprofessional teams.

Thus, investing in team-development initiatives and preparing for an interprofessional leadership model for the future is critical. This includes not only understanding the dynamics, role scope, professional boundaries and philosophies of practice of other professions but also investing in the attitudes of mutual respect, mutual trust and cooperation; behaviours of conflict management, communication, collaborative leadership and decision-making; and cognitions of situational awareness, shared understanding of roles and responsibilities, and shared mental models to work effectively together (Ingels et al., 2023). Without a personal investment in developing successful team dynamics, healthcare leaders will not succeed at leading interprofessional teams.

THE COMPLEXITIES OF INTERPROFESSIONAL TEAMS

In a small Australian metropolitan residential aged-care facility, Mirela, the care coordinator, is paired to work with Susan, the lifestyle manager, in a dyad leadership model. However, while Susan has a background in clinical work as a registered nurse (still registered), she does not want to be burdened with extra tasks outside her new and exciting position. Upon working with Mirela on managing 12 clients within her area, it becomes clear that Mirela (to whom Susan previously reported) is assigning her with clinical duties to help Mirela manage her workload. These additional tasks lead to Susan constantly having to work at home to catch up with her reporting and having to stay back at work to complete her tasks. The CEO notes that Susan is working late and, after a performance meeting, it becomes clear that some role-boundary management is needed across the company. The CEO provides Mirela and Susan some time to 'work it out' together before realising after 4 weeks that some intervention is needed. The CEO does not want to lose either staff member and wants to support both in their leadership roles, so they implement a team-building activity that includes both positions shadowing each other for a week, with backfill for the other role during the time of shadowing using corporate staff. Within a few weeks, Susan and Mirela form a unique bond, and Susan is no longer doing 'extra tasks' for Mirela as Mirela now understands how busy Susan's new role is.

Summary

- Interprofessional teams are defined as 'health professionals working collaboratively in integrated teams to draw on individual and collective skills and experiences across disciplines' (Clarke & Hassmiller, 2013, p. 334).
- Principles of successful interprofessional teams include effective communication, autonomy, equality of resources, blending of professional cultures, integrated care and mutual respect.
- Leading interprofessional teams is a difficult and challenging experience, especially as communication styles differ and leadership styles need to be flexible in order to support such diverse teams.
- There are enablers and barriers to leading interprofessional teams.

Reflective questions

1. Why are interprofessional teams important in healthcare organisations?
2. How is leading interprofessional teams different from leading other teams?
3. List three different models of interprofessional teams that could be used in healthcare organisations.
4. How can the roles of team members affect team dynamics?
5. Why are interprofessional teams hard to manage?

Self-analysis question

What is your understanding of the differences between the values and the beliefs of team members, and how much do these affect your leadership?

References

American Hospital Association (2018). *A Model for Clinical Partnering: How Nurse and Physician Executives Use Synergy as Strategy*. https://www.aha.org/system/files/2018-08/plf-issue-brief-clinical-partnering.pdf

Biga, C. (2024). Synergizing success: The power of dyad leadership in cardiology. *Journal of the American College of Cardiology, 83*(21), 2128–2129.

Bridges, D., Davidson, R. A., Odegard, P. S., Maki, I. V. & Tomkowiak, J. (2011). Interprofessional collaboration: Three best practice models of interprofessional education. *Medical Education Online, 16*(6035). https://doi.org/10.3402/meo.v16i0.6035

Burzotta, L. & Noble, H. (2011). The dimensions of interprofessional practice. *British Journal of Nursing, 20*(5), 310–315. https://doi.org/10.12968/bjon.2011.20.5.310

Clarke, P. & Hassmiller, S. (2013). Nursing leadership: Interprofessional education and practice. *Nursing Science Quarterly, 26*(4), 333–336. https://doi.org/10.1177/0894318413500313

Edwards, N., Kornacki, M. & Silversin, J. (2002). Unhappy doctors: What are the causes and what can be done? *British Medical Journal, 324*(7341), 835–838. https://doi.org/10.1136/bmj.324.7341.835

Edwards, N., Marshall, M., McLellan, A. & Abbasi, K. (2003). Doctors and managers: A problem without a solution? *British Medical Journal, 326*(7390), 609–610. https://doi.org/10.1136/bmj.326.7390.609

Fitzgerald, A. (2002). Doctors and nurses working together: A mixed method study into the construction and changing of professional identities [Unpublished doctoral dissertation], University of Western Sydney. http://uwsprod.uws.dgicloud.com/islandora/object/uws%3A789

Gopee, N. & Galloway, J. (2009). *Leadership and management in healthcare*. Sage.

Ingels, D. J., Zajac, S. A., Kilcullen, M. P., Bisbey, T. M. & Salas, E. (2023). Interprofessional teamwork in healthcare: Observations and the road ahead. *Journal of interprofessional care, 37*(3), 338–345.

Interprofessional Education Collaborative Expert Panel (ECEP). (2011). *Core competencies for interprofessional collaborative practice: Report of an expert panel*. ECEP.

Landsdale, B. M. (2002). *Cultivating inspired leaders*. Kumarian.

Morrison, S. (2007). Working together: Why bother with collaboration? *Work Based Learning in Primary Care, 5*, 65–70.

Mumma, C. M. & Nelson, A. (2002). Theory and practice models for rehabilitation nursing. In S. P. Hoeman (ed.), *Rehabilitation nursing: Process, application and outcomes* (pp. 20–36). Mosby.

Parkin, P. (2009). *Managing change in health care*. Sage.

Radford, K. & Meissner, E. (2024). Debate: Tackling the aged care workforce. *Public Money & Management, 44*(5), 341–342. https://doi.org/10.1080/09540962.2024.2338998

Radford, K., Meissner, E., Church, M., Kosiol, J., Chai, A., Maddern, J., Perkins, D. & Pearson, N. (2024). *Developing and piloting a role matrix that empowers careers across aged care: Final report*. St Basil's Homes and Griffith University. Retrieved from: https://ariia.org.au/projects/st-basils-homes-sa-and-griffith-university-developing-and-piloting-role-matrix-empowers

Reese, D. J. & Sontag, M. A. (2001). Successful interprofessional collaboration on the hospice team. *Health and Social Work, 26*(3), 167–175. https://doi.org/10.1093/hsw/26.3.167

Rost, J. C. & Barker, R. A. (2000). Leadership education in colleges: Toward a 21st century paradigm. *Journal of Leadership Studies, 7*(1), 3–12. https://doi.org/10.1177/107179190000700102

Sanford, K. (2015). *Dyad leadership in healthcare: When one plus one is greater than two*. Lippincott Williams & Wilkins.

Schein, E. H. (1978). *Career dynamics: Matching individual and organizational needs*. Addison-Wesley.

Seaton, J., Jones, A., Johnston, C. & Francis, K. (2024). Promoting effective interprofessional collaborative practice in the primary care setting: Recommendations from Queensland physiotherapy private practitioners. *Australian Journal of Primary Health, 30*(1).

Spurgeon, P., Clark, J. & Ham, C. (2011). *Medical leadership: From the dark side to centre stage*. Radcliffe.

Trivedi, D., Goodman, C., Gage, H., Baron, N., Scheibl, F., Illiffe, S. Manthorpe, J., Bunn, F. & Drennan, V. (2013). The effectiveness of inter-professional working for older people living in the community: A systematic review. *Health and Social Care in the Community, 21*(2), 113–128. https://doi.org/10.1111/j.1365-2524.2012.01067.x

Clinical governance

Cathy Balding

12

Learning objectives

How do I:

- understand the origins of clinical governance?
- identify the core components of clinical governance required to support good care?
- make the connection between corporate governance and clinical governance?
- explain responsive regulation?
- develop skills to lead clinical governance in my organisation?

Introduction

The past three decades have seen the rise of clinical governance, firstly as a concept and ultimately as a system. Increasing knowledge of the scope of iatrogenic harm to consumers, coupled with public inquiries into poor care around the world, is driving the development of governance of clinical care into an established component of corporate governance. Many gains are being realised in Australia, including a reduction in infections and preventable in-hospital cardiac arrests, improved experiences and outcomes for patients, better governance of clinical care and more meaningful involvement of patients and consumers in health care (Australian Commission on Safety and Quality in Health Care (ACSQHC), 2019).

Despite the gains, clinical governance systems are still not achieving universally consistent quality care (Leggat & Balding, 2017a). Accreditation is still viewed by many as an administrative burden designed to achieve accreditation. Some quality-related metrics have plateaued over time; according to Braithwaite, Glaziou and Westbrook (2020), 60 per cent of care, on average, is in line with evidence-based or consensus-based guidelines, while 30 per cent is some form of waste or of low value, and 10 per cent causes harm.

Unsafe and suboptimal care also impose heavy financial burdens, estimated in developed countries at 12.6 per cent of health expenditure, comprising: 5.4 per cent in acute care, 3.3 per cent in primary care and 3.9 per cent in long-term care (Slawomirski & Klazinga, 2022). The ACSQHC (2019) notes that in the financial year 2017–18, hospital-acquired complications cost the public sector an estimated $4.1 billion or 8.9 per cent of total hospital expenditure. On average, a complication costs a hospital more than three times the extra revenue it received for the complication (Duckett, Jorm, Moran & Parsonage, 2018).

Clinical governance: 'Clinical governance is the set of relationships and responsibilities established by a health service organisation between its state or territory department of health, governing body, executive, clinicians, patients, consumers and other stakeholders to ensure good clinical outcomes. It ensures that the community and health service organisations can be confident that systems are in place to deliver safe and high-quality health care, and continuously improve services.' (ACSQHC, 2017, p.1).

Corporate governance: '[T]he framework of rules, roles, relationships, systems and processes within and by which authority is exercised and controlled in corporations' (AICD, 2011, p. 2).

History

Genesis

Over time, governments, consumers, boards, managers and clinicians have realised the value, and necessity, of addressing clinical care with the same focus that corporate issues receive. 'If clinical governance is to be successful it must be underpinned by the same strengths as corporate governance: it must be rigorous in its application, organisation-wide in its emphasis, accountable in its delivery, developmental in its thrust, and positive in its connotations' (Scally & Donaldson, 1998, p. 62).

Healthcare is a complex and high-risk industry (Plsek & Greenhalgh, 2001). Considering the explosion of new technologies and the constant growth in knowledge, seemingly limitless demand and rising community expectation, along with the vagaries of state and federal politics and funding, it is no surprise that containing clinical risk and providing consistently good care is a continuing challenge (Balding, 2008). Within this environment, self-regulation and individual approaches are not sufficient to ensure quality care.

Clinical governance puts a system of monitoring, support and accountability around the historical individualism of health care to assist staff to provide quality care within a complex environment. Clinical governance is a subset of corporate governance in human services.

The Australian Stock Exchange Corporate Governance Principles describe **corporate governance** as 'the framework of rules, roles, relationships, systems and processes within and by which authority is exercised and controlled in corporations' (Australian Institute of Company Directors (AICD), 2011, p. 2).

A **clinical governance framework** sets out the organisational systems and processes that need to be in place to ensure that patients receive the best possible care. In Australia, the framework is based on the National Safety and Quality Health Service Standards, which are outlined in the section that follows (ACSQHC, 2017).

Health professionals the world over have traditionally pursued high standards through monitoring and improving the quality of their own care, and membership of professional associations that encourage peer review and professional development. Unwarranted variation in care practice remains stubbornly embedded, however (Leggat & Balding, 2017b). In the past, when things went wrong and resulted in patient harm, there were few mechanisms for identifying, discussing and learning from issues, with blame and shame being the most likely outcome. This culture, a lack of reliable data and heavy reliance on individual experts to provide consistently good care masked many clinical and systems inadequacies (Spear & Schmidhofer, 2005). Fear of legal consequences and a culture that blamed error on human failing ensured that health care was slow to acknowledge and learn from mistakes (Balding, 2008). Robust governance and leadership were required to support individuals who could not, through good intent and hard work alone, overcome the inadequate or non-existent systems they were working with, within an increasingly complex environment.

Clinical governance framework: The 'rules, roles, relationships, systems and processes that support safe, quality care within an organisation' (ACSQHC, 2017, p.1).

Turning point

The first large-scale Australian study of hospital-acquired adverse events provided much-needed focus and clarity. The 1995 Quality in Australian Health Care Study revealed that 16.6 per cent of reviewed admissions was associated with an adverse event, with 51 per cent of these considered preventable (Wilson et al., 1995). Australia responded in 2000 by setting up the ACSQHC, which was charged with developing Australia's first national approach to system-wide quality issues (Wilson & Van Der Weyden, 2005).

In Aotearoa New Zealand, concerns about inconsistencies in healthcare quality and unequal access to healthcare services gained public and political attention in the 1970s. Since then, several reforms have attempted to address these issues, including implementation of various funding approaches and restructures of health service operations and governance, which continue to the present day (NZ Parliamentary Library, 2009). Aotearoa New Zealand also instituted national certification of health and aged-care services in 2001, when the Health and Disability Services Standards (HDSS) were first introduced. The Ministry of Health led their development as part of its broader regulatory role in overseeing health and disability services in the country. In 2010, to lead a national safety and quality approach, the New Zealand Health Quality & Safety Commission (NZHQSC, 2013) was established.

The statistics were soon followed by a series of public inquiries into safety and quality of care in hospitals, firstly in the United Kingdom, with the Bristol Royal Infirmary case (United Kingdom Department of Health, 2001), and then in several Australian hospitals (Dunbar, Reddy, Beresford, Ramsey & Lord, 2007). The United Kingdom's National Health Service (NHS) introduced clinical governance after the Bristol Royal Infirmary inquiry in 1998, defining it as 'a system through which NHS organisations are accountable for continuously improving the quality of their services and safeguarding high standards of care by creating an environment in which excellence in clinical care will flourish' (Scally & Donaldson, 1998, p. 62). Other countries then followed suit.

Australia has also had its share of investigations into poor care, including at Camden and Campbelltown Hospitals in New South Wales, Canberra Hospital, King Edward Memorial Hospital in Western Australia and Bundaberg Hospital in Queensland, to name a few. Each review arose after internal mechanisms failed to detect and resolve the issues, and it was frequently left to whistleblowers to shine a light on continuing problems. The Royal Commission into Aged Care Quality in Australia (Commonwealth of Australia, 2021) explored hundreds of instances of poor care and neglect in residential and home care. Improving clinical governance was relevant to around half of the 148 recommendations of the Royal Commission.

Consistent organisational and management issues have been identified from analysis of public inquiries and Royal Commissions into poor care; these include:

- a culture of blame and inattention to care quality
- focus on meeting external key performance indicators and targets at the expense of internal standards of care
- lack of leadership of, clear lines of accountability for, and reporting on, the quality and safety of the services provided
- insufficient consideration of patients and their families
- tolerance of substandard care
- ineffective credentialling, training and support for staff
- preoccupation with corporate matters at the expense of focus on clinical care
- ineffective reporting and action relating to clinical care. (Mid Staffordshire NHS Foundation Trust Public Inquiry, 2013; Walshe & Shortell, 2004; Commonwealth of Australia, 2021).

The studies and public inquiries reinforced that continuing reliance on hardworking and well-intentioned individuals, and clinical governance implemented for accreditation compliance, are not enough to guarantee consistently good care in the complexity of health, aged and human services. While each inquiry and commission addresses its own context and terms of reference, the common actions required for change are clear: leadership of safety and quality from the top of the organisation, engagement of patients and families in care, a culture of openness and transparency, rigorous implementation and monitoring of basic care standards, specific support for staff to provide quality care and robust reporting and action for improvement (Travaglia, Hughes & Braithwaite, 2011). These drivers have gradually been absorbed into the foundations of clinical governance, but their application remains variable.

Despite the lessons learned, it took another public inquiry, this time in the United Kingdom, to demonstrate the need for greater robustness in clinical governance design and implementation.

THE MID STAFFORDSHIRE NHS FOUNDATION TRUST PUBLIC INQUIRY

This inquiry is considered internationally as the 'go-to' case study for gaining an understanding of clinical governance. The scale of patient neglect and the clarity with which Robert Francis QC (2013) distils and presents the problems and solutions has made it a recognised model for demonstrating how poor care can occur in health care – and what is required to prevent it.

The Mid Staffordshire hospitals underwent two public inquiries investigating poor care during the period from 2005 to 2009. The case clearly demonstrates what can happen without a system of leadership, accountability and monitoring. It caught international attention in a way that many other public inquiries have not, possibly because it was about the denial of basic standards of care. The clinical governance failures and lessons learned are universal and applicable across systems and countries.

At these hospitals, elderly and vulnerable patients were left unwashed, unfed and without fluids. Some were left in excrement-stained sheets and beds. Patients who could not eat or drink without help did not receive it. Medicines were prescribed but not given.

How could this happen in a modern hospital in 21st-century England? The chair of the inquiry, Robert Francis QC, is clear: it happened because of a complete breakdown of clinical governance. According to Francis, the hospital trust board 'did not listen sufficiently to its patients and staff or ensure the correction of deficiencies [that were] brought to [their] attention' (Mid Staffordshire NHS Foundation Trust Public Inquiry, 2013, p. 3) and '… failed to tackle a culture involving tolerance of poor standards and disengagement from managerial and leadership responsibilities' (p. 3). The board and executive were preoccupied with achieving access and budget targets rather than focusing on the standard of care they were providing. The hospitals met their external compliance requirements, but these were focused more on corporate than on clinical matters (Mid Staffordshire NHS Foundation Trust Public Inquiry, 2013).

Clinical governance evolution

Clinical governance evolved again after the Mid Staffordshire case and continues to develop. It was obvious from that Inquiry that the pursuit of consistently good care requires clinical governance that is more than compliance and 'box-ticking'. Boards now accept that they are accountable for the quality of clinical care provided by their organisation, although the skills with which this accountability is enacted varies considerably. Clinical governance is now positioned within existing corporate governance systems, with boards overseeing it as they do financial and strategic governance. Leaders understand that clinical governance is essential to ensuring not just that accreditation will be maintained, but that the organisation will prosper over the long term and that insurance may not cover negligence if adequate clinical governance is not in place (AICD, 2011). Board and operational committees are now well established and undertake the 'heavy lifting' of examing the detail of how clinical risk, care quality and compliance are managed, so as to oversee and drive progress. This sometimes puts board directors at odds with their executives, as executives may feel the board is interfering in operations. However, boards must assure themselves that executives are putting effective systems in place to support staff, and that these enable good care, without telling the executives how to make this happen. The reliability and validity of quality data to support governance is slowly improving, and new clinical governance frameworks are emerging, based on improved knowledge of what it takes to support consistently good care, with the Aotearoa New Zealand clinical governance framework released in 2024 (NZHQSC, 2024).

Australian system

The introduction of clinical governance in Australia received a significant boost with the requirement from 2013 for health services to meet a national mandatory set of 10 national safety and quality standards, the first two of which provide a comprehensive clinical governance platform for health services.

National Safety and Quality Health Service Standard 1, which is concerned with 'governance for safety and quality in health service organisations', provides detailed information on the requirements of an effective health-service governance system, incorporating 'the set of processes, customs, policy directives, laws and conventions affecting the way an organisation is directed, administered or controlled' (ACSQHC, 2012a, p. 6).

As an overview, Standard 1 requires (ACSQHC, 2012a):

- an integrated system of governance that actively manages patient safety and quality risks and supports a culture of safety and transparency
- the governance system to set out safety and quality aspirations, policy, procedures and protocols, and assign staff and committee roles, responsibilities and accountabilities for patient safety and quality
- the clinical workforce to be guided by current best practice and evidence-based clinical guidelines
- managers and the clinical workforce to have the right qualifications and skills to provide high-quality health care
- patient safety incidents to be reported and analysed, and this information used to improve safety systems.

Standard 2, which describes requirements for 'partnering with consumers', aims to ensure that health services are 'responsive to patient, carer and consumer input and needs' (ACSQHC, 2012b, p. 6). According to the standard, significant benefits to clinical quality and outcomes, the experience of care and the business and operations of delivering care are realised through these partnerships (ACSQHC, 2012b).

Other sectors, such as primary care, mental health care and community health and aged care, have developed their own approaches, embedded in accreditation requirements. These clinical – or quality – governance models may look different from one another, but the core components are essentially the same, although the national healthcare safety and quality standards lay out the most comprehensive requirements for clinical governance of all human service standards.

Responsive regulation

The National Safety and Quality Health Service Standards form part of a broader national accreditation reform agenda across all sectors based on a responsive regulatory approach to clinical governance. Responsive regulation is a hierarchical approach with mechanisms that range from persuasion to command and control, as shown in the following list (Healy & Dugdale, 2009):

- voluntarism: clinical protocols, new technology, personal monitoring, continuing education
- market mechanisms: competition, performance payments and contracts, consumer information
- self-regulation: voluntary accreditation, reporting on performance targets, benchmarking, peer review, open disclosure

- meta-regulation: mandated accreditation, clinical governance and continuous improvement, incident-reporting and root cause analysis, protection for whistleblowers, published performance indicators, consumer complaints commissioner, funding agreements
- command and control: criminal or civil penalty, licence revocation or suspension, physician revalidation.

Australian health professionals and services have traditionally practised a mix of voluntarism and self-regulation for the standard of care they provide. Each jurisdiction also uses market mechanisms, such as the requirement that health services report certain data (e.g. infection rates) to the relevant government and commission as part of performance contracts and payments (Healy & Dugdale, 2009).

The rise of care complexity has seen federal and jurisdictional governments increase the use of meta-regulation and command and control mechanisms. The steady increase in mandatory requirements for accreditation of high-risk services covers each level of the regulation hierarchy and brings command and control into play in a way not previously seen. Jurisdictions and commissions employ a regulatory response to health and aged-care services that fail to meet standards, based on the level of risk to consumers. Continuing and serious breaches of the standards may incur financial penalties and result in services being temporarily closed. Licence removal or service closures are last resorts (Healy & Dugdale, 2009).

Leading effective clinical governance into the future

Clinical governance is evolving to address missing links in ineffective approaches as knowledge of what works matures. But progress is slow, with continuing care problems and substantial cost of poor care still evident. Some leadership actions identified by the research as essential for effective clinical governance are not routinely included in clinical governance frameworks. Ideally, clinical governance should act as the bridge between an organisation's aspirations for care quality in its strategic plan and the reality at point of care (Leggat & Balding, 2017a), but this is not yet a consistent cornerstone of clinical governance. Achieving quality care across an organisation requires the implementation of clinical governance as a coherent strategy, focused on achieving a concrete definition of success (Dixon-Woods et al., 2014), and yet a shared understanding of quality care, expressed in terms of benefits for both staff and consumers, is not yet universally recognised as essential to success (Balding & Leggat, 2021).

There is growing evidence and acceptance that the quality of organisational (and sector) leadership and management are significant predictors of care quality (Sfantou et al., 2017), and that an engaged and supported workforce is critical to achieving high-quality care (Curry et al., 2015), but specific strategies to achieve these are not yet common across health services.

Clinical governance framework foundations

Many staff are still required to work with bureaucratic clinical governance systems that disengage rather than support them. Despite the intention of clinical governance as a support for staff to provide quality care, staff often experience it the other way around: that they exist to support clinical governance and improvement initiatives that may not be useful, are poorly implemented, or both (Lawton & Thomas, 2022). Clinical governance mechanisms are likely to be more effective when they support increased satisfaction for both consumers and staff, but adding administrative burdens with no clear advantage contributes to staff dissatisfaction, with studies showing a significant association between burnout and patient safety (Hall, Johnson, Watt, Tsipa & O'Connor, 2016).

The rise of artificial intelligence (AI) will add a next-level dimension to clinical governance systems. Clinicians will be freed from routine administrative tasks to focus on care. Data collection and analysis will occur in real time and will be used to guide clinical decision-making and practice, both at the bedside and in the bigger-picture design of clinical systems. Risks will be identified earlier or avoided altogether through process automation and early warning systems. Clinical governance mechanisms, such as incident reporting, will no longer require staff to remember to use them but will be built into work systems. Consumers will contribute to their care and service improvement through better information and helpful tools that streamline choices, decision-making and participation (Alowais et al., 2023). Reduction in waste and harm will improve care and save resources. Decision-making, diagnosis and treatment support will be augmented, if not fully automated.

But AI, like all tools, is only as useful as it is designed to be, and the focus with which it is governed. AI in health care presents significant risks as well as enormous benefits. In this environment, it could be argued that there is greater need for leaders to bring purpose and clarity to clinical governance. Concentrating AI on supporting point-of-care quality, avoiding pitfalls and motivating and encouraging staff and consumers to work with new technology to strive for shared quality goals will require robust oversight.

The next stage of clinical governance must get the mix of technology and people right to support good care and to reduce the human and financial costs of poor care. Developing clear purpose, shaping leaders and achieving staff and consumer satisfaction in the pursuit of quality care, supported, rather than dominated by AI, will be central to success. Chief executives and boards must translate strategic intent for good care into meaningful, supported implementation in operations. Whatever evolutions in governance and technology the future has in store, people create quality care, and supporting staff to work to their potential will always be a measure of effectiveness in clinical governance. Ultimately, clinical governance is judged not by whether it ticks an accreditation box, but by its effectiveness in realising a shared vision of quality care in practice.

Summary

- Clinical governance is a key component of the governance of any health service and should be given the same priority as corporate governance.
- Clinical governance systems should support all staff – direct care, managers and support staff – to enact their accountabilities for quality of care.
- The key components of clinical governance are goal-setting, leadership, skilled workforce, clinical risk management, evidence-based care and learning from data, harm and suboptimal care to improve.

- Responsive regulation in this context is a hierarchy of approaches used to regulate the safety and quality of health care, from persuasion to command and control.
- Leading clinical governance requires the board and executive to develop a clear vision for quality care, to implement governance systems as a useful support for staff to achieve it in their daily work, to closely monitor and drive progress, and to respond to high-risk situations.

Reflective questions

1. Why does a healthcare organisation need a system of clinical or care governance?
2. Why did clinical governance not evolve naturally as part of corporate governance in health services?
3. What would happen in your health service if the clinical governance system was terminated?
4. What dissuades staff from engaging with the clinical governance system?
5. Who is ultimately accountable for the quality of the care provided in a health service?

Self-analysis questions

A local hospital has advertised for a new board director, who will also be a member of the board's clinical governance subcommittee. You are responding. Write a one-paragraph application outlining your clinical governance skills and knowledge. Following this, write one paragraph describing the gaps in your knowledge and experience, and how you will fill them.

References

Alowais, S.A., Alghamdi, S.S., Alsuhebany, N. et al. (2023). Revolutionizing healthcare: The role of artificial intelligence in clinical practice. *BMC Medical Education*, 23, 689. https://doi.org/10.1186/s12909-023-04698-z

Australian Commission on Safety and Quality in Health Care (ACSQHC). (2019). *The state of patient safety and quality in Australian hospitals*. ACSQHC. Retrieved from: https://www.safetyandquality.gov.au/publications-and-resources/resource-library/state-patient-safety-and-quality-australian-hospitals-2019

——— (2017) *National model clinical governance framework*. ACSQHC.

——— (2014). *Accreditation and the NSQHS standards*. ACSQHC. Retrieved from: http://www.safetyandquality.gov.au/our-work/accreditation-and-the-nsqhs-standards

——— (2012a). *Safety and quality improvement guide standard 1: Governance for safety and quality in health service organisations*. ACSQHC. Retrieved from: http://www.safetyandquality.gov.au/wp-content/uploads/2012/10/Standard1_Oct_2012_WEB1.pdf

——— (2012b). *Safety and quality improvement guide standard 2: Partnering with consumers*. ACSQHC. Retrieved from: http://www.safetyandquality.gov.au/wp-content/uploads/2012/10/Standard2_Oct_2012_WEB.pdf

Australian Institute of Company Directors (AICD). (2011). *The board's role in clinical governance*. AICD. Retrieved from: http://www.companydirectors.com.au/Director-Resource-Centre/Publications/Book-Store/PUB59

Balding, C. (2008). From quality assurance to clinical governance. *Australian Health Review*, 32(3), 383–391. https://doi.org/10.1071/AH080383

Balding, C. & Leggat, S.G. (2021). Making high quality care an organisational strategy: Results of a longitudinal mixed methods study in Australian hospitals. *Health Services Management Research*, 34(3): 148–157.

Braithwaite, J., Glasziou, P. & Westbrook, J. (2020). The three numbers you need to know about healthcare: The 60–30-10 Challenge. *BMC Medicine, 18*, 102. https://doi.org/10.1186/s12916-020-01563-4

Commonwealth of Australia. Royal Commission into Aged Care Quality and Safety (RCACQS). (2021). *Final report: Care, dignity and respect*. RCACQS. Retrieved from: http://nla.gov.au/nla.obj-2928215218

Curry, L. A., Linnander, E. L., Brewster, A. L., Ting, H., Krumholz, H. M. & Bradley, E. H. (2015). Organizational culture change in U.S. hospitals: A mixed methods longitudinal intervention study. *Implementation Science* 2015; 10: 29–41.

Dixon-Woods, M., Baker, R., Charles, K., Dawson, Jerzembek, G., Martin, G., McCarthy, I., McKee, L., Minion, J., Ozieranski, P., Willars, J., Wilkie, P. & West, M. (2014). Culture and behaviour in the English National Health Service: overview of lessons from a large multimethod study. *BMJ Quality & Safety, 23*(2),: 106–115.

Duckett, S., Jorm, C., Moran, G. & Parsonage, H. (2018). *Safer care saves money: How to improve patient care and save public money at the same time*. Grattan Institute. Retrieved form: https://grattan.edu.au/report/safer-care-saves-money/

Dunbar, J., Reddy, P., Beresford, B., Ramsey, W. & Lord, R. (2007). In the wake of hospital inquiries: Impact on staff and safety. *Medical Journal of Australia, 186*(2), 80–83.

Francis, R. (2013). *Press statement*. Retrieved from: https://www.gov.uk/government/publications/report-of-the-mid-staffordshire-nhs-foundation-trust-public-inquiry

Hall, L. H., Johnson, J., Watt, I., Tsipa, A. & O'Connor, D. B. (2016). Healthcare staff wellbeing, burnout, and patient safety: A systematic review. *PLOS One, 11*(7), e0159015. https://doi.org/10.1371/journal.pone.0159015

Healy, J. & Dugdale, P. (2009). Regulatory strategies for safer patient health care. In J. Healy & P. Dugdale (eds), *Patient safety first: Responsive regulation in health care* (pp. 1–23). Allen & Unwin.

Lawton, R. & Thomas E.J. (2022). Overcoming the 'self-limiting' nature of QI: Can we improve the quality of patient care while caring for staff? *BMJ Quality & Safety, 31*(12), 857–859. https://doi.org/10.1136/bmjqs-2022-015272

Leggat, S.G. & Balding, C. (2017a). Bridging existing governance gaps: Five evidence-based actions that boards can take to pursue high quality care. *Australian Health Review, 43*(2), 126–132. https://doi.org/10.1071/AH17042

——— (2017b). A qualitative study on the implementation of quality systems in Australian hospitals. *Health Services Management Research, 30*(3), 179–186. https://doi.org/10.1177/0951484817715594

Mid Staffordshire NHS Foundation Trust Public Inquiry. (2013). *Report of the Mid Staffordshire NHS Foundation Trust Public Inquiry: Executive summary* (Chaired by R. Francis QC). Retrieved from: https://www.gov.uk/government/uploads/system/uploads/attachment_data/file/279124/0947.pdf

New Zealand Health Quality & Safety Commission (NZHQSC). (2024). *Collaborating for quality: A framework for clinical governance*. Health Quality & Safety Commission. Wellington, NZ. Retrieved from: https://www.hqsc.govt.nz/assets/Our-work/Leadership-and-capability/Building-leadership-and-capability/Publications-resources/Clinical-governance-framework.pdf

——— (2013). *Annual report 2012–13*. Retrieved from: https://www.hqsc.govt.nz/assets/Core-pages/About-us/Annual-reports/HQS_AnnualReport2013LR_LOCKED.pdf

Parliamentary Library. (2009). New Zealand Health System Reforms Research Paper 09/03.

Plsek, P. & Greenhalgh, T. (2001). The challenge of complexity in health care. *British Medical Journal, 323*, 625–628. https://doi.org/10.1136/bmj.323.7313.625

Scally, D. & Donaldson, L. (1998). Clinical governance and the drive for quality improvement in the new NHS in England. *British Medical Journal, 317*, 61–65. https://doi.org/10.1136/bmj.317.7150.61

Sfantou, D. F., Laliotis, A., Patelarou, A. E., Sifaki-Pistolla, D., Matalliotakis, M. & Patelarou, E. (2017). Importance of leadership style towards quality of care measures in healthcare settings: A systematic review. *Healthcare (Basel, Switzerland)*, *5*(4), 73. https://doi.org/10.3390/healthcare5040073

Slawomirski, L. & Klazinga, N. (2022). The economics of patient safety: From analysis to action. *Health working papers* [No. 145]. Directorate for Employment, Labour and Social Affairs Health Committee, OECD.

Spear, S. & Schmidhofer, M. (2005). Ambiguity and workarounds as contributors to medical error. *Annals of Internal Medicine*, *142*(8), 627–630. https://doi.org/10.7326/0003-4819-142-8-200504190-00011

Travaglia, J., Hughes, C. & Braithwaite, J. (2011). Learning from disasters to improve patient safety: Applying the generic disaster pathway to health system errors. *Quality and Safety in Health Care*, *20*(1), 1–8. https://doi.org/10.1136/bmjqs.2009.038885

United Kingdom Department of Health. (2001). The report of the public inquiry into children's heart surgery at the Bristol Royal Infirmary 1984–1995: Learning from Bristol. Stationery Office.

Walshe, K. & Shortell, S. (2004). When things go wrong: How health care organizations deal with major failures. *Health Affairs*, *23*(3), 103–111. https://doi.org/10.1377/hlthaff.23.3.103

Wilson, R., Runciman, W., Gibberd, R., Harrison, B., Newby, L. & Hamilton, J. (1995). The quality in Australian health care study. *Medical Journal of Australia*, *163*(9), 458–471.

Wilson, R. & Van Der Weyden, M. (2005). The safety of Australian healthcare: 10 years after QAHCS. *Medical Journal of Australia*, *182*(6), 260–261.

13 Partnering with stakeholders

Sharon Brownie and Audrey Holmes

Learning objectives

How do I:

- understand definitions, rationale, key concepts and public policy associated with stakeholder partnerships in healthcare settings?
- identify stakeholder groups essential to quality health-service delivery?
- apply success factors associated with effective partnerships?
- evaluate real-world situations, undertake stakeholder analyses and make recommendations for stakeholder engagement?
- reflect on the skills associated with developing, formalising and maintaining effective stakeholder partnerships?

Introduction

This chapter outlines the importance of partnering with stakeholders for quality health-service management and delivery and highlights common patterns driving partnership-based public policy. It introduces concepts associated with partnering in health services, defines key terms and discusses managerial skills or competencies needed to engage with stakeholders and implement partnership-based policy. The interests of key health-sector stakeholders are discussed, and important steps are outlined for managers undertaking stakeholder analyses. Finally, the chapter explores essential factors for successful partnerships and the competencies managers need to successfully develop and maintain stakeholder partnerships.

Definitions

The roots of partnership-based public policies are evident in economic development theory dating back more than 25 years (Brownie, 2007). During the 1990s, leading economic development theorists considered networked and associational approaches to be essential in local development and economic success (Cooke & Morgan, 1998). The focus on partnerships across healthcare professions and sectors has increased given their potential to address complex problems, optimise innovation and decrease costs associated with rising demand for healthcare services (Gray & Purdy, 2018; Regenstein, Trott, Williamson & Theiss, 2018; Schot, Tummers & Noordegraaf, 2020).

Partnership-based public policy can be found in all government health and social services. **Partnership** models are promoted to manage **stakeholder** relationships (Corbin et al., 2018). They have potential to achieve an **alchemical effect**, or **synergy**, which occurs when stakeholders achieve better outcomes working together than when working individually (Corbin, Jones & Barry, 2018; Loban, Scott, Lewis & Haggerty, 2021). For example, partnership between Australian state governments and the construction industry through the 'MATES in Construction' initiative launched new strategies to support construction workers struggling under COVID-19 stay-at-home orders (https://mates.org.au/about-us).

The importance of stakeholder partnerships

Increasing demand for health services is attributable to factors such as population ageing, increasing rates of chronic diseases and non-communicable diseases (including comorbidities), rising costs, environmental health concerns, social and technological changes, and public expectations to live longer, healthier lives (Karam, Brault, Van Durme & Macq, 2018; Regenstein et al., 2018). **Collaboration** through partnerships can effectively address complex healthcare problems, service coordination issues and increasing healthcare demands and costs when human and financial resources are limited (Brownie, Thomas, McAllister & Groves, 2014; Loban et al., 2021). Collaboration can also optimise technological advancements and innovations, enhance knowledge sharing, improve service delivery and wellbeing, and support the realisation of infrastructure projects (Nederhand & Klijn, 2019; Nyström, Karltun, Keller & Andersson Gäre, 2018; Towe et al., 2016). Importantly,

Partnership: Two or more organisations working collaboratively to pursue and achieve common goals and objectives

Stakeholder: 'Anybody who can affect or is affected by an organisation, strategy or project' (Morphy, n.d., para. 2)

Alchemical effect/ Synergy: Synergy is a key mechanism whereby partnerships gain advantages over individual stakeholders working independently towards the same goals (Loban, Scott, Lewis & Haggerty, 2021)

Collaboration: 'A process through which parties who see different aspects of a problem can constructively explore their differences and search for solutions that go beyond their own limited vision [and/or resources] of what is possible' (Gray, 1989, p. 5)

collaborative partnerships play a role in the development of strategies to mitigate large-scale public health concerns such as the COVID-19 pandemic (Baxter & Casady, 2020).

Improving service coordination is a key driver of health-service reform (Brownie et al., 2014; Nederhand & Klijn, 2019; Towe et al., 2016). Public health institutions are under increasing pressure to efficiently and effectively deliver quality services (Morely & Cashell, 2017). However, barriers include complex health problems that can cross boundaries into sectors outside traditional healthcare (e.g. housing, environmental concerns) and the socioeconomic impact of increasing patient complexity (Chandra et al., 2017; Regenstein et al., 2018; Karam et al., 2018). The term '**wicked problems**' describes multifaceted health and social problems that are hard to define unstable, lack clear solutions and are socially and politically complex. Connections to other problems within and across sectors, diverse stakeholder perspectives and financial implications mean they often appear 'unsolvable' (Keijser, Huq & Reay, 2020; Petrie & Peters, 2020). Wicked problems have proliferated in the increasingly complex healthcare environment (e.g. modernisation, technological advancements), and affect the delivery of quality health services (Petrie & Peters, 2020). Resolving these problems requires significant changes in individual and population behaviours (Head & Alford, 2013).

Solving wicked problems requires the cooperation and input of multiple parties and depends on the capacity and willingness of different partners to work together (Morely & Cashell, 2017; Nederhand & Klijn, 2019), including partnering with consumers (Pomey et al., 2015). Cross-sector collaboration can help improve population health and wellbeing by maximising contributions from multiple sectors, including those outside health (e.g. housing, law) (Chandra et al., 2017). Benefits of partnering with stakeholders include increased and streamlined access to services, cost efficiencies and avoidance of duplication. By working together, partners can develop creative solutions to barriers or obstacles. Partnerships enable programs to be more flexible, health services to be more responsive to community and individual needs, and innovative and multifaceted solutions for complex problems (Gray & Purdy, 2018; Loban et al., 2021).

> **Wicked problems:**
> These are 'fundamental, challenging problems that exist within and between social sectors, are not solvable through linear planning or the application of causal models and tools, have no definitive problem formulations or solutions, and are impacted and changed when their intended solutions are implemented' (Keijser, Huq & Reay, 2020, p. 12)

NESTS OF WELLNESS

Providing consistent access to high-quality, timely and affordable care is challenging in rural communities and communities struggling in the post-pandemic inflationary context. Innovative, collaborative partnerships can overcome demographic, geographic, socioeconomic and financial barriers to enhance access to health and social services.

In Australia, a family owned pharmaceutical company, Boehringer Ingelheim, partnered with Heart of Australia to address rural health workforce issues. They developed the 'Heart of Australia NextGen Medics Program' (https://www.boehringer-ingelheim.com/au/press-release/heart-of-australia), which is enabling allied health and medical students to undertake immersive rural-based training. Students have the unique opportunity to experience rural health-service delivery and community life, and to gain firsthand insights into challenges and disparities in rural health-service delivery. Many students commit to rural jobs upon graduation, which achieves the partnership's objective of improving the supply and sustainability of the rural health workforce.

Partnerships for health can involve diverse players. In Aotearoa New Zealand, a new partnership has been established whereby government departments offer partnership-based activities to improve the lives of people in the Wellington region. The focus is on innovations in community health and wellbeing initiatives to address inequality, sanitation and provision of clean water, housing and mental health services. The partnership provides a 3-year sponsorship through the Westpac Government Innovation Fund to join annual 13-week programs hosted by the New Zealand GovTech Accelerator (https://www.miragenews.com/new-innovation-partnership-to-help-improve-new-586560/). This partnership encompasses many innovative social-welfare programs and has identified simple solutions to seemingly complex issues. For example, during one program, participating case workers found many clients were unsuccessful in seeking financial assistance because of missing or incorrect paperwork, and supporting them to understand and provide the correct paperwork decreased frustration and solved many issues (https://oecd-opsi.org/innovations/govtech-innovative-social-welfare-programme-with-nz-and-ph/).

Stakeholder groups in healthcare

Consumers

A key healthcare partnership is that between service providers and those who use health services. Varying terminology is used to describe health service users, including 'patients', 'clients', 'service users' and 'consumers'. In this chapter, health service users are referred to as consumers.

Quality health services should establish meaningful partnerships with consumers, with patient engagement considered a cornerstone for improving care quality (Pomey et al., 2015). The concept of patient-centred care has been extended to a model in which consumers are considered partners in care (Petrie & Peters, 2020; Pomey et al., 2015). Effective partnerships enable consumers to be active in their care and to participate in decision-making. However, for these partnerships to be truly collaborative, consumers may need to be supported to take active roles (Pomey et al., 2015). Transparency and communication between organisations or care teams and consumers are essential (Petrie & Peters, 2020).

Establishing and maintaining partnerships between health professionals and consumers takes time and effort on both sides, including building personal connections, sharing decision-making and understanding differing motivations and goals (Morely & Cashell, 2017; Wolf et al., 2017). Collaboration is based on shared understanding, trust and respect, and effective and appropriate communication is essential. Considerations include incorporating consumer perspectives, experiences, knowledge and values into planning and delivering care; sharing information openly and in a way that encourages participation; supporting consumers and their families or caregivers to participate; and understanding barriers to participation and frustrations from consumers' perspectives (Canberra Health Services, 2022; Pomey et al., 2015). Meaningful partnerships also involve inviting consumer collaboration in developing and implementing health policy and programs (Merner et al., 2023), and service design and delivery. This can encourage quality improvement and is effective at local, national and global levels (Merner et al., 2023). Committed providers should develop ways for consumers and families to be involved at different levels and should consider offering relevant support for individual consumers.

Families and caregivers

Meeting consumers' health needs often requires extensive support from family members and other caregivers, which requires a partnership approach (Parmar et al., 2022; Scales, King & Dieppa, 2023). Such collaborative partnerships can be particularly important for vulnerable and dependent consumers, including children, older people and consumers living with chronic health problems, mental illness or intellectual disability (Wallcraft et al., 2011). Key components of successful partnerships with families and caregivers include mutual respect and consideration, good communication, sharing information and joint decision-making.

Well-developed healthcare partnerships with families and caregivers can improve health outcomes. For example, partnership between health professionals and a child's family plays a critical role in facilitating the child's development (Australian Education Research Organisation, 2022). Partnering with family and caregivers can increase understanding of individual consumer's needs, develop knowledge of their specific health concerns and enable participation in care and decision-making. Families also have unique knowledge about the consumer's personal and social context and how their health concerns affect their daily life. They can assist in communication between the consumer and health professionals (Rendalls, Spigelman, Goodwin & Daniel, 2019), resulting in the consumer being better supported throughout their healthcare experience.

Research collaborators

Traditionally, hospital-based research tended to have a clinical focus; the research focus has shifted to health services and outcomes (Dimick & Greenberg, 2014). The phrase 'better research – better healthcare' is well known (Evans, Thornton, Chalmers & Glasziou, 2011), and active partnerships between academic researchers, health service providers and policy-makers are increasing. Research collaboration supports the translation and co-production of knowledge, facilitates evidence-based practice and generates research relevant to end users (Nyström et al., 2018; Rycroft-Malone et al., 2016). Development of long-term relationships between researchers and decision-makers may contribute to bridging gaps between research and practice (Nyström et al., 2018).

The development and implementation of guidelines is another area in which stakeholder engagement or partnership is increasingly important (Petkovic et al., 2020). A strong clinical evidence base is necessary to ensure patient safety and to promote effective practice across different healthcare settings (Adams, Sommers & Robinson, 2013). Furthermore, some funding organisations require research proposals to include collaborative research teams involving various stakeholders (e.g. community representatives) and researcher–decision-maker partnerships (Nyström et al., 2018).

Whole-of-government collaborators

Collaborative interagency partnerships are important in addressing healthcare complexity and entwined health and social issues (Head & Alford, 2013). Slogans such as 'Mental Health Is Everybody's Business' highlight the need for collaboration and coordination across government departments, including health, housing, police and social welfare. These collaborative efforts include formal partnerships that span the public and private sectors (e.g. non-governmental organisations) and enable coordination of stakeholders at international,

national and local levels (Baxter & Casady, 2020). Interconnections between community development and public health enable effective partnerships that facilitate coordinated approaches to health and wellbeing (Towe et al., 2016). Joint action and clear policy are essential in promoting population health and equity (Corbin et al., 2018). Recent Australian health reforms reflect the understanding that well-coordinated and integrated continuity of care is central to effective health systems, especially for those serving consumers with multiple, ongoing and complex conditions (Angeles, Crosland & Hensher, 2023). The Strengthening Medicare Taskforce was established to ascertain how interprofessional collaboration in health care could be funded to promote healthy lifestyles and healthy ageing, and support people with complex needs (Australian Government, 2022).

Despite a clear mandate for whole-of-government partnerships and collaboration, implementing such partnerships is complex and challenging, especially given the importance of leadership across different sectors (Brownie et al., 2014; Towe et al., 2016). Structural reform, including changes to funding mechanisms (Chiarella & Griffin, 2022; Australian Government, 2022), are part of the solution, but success also depends on health professionals forming working partnerships to deliver services.

First Nations and other marginalised groups

Health services have been reported as failing indigenous peoples, many of whom experience significant disparity in health access and outcomes (World Health Organization, 2022). Mathias and Lovell (2022) note that partnership-based co-design and delivery of health services with indigenous peoples in local communities can achieve better alignment with local need, thereby improving health service quality and outcomes; be responsive and appropriate for local cultures and needs; effectively use and enhance local strengths and assets; and engage people in a way that focuses on health and improves wellbeing.

In the Australian context, non-Indigenous leaders should undertake training to build understanding of partnering with Indigenous peoples (Anderson et al., 2022). Partnership approaches should involve culturally grounded leadership in which cultural safety is openly practised and includes factors such as First Nations branding, community engaged ethics approval, cultural understanding about the need for flexible and iterative processes, and fair remuneration. Additional principles include respect that formalises First Nations sovereignty and ownership, inclusive partnerships that foster collaboration and support self-determination, transparent processes and continuous evaluation of relationships and outcomes with shared space for two-way learning. These partnerships should include statements of clear benefit to the community, with tangible, measurable and sustainable outcomes (Anderson et al., 2022). Guidelines developed by Canada's Indigenous Primary Healthcare Council (2023) detail four engagement principles:

> Principle 1: Appropriate and meaningful consultation
> Principle 2: True and equal partners
> Principle 3: Right to self-governance
> Principle 4: Indigenous health in Indigenous hands

Indigenous reference groups offer a starting point in progressing research that enables the voice of indigenous peoples to be heard and factored into health-service design and delivery. O'Brien and colleagues (2022) partnered with an Aboriginal and Torres Strait

Islander reference group to develop a culturally relevant model of osteoarthritis care in Australia. Critical components for service delivery included cultural alignment, building trusting relationships, inclusion of home visits and call-out features, and the involvement of Indigenous health professionals. Partnering to co-design health services that effectively meet indigenous health needs and reduce health disparities requires cultural competence, which extends beyond cultural awareness. It is a collection of principles, attitudes, policies, behaviours and planning strategies that are combined in an authentic and transparent manner, with continuous, results-based evaluation (Bainbridge, McCalman, Clifford & Tsey, 2015).

Success factors in stakeholder partnerships

The success of a partnership depends on several factors. Strong leadership, a clearly defined purpose, realistic goals and objectives, and high levels of participation and input from all partners are essential. Clear and timely communication is particularly important. Communication channels or mechanisms need to reflect each partner's internal structures and information needs, which means that communication may need to be in multiple forms or styles. A strategic communication plan is essential to ensure that information flows within and between partnering organisations, and to and from external stakeholders.

Trust, respect and learning from other partners' experiences are also important for successful partnerships (Gray & Purdy, 2018; Nederhand & Klijn, 2019). They enable partners to work towards common goals, encourage input and participation, and facilitate the sharing of resources and responsibilities. Genuine partnerships reflect an understanding that each partner has something to contribute and that risks and benefits are shared. Mutual trust and respect enable partnering organisations to gain from the partnership without compromising partnership goals. However, all partners must be committed to shared responsibility and authority, cooperation, a shared mission aligned with stakeholders' (individual or institutional) goals and clear communication (Corbin et al., 2018; Schot et al., 2020).

A partnership structure must be robust and sufficiently flexible to enable it to be adaptable to changing needs as the partnership progresses. Frequent interactions between partners, and clear definition of roles and expectations, both internal and external, are paramount (Rycroft-Malone et al., 2016). All partners must be committed to the partnership and must establish a shared understanding of the partnership's purpose. Partnership structures need to be transparent. To enable shared planning, implementation and evaluation, partnerships need sufficient resources (time, human and financial) (Corbin et al., 2018; Morely & Cashell, 2017). Partners must also understand how to jointly make decisions within the partnership structure (Grudinschi et al., 2013).

Management and stakeholder partnerships

The concept of stakeholder partnerships is easy to discuss but difficult to implement. Partnerships can be frustrating, especially as different stakeholders may have different priorities despite their shared purpose. Successful partnerships require clear leadership and governance, and the processes may differ from those applied in independent organisations

(Loban et al., 2021). A challenge for collaborative partnerships in healthcare and community contexts is implementing effective leadership models involving shared authority and decision-making, with leaders drawn from across stakeholder groups (Chelminski, 2020; Towe et al., 2016). Traditional management competencies alone are not sufficient to achieve increased interagency collaboration and partnerships.

In his seminal book, *Getting agencies to work together: The practice and theory of managerial craftsmanship*, Eugene Bardach (1998) outlined the individual and organisational interagency, collaborative capacity needed by managers. This concept has since been expanded to include mapping changing structures and relationship patterns among stakeholders and partnering agencies. 'Getting things done' and being able to influence without authority are additional management competencies necessary for effective stakeholder engagement. Power held through a role in one organisation may not be relevant in a partnership context; therefore, relationship and negotiation skills are needed to influence action in the absence of direct line authority (Chelminski, 2020). This requires communication, open and transparent processes and trust-building at community, entity and individual levels (Chelminski, 2020; Corbin et al., 2018).

Termeer, Dewulf, Breeman and Stiller (2013) outline four key skills needed by health service managers to address complex or wicked problems:

1. **reflexivity** – the capability to deal with multiple issues
2. **resilience** – the capability to adjust in demanding and changing circumstances
3. **responsiveness** – the capability to respond to changing expectations and agendas
4. **revitalisation** – the capability to unblock stagnations.

Managers also require 'cultural intelligence', or the ability to work across geographic and cultural boundaries, with different age groups and with people of different ethnicities and beliefs (Middleton, 2014).

A good manager recognises stakeholders' potential impact in helping or hindering service development and delivery. They understand that knowing their stakeholders and establishing sound communication plans increase the likelihood of achieving their objectives. Stakeholder analysis and management are therefore key tools for managers. Morphy (n.d.) recommends a systematic, four-step approach to identifying and engaging with stakeholders: stakeholder identification, stakeholder analysis, communication-planning and engagement.

When identifying stakeholders, it helps to clarify whether they are internal or external stakeholders (see Figure 13.1). Specific strategies may be needed to gain the interest, involvement and commitment of different stakeholders (Debono, Travaglia, Sarrami-Foroushani & Braithwaite, 2013), including recognising that stakeholders' motivations for partnering may differ and their willingness to engage may depend on their understanding of potential benefits (Gray & Purdy, 2018; Rycroft-Malone et al., 2016). Therefore, it is important to consider each stakeholder's needs and characteristics. Furthermore, some degree of formalisation may be necessary to ensure a partnership remains sustainable and resilient (Baxter & Cassady, 2020).

Health service managers need to understand each stakeholder's characteristics, including their level of influence. A simple stakeholder analysis involves asking the following questions: *What are they most interested in? What are their biggest concerns? Who can they influence and what is their potential impact? What do we need to do to get their support?*

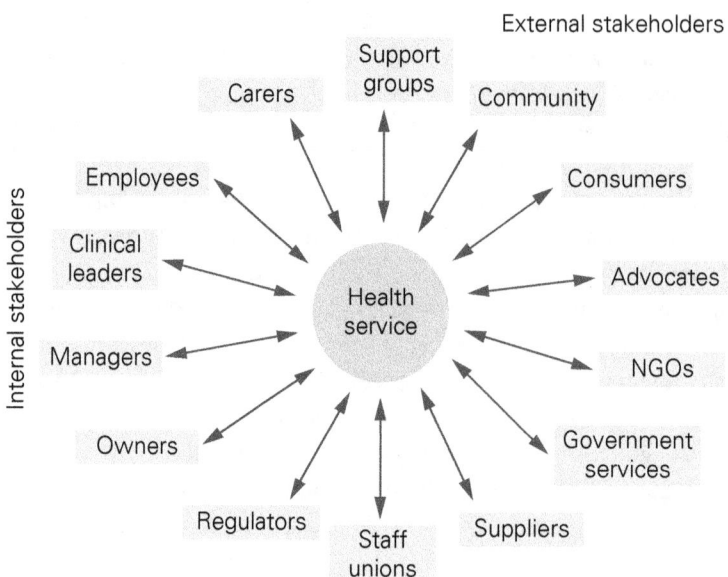

Figure 13.1 Internal and external stakeholders

Leadership and stakeholder partnerships

Collaborative partnerships function differently from traditional organisations (Loban et al., 2021), including their leadership (Cooke, Langley, Wolstenholme & Hampshaw, 2017; Karam et al., 2018). Partnerships are centred on cooperation between organisations and often aim to address complex problems. Different sectors (e.g. health, social services, education) and different stakeholder groups (e.g. government, service providers, community) may need to be involved, meaning different cultures, needs and perspectives must be considered and aligned.

Leadership within a partnership draws together stakeholders with different resources and expertise. Leaders must 'keep the big picture in mind' and maintain the focus on the shared vision or goals. Leaders must be able to clearly communicate these goals, direct partnership resources and action, and obtain any necessary external support. Effective leaders should also understand the dynamics of power-sharing, whereby all partners can influence goals and outcomes by contributing expertise. This shared authority fosters joint ownership and collective responsibility (Towe et al., 2016).

Leadership within a partnership can be neutral, with leaders having few ties to partner organisations and no agenda outside the partnership goals. This means partners have an equal voice and representation, irrespective of differences in resources or community standing. The leadership can also be based on a distributed model in which all partners participate, or an equity-based model in which all partners' views are respected but influence depends on each partner's financial support of the partnership. To be effective and ensure engagement, leaders need to develop a unique skillset, including strong interpersonal and communication skills, to encourage input and participation across partners.

Summary

- Partnering with stakeholders is essential for quality health-service delivery.
- Partnership success factors include strong leadership, a clearly defined purpose, realistic goals and objectives, and a high level of participation with input from all partners.
- Identifying key stakeholders in the health service, department or organisation is essential, as is determining the various interests of these stakeholders and how best to interact with them.
- Leaders and managers must possess reflexivity, resilience, responsiveness, revitalisation, and cultural intelligence skills and attitudes in order to work well with stakeholders.

Reflective questions

1. How much do you know about your stakeholders, their priority issues or concerns, level of influence and their potential effect on the viability and effectiveness of your service?
   Do you have the knowledge to complete a simple stakeholder-analysis worksheet?
2. How can you learn about your stakeholders' concerns and interests and reflect these in your practice?
3. Can you think of a time when you were working on an issue with a stakeholder but using different terminology to refer to the same concept? How did it affect the achievement of mutual goals? How did you work through it?
4. Can you think of a time when your relationship with a key stakeholder went wrong? What were the contributing factors and how did you respond to, and salvage, the situation?
5. Have you observed examples of partnership-based innovation in your area of practice?
   If so, could you undertake a critical review to identify key factors that underpinned success or otherwise?

Self-analysis questions

As a health service manager, are you satisfied with the level and quality of your engagement with internal and external stakeholders? When considering your skills in stakeholder identification, analysis and engagement, which areas of competency are you able to identify for improvement, and how will you address these?

References

Adams, J., Sommers, E. & Robinson, N. (2013). Public health and health services research in integrative medicine: An emerging, essential focus. *European Journal of Integrative Medicine*, *5*(1), 1–3. https://doi.org/10.1016/j.eujim.2012.11.004

Anderson, K., Gall, A., Butler, T., Ngampromwongse, K., Hector, D., Turnbull, S., Lucas, K., Nehill, C., Boltong, A., Keefe, D. & Garvey, G. (2022). Development of key principles and best practices for co-design in health with First Nations Australians. *International Journal of Environmental Research in Public Health*, *20*(1). https://doi.org/10.3390/ijerph20010147

Angeles, M. R., Crosland, P. & Hensher, M. (2023). Challenges for Medicare and universal health care in Australia since 2000. *Medical Journal of Australia*, *218*(7), 322–329.

Australian Education Research Organisation. (2022). *Engaging with families of children with disability to support early learning and development in early childhood education and care* (ECEC). Retrieved from: https://www.edresearch.edu.au/sites/default/files/2022-11/family-engagement-disability-guide-ecec-aa.pdf

Australian Government. (2022). *Strengthening Medicare Taskforce report*. Retrieved from: https://www.health.gov.au/sites/default/files/2023-02/strengthening-medicare-taskforce-report_0.pdf

Bainbridge, R., McCalman, J., Clifford, A. & Tsey, K. (2015). Cultural competency in the delivery of health services for Indigenous people. *Closing the Gap Clearing House, 13*, 1–44. Retrieved from: https://www.aihw.gov.au/getmedia/4f8276f5-e467-442e-a9ef-80b8c010c690/ctgc-ip13.pdf

Bardach, E. (1998). *Getting agencies to work together: The practice and theory of managerial craftsmanship*. Brookings Institution.

Baxter, D. & Casady, C. B. (2020). Proactive and strategic healthcare public-private partnerships (PPPs) in the coronavirus (Covid-19) epoch. *Sustainability, 12*, 5097.

Brownie, S. (2007). *From policy to practice: The New Zealand experience in implementation partnership-based local development policy* [Doctoral dissertation]. Charles Sturt University.

Brownie, S., Thomas, J., McAllister, L. & Groves, M. (2014). Australian health reforms: Enhancing interprofessional practice and competency within the health workforce. *Journal of Interprofessional Care, 28*(3), 252–253. https://doi.org/10.3109/13561820.2014.881790

Canberra Health Services. (2022). *Partnering for exceptional care*. Retrieved from: https://www.canberrahealthservices.act.gov.au/__data/assets/pdf_file/0003/2200296/CHS-Exceptional-Health-Care-Report-2022_V10_AADIGITALFA.pdf

Chandra, A., Acosta, J., Carman, K. G., Dubowitz, T., Leviton, L., Martin, L. T., Miller, C., Nelson, C., Orleans, T., Tait, M., Trujillo, M., Towe, V., Yeung, D. & Plough, A. L. (2017). Building a national culture of health: Background, action framework, measures, and next steps. *Rand Health Q, 6*(2), 3.

Chelminski, P. R. (2020). Leading without line authority. In A. J. Viera & R. Kramer (eds), *Management and leadership skills for medical faculty and healthcare executives* (p. 191). Springer International Publishing.

Chiarella, M. & Griffin, K. (2022). Strengthening Medicare taskforce: How to modernise primary health care. *APNA Primary Times Summer 2022–23, 22*(2). Retrieved from: https://www.apna.asn.au/hub/primary-times-articles/primary-times--summer-2022-23/strengthening-medicare-taskforce--how-to-modernise-primary-health-care

Cooke, P. & Morgan, K. (1998). *The associational economy: Firms, regions, and innovation*. Oxford University Press.

Cooke, J., Langley, J., Wolstenholme, D. & Hampshaw, S. (2017). 'Seeing' the difference: The importance of visibility and action as a mark of 'authenticity' in co-production comment on 'Collaboration and co-production of knowledge in healthcare: Opportunities and challenges.' *International Journal of Health Policy Management, 6*(6), 345–348.

Corbin, J. H., Jones, J. & Barry, M. M. (2018). What makes intersectoral partnerships for health promotion work? A review of the international literature. *Health Promotion International, 33*, 4–26.

Debono, D., Travaglia, J., Sarrami-Foroushani, P. & Braithwaite, J. (2013). *Consumer engagement in the Agency for Clinical Innovation (ACI): Key stakeholder perspectives*. Retrieved from: https://www.researchgate.net/publication/304348824_Consumer_engagement_in_the_Agency_for_Clinical_Innovation_ACI_Key_stakeholder_perspectives

Dimick, J. B. & Greenberg, C. C. (2014). An introduction to health services research. In J. B. Dimick & C. C. Greenberg (eds), *Success in academic surgery* (pp. 3–8). Springer.

Evans, I., Thornton, H., Chalmers, I. & Glasziou, P. (2011). *Testing treatments: Better research for better health care*. Pinter & Martin.

Gray, B. (1989). *Collaborating: Finding common ground for multiparty problems*. Jossey-Bass.

Gray, B. & Purdy, J. (2018). *Collaborating for our future. Multistakeholder partnerships for solving complex problems*. Oxford University Press.

Grudinschi, D., Kaljunen, L., Hokkanen, T., Hallikas, J., Sintonen, S. & Puustinen, A. (2013). Management challenges in cross-sector collaboration: Elderly care case study. *The Innovation Journal*, *18*(2), 1–22.

Head, B. W. & Alford, J. (2013). Wicked problems: Implications for public policy and management. *Administration & Society*, *20*(10), 1–29. https://doi.org/10.1177/0095399713481601

Indigenous Primary Healthcare Council. (2023). *Indigenous health systems transformation: Foundations for IPHCC's OHT provincial framework*. Retrieved from: https://iphcc.ca/wp-content/uploads/2022/09/Indigenous-HST_Booklet.pdf

Karam, M., Brault, I., Van Durme, T. & Macq, J. (2018). Comparing interprofessional and interorganizational collaboration in healthcare: A systematic review of the qualitative research. *International Journal of Nursing Studies*, *79*, 70–83.

Keijser, W., Huq, J.-L. & Reay, T. (2020). Enacting medical leadership to address wicked problems. *BMJ Leader*, *4*, 12–17.

Loban, E., Scott, C., Lewis, V. & Haggerty, J. (2021). Measuring partnership synergy and functioning: Multi-stakeholder collaboration in primary health care. *PLOS One*, *16*(5), e0252299.

Mathias, K. & Lovell, S. (2022). *NZ's health service is failing some communities: Building a better national system requires local partnerships*. Retrieved from: https://theconversation.com/nzs-health-service-is-failing-some-communities-building-a-better-national-system-requires-local-partnerships-180774

Merner, B., Schonfeld, L., Virgona, A., Lowe, D., Walsh, L., Wardrope, C., Graham-Wisener, L., Xafis, V., Colombo, C., Refahi, N., Bryden, P., Chmielewski, R., Martin, F., Messino, N. M., Mussared, A., Smith, L., Biggar, S., Gill, G., Menzies, D., Gaulden, C. M. ... Hill. S. (2023). Consumers' and health providers' views and perceptions of partnering to improve health services design, delivery and evaluation: A co-produced qualitative evidence synthesis. *Cochrane Database of Systematic Reviews*, CD013274.

Middleton, J. (2014). *Cultural intelligence: CQ: The competitive edge for leaders crossing borders*. Bloomsbury.

Morely, L. & Cashell, A. (2017). Collaboration in health care. *Continuing Medical Education*, *48*(2), 207–216.

Morphy, T. (n.d.). *Stakeholder definition*. Retrieved from: http://www.stakeholdermap.com/stakeholder-definition.html

Nederhand, J. & Klijn, E. H. (2019). Stakeholder involvement in public–private partnerships: Its influence on the innovative character of projects and on project performance. *Administration & Society*, *51*(8), 1200–1226.

Nyström, M. E., Karltun, J., Keller, C. & Andersson Gäre, B. (2018). Collaborative and partnership research for improvement of health and social services: researcher's experiences from 20 projects. *Health Research Policy and Systems*, *16*, 46.

O'Brien, P., Prehn, R., Rind, N., Lin, I., Choong, P. F. M., Bessarab, D., Coffin, J., Mason, T., Dowsey, M. M. & Bunzli, S. (2022). Laying the foundations of community engagement in Aboriginal health research: Establishing a community reference group and terms of reference in a novel research field. *Research Involvement and Engagement*, *8*(1), 40. https://doi.org/10.1186/s40900-022-00365-7

Parmar, J., Anderson, S., Duggleby, W., Lobchuk, M., Drance, E., L'Heureux, T., Lowther, J. & Crowder, K. (2022). Steps toward raise: Co-design of competency-based education to engage family caregivers as partners. *Innovation in Aging*, *6*(Supplement 1), 54–55.

Petkovic, J., Riddle, A., Akl, E. A., Khabsa, J., Lytvyn, L., Atwere, P., Campbell, P., Chalkidou, K., Chang, S. M., Crowe, S., Dans, L., El Jardali, F., Ghersi, D., Graham, I. D., Grant, S., Greer-Smith, R., Guise, J-. M., Hazlewood, G., Jull, J. ... Tugwell, P. (2020). Protocol for the development of guidance for stakeholder engagement in health and healthcare guideline development and implementation. *Systematic Reviews*, *9*, 21.

Petrie, S. & Peters, P. (2020). Untangling complexity as a health determinant: Wicked problems in healthcare. *Health Science Inquiry*, *11*(1). https://doi.org/10.29173/hsi299

Pomey, M., Hihat, H., Khalifa, M., Lebel, P., Néron, A. & Dumez, V. (2015). Patient partnership in quality improvement of healthcare services: Patients' inputs and challenges faced. *Patient Experience Journal*, *2*(1), 29–42.

Regenstein, M., Trott, J., Williamson, A. & Theiss, J. (2018). Addressing social determinants of health through medical-legal partnerships. *Health Affairs*, *37*(3), 378–385.

Rendalls, S., Spigelman, A. D., Goodwin, C. & Daniel, N. (2019). Health service engagement with consumers and community in Australia for issue: Engagement and accountability with your community. *Clinical Governance*, *24*(4), 274.

Rycroft-Malone, J., Burton, C. R., Bucknall, T., Graham, I. D., Hutchinson, A. M. & Stacey, D. (2016). Collaboration and co-production of knowledge in healthcare: Opportunities and challenges. *International Journal of Health Policy Management*, *5*(4), 221–223.

Scales, K., King, J. & Dieppa, E. (2023). Partnering to improve care: Strengthening the family caregiver and home care worker relationship. *Innovation in Aging*, *7*(Supplement 1), 462.

Schot, E., Tummers, L. & Noordegraaf, M. (2020). Working on working together. A systematic review on how healthcare professionals contribute to interprofessional collaboration. *Journal of Interprofessional Care*, *34*(3), 332–342.

Termeer, C., Dewulf, A., Breeman, G. & Stiller, S. J. (2013). Governance capabilities for dealing wisely with wicked problems. *Administration & Society*, (January). https://doi.org/10.1177/0095399712469195

Towe, V. L., Leviton, L., Chandra, A., Sloan, J. C., Tait, M. & Orleans, T. (2016). Cross-sector collaborations and partnerships: Essential ingredients to help shape health and well-being. *Health Affairs*, *35*(11), 1964–1969.

Wallcraft, J., Amering, M., Freidin, J., Davar, B., Froggatt, D., Jafri, H., Javed, A., Katontoka, S., Raja, S., Rataemane, S., Steffen, S., Tyano, S., Underhill, C., Wahlberg, H., Warner, R. & Herrman, H. (2011). Partnerships for better mental health worldwide: WPA recommendations on best practices in working with service users and family carers. *World Psychiatry*, *10*(3), 229–236.

Wolf, A., Moore, L., Lydahl, D., Naldemirci, Ö., Elam, M. & Britten, N. (2017). The realities of partnership in person-centred care: a qualitative interview study with patients and professionals. *BMJ Open*, *7*, e016491.

World Health Organization (WHO). (2022). *Indigenous peoples and tackling health inequities* [WHO side event at the 21st session of the UN Permanent Forum on Indigenous Issues]. Retrieved from: https://www.who.int/news-room/events/detail/2022/05/03/default-calendar/indigenous-peoples-and-tackling-health-inequities--who-side-event-at-the-2022-session-of-the-un-permanent-forum-on-indigenous-issues

Power and political astuteness

14

Nicola McNeil

Learning objectives

How do I:

- understand the use of power in organisations?
- identify the main sources of power in organisations?
- critically analyse the positive and negative aspects of power and influence?
- understand how political processes operate in organisations?
- understand the consequences of political activities in organisations?
- enhance my skills in the various tactics that can be used to shape political outcomes in organisations?

Introduction

Politics is an inevitable feature of organisational life, particularly in large bureaucratic organisations such as hospitals and government departments. Political activities arise when there is a lack of consensus about how an organisation should be managed. They are typically employed to reconcile these divergent interests, which may be the result of competition for resources within the organisation, the pursuit of personal goals by individuals or a high level of uncertainty within the organisation.

Traditionally, political activities have been concerned with obtaining, developing and exploiting power to influence others in order to achieve desired outcomes (Pfeffer, 1981). Consequently, decisions shaped by political activities are not always rational – they do not always produce optimal outcomes, as individuals may seek to satisfy their own wants and needs, often at the expense of others (Kumar & Ghadially, 1989). However, more recently, organisational behaviourists have conceptualised organisational politics as the *perception* that an individual or group is using influence and tactics to serve a personal agenda (Ferris & Kacmar, 1992). One person may consider a co-worker's behaviour to be a typical and rational response, whereas another colleague may view the same behaviour as self-serving and highly political. Therefore, what is deemed to be political or normal behaviour ultimately depends on the opinion of the observer.

Definitions

At the core of any political activity is the exercise of power and influence. Researchers argue that an understanding of power – where it comes from and how it can be used – is crucial to achieving both personal and organisational goals (Runde & Flanagan, 2007). There are several ways of viewing the idea of **power**: it can be seen as a characteristic that an individual possesses or as something that is generated by social relations. However, power is most commonly defined as the ability to change another's behaviour or to influence others: holders of power generally exert their power to attain an outcome they desire (Astley & Sachdeva, 1984). That is, a person has power over another when they can get that person to do something they would not otherwise have done (Dahl, 1957).

Power: An agent's ability to influence the target

Relationships of power exist where there is a perceived dependency between two or more people in an organisation. For example, a manager may appear to control vital information or resources that are needed by others in the organisation. This need for information or resources creates a dependency on the manager, which in turn leads to the manager having power over the others.

Authority

Authority: A unique manifestation of power attached to a position in the hierarchy rather than to an individual (Pfeffer, 1978)

Power is not the same as **authority**. Pfeffer (1978) argues that authority is a unique manifestation of power. He suggests that authority stems from an individual's place in the hierarchy; therefore, authority is attached to a position in the hierarchy, rather than to an individual. Thus, position-holders within an organisation can use the authority vested in their positions to make decisions and shape outcomes.

There are a few important points to note about authority. Firstly, subordinates typically comply with the instructions of their supervisors or managers because they recognise that the authority they hold is legitimate. Secondly, authority is reflected in the organisational hierarchy and is devolved down the chain of command of an organisation, with more authority being vested in positions at the top of the hierarchy. Power is not confined to positions of authority. For example, a nurse may exercise power over their supervisor: there may be a relationship of dependence between the two that results in the nurse being able to shape the behaviour of her supervisor. Thus, power can be exercised in any direction in the hierarchy – up, down or horizontally – that is, between units in the organisation.

Sources of power

French and Raven (1959) identify two main sources of individual power: power that is derived from the position an individual holds in the organisational hierarchy, or position power (which includes legitimate, reward and coercive power); and power that stems from an individual's characteristics, or their personal power (which includes expert and referent power).

Legitimate power

Legitimate power is derived from the authority vested in an individual by virtue of the position they hold within the organisation. The source of this power is based on the idea of legitimate authority, which is conferred on an individual who occupies a particular position. For example, a charge nurse will typically have legitimate power over subordinates, as part of their job description will require them to direct and monitor the behaviour of the nursing staff they supervise.

However, the effective exercise of this power relies upon the willingness of the subordinates to accept or comply with someone's authority over them (Giddens, 1997; Hardy & Clegg, 1996). For example, the power of a nurse manager to make a nurse change their working hours to suit a roster depends on the willingness of the nurse to agree to such an arrangement.

There are several aspects to consider regarding legitimate power. Firstly, as the position in the hierarchy holds the power, the individual will surrender this source of power when they vacate the position. Secondly, legitimate power is limited in its scope, as it applies to work-related situations. A chief executive officer would not have legitimate power over how an employee spent their leisure time or how they might spend their discretionary income.

Legitimate power: Power derived from the authority vested in an individual by virtue of the position they hold within the organisation

Reward power

Reward power concerns the capacity to reward employees (or to withhold rewards or privileges). It is held by an individual who can confer promotions, financial rewards, leave or praise to employees. For example, the dean of a faculty of medicine holds reward power: they have the ability to grant bonuses to high-performing staff, award citations for high-quality teaching and research, and promote or provide opportunities to deserving staff.

In some respects, reward power is similar to legitimate power, in that the ability to reward individuals is often tied to a position in the hierarchy; for example, a chief executive officer or general manager can provide monetary incentives, but these formal rewards are not typically within the purview of a co-worker.

Reward power: The capacity to reward employees

However, reward power is not solely dependent on hierarchy. Employees can exercise informal reward power by offering recognition, appreciation or social inclusion to their peers. For instance, a colleague might express gratitude for a team member's contribution, nominate them for peer-driven awards or create opportunities for collaborative projects that align with the team member's interests. These forms of informal rewards can be highly motivating and can contribute to a positive workplace culture.

The use of both formal and informal reward power is an important element in understanding how to motivate employees. If the reward being offered – whether extrinsic or intrinsic – is highly valued by individuals, reward power will be strong. Conversely, reward power will be weakened when the rewards have little appeal for the recipients.

Coercive power

Coercive power: Power resulting from the use of threats, punishment or force to gain compliance or control over others

Coercive power is a form of influence in which an individual uses threats, punishment or force to gain compliance or control over others. Exercising this power can result in negative consequences, such as chastising, demoting or terminating the employment of subordinates, to ensure that people adhere to policies and processes and follow orders. In certain circumstances it may be necessary to use coercive power to stem inappropriate, unethical or illegal behaviour of employees. For example, if an employee repeatedly refuses to follow health and safety protocols, which endangers not only themselves but also patients and other co-workers, it may be appropriate for a supervisor to exert their coercive power to quash such behaviours.

Expert power

Expert power: Power stemming from a person's acknowledged expertise and skill in a given area

Expert power stems from a person's acknowledged expertise and skill in a given area. When an individual demonstrates their proficiency, their thoughts and recommendations will be regarded as credible, and they are likely to be trusted and respected by others. People may be persuaded to follow suggestions and instructions because they defer to a higher level of understanding.

Marie Curie, who discovered the chemical elements radium and polonium and pioneered research into the treatment of tumours using radiation, had expert power. Her contributions to chemistry and medical research were recognised by the award of a Nobel Prize in both chemistry and physics. Prior to her death in 1934, Curie was able to use her expert power to attract funding and other resources to continue her important work, and she also changed the way other researchers conducted their studies (*Marie Curie – Biographical*, 2015).

Referent power

Referent power: Power stemming from a person's charisma, likeableness or appeal

Referent power stems from a person's charisma, likeableness or appeal and the resultant influence this has on others. A prime example of referent power is the influence that celebrity endorsements have on our purchasing behaviour. For example, consider the recent growth in celebrity branded fragrances, including perfumes with branding by Beyoncé, David Beckham, Taylor Swift, Britney Spears and Jennifer Lopez. Consumers may strongly identify with these celebrities and be persuaded to purchase the perfumes they endorse.

In the work environment, an employee with charisma or appeal may find they have considerable influence over others who respect or wish to please them. The obvious danger of referent power is that someone who is affable or charismatic may acquire significant power in the organisation without having the requisite authority or knowledge to use this power effectively.

While French and Raven's (1959) model is helpful for analysing interpersonal power dynamics, it does not fully illuminate how power operates at the systemic level, nor its evolution over time. It treats power as relatively static and tied to the individual's role or actions, thereby overlooking the broader social, cultural and historical contexts that shape power relations. In contrast, Bourdieu's (1977) *Outline of a theory of practice* shifts the focus from individual acts of influence to more systemic and relational aspects of power. This framework explores how power is embedded within social structures, is reproduced through cultural norms and practices, and operates in dynamic interactions between individuals and institutions. By exploring the interconnected concepts of *habitus*, *field* and *capital*, Bourdieu offers a deeper and more nuanced perspective on the dynamics of power within complex healthcare environments (Lewer, 2023).

In the healthcare field, professionals operate within a structured environment shaped by hierarchical roles, established rules and standardised practices. Physicians, nurses and administrators interact within this space, vying for resources, recognition and influence, and leveraging different forms of capital, including:

- cultural capital – physicians possess medical expertise and credentials that confer a certain level of authority to them
- social capital – healthcare professionals rely on teamwork and interpersonal relationships to influence care delivery
- symbolic capital – titles, such as 'surgeon' and 'chief medical officer', confer prestige and legitimised power.

Habitus refers to the behaviours, dispositions and attitudes shaped by professional training and workplace culture (Bourdieu 1977). It guides how individuals interact with colleagues and patients, how they perceive their roles and make decisions. For example, a healthcare administrator's habitus might include valuing operational efficiency, influenced by management training and budgetary constraints. This can shape how they allocate resources, schedule staff or prioritise investments in infrastructure. A surgeon's habitus, formed through rigorous training and decision-making under pressure, might include the ability to remain composed and make decisive judgements, reflecting a blend of technical skill and mental resilience.

Power dynamics in health care are intricately tied to the distribution of capital among professionals. Individuals and groups with greater capital often influence and define the norms and practices within the field. Physicians often hold a strong position within the field due to their significant cultural capital, derived from specialised knowledge and training, as well as symbolic capital, such as the prestige associated with their role. In contrast, nurses contribute influence through their expertise, patient advocacy and coordination of care, which are vital to achieving positive patient outcomes. These hierarchical structures are frequently accepted as 'natural', shaped by the habitus developed through professional training and workplace culture.

However, power is not static. Individuals and groups can challenge and reshape power structures. For instance, interprofessional collaboration initiatives aim to redistribute authority, emphasising teamwork over hierarchy. Similarly, movements toward patient-centred care shift symbolic capital toward patients, recognising their lived experiences as valuable contributions to decision-making.

Use of power

While an individual may possess power, it does not mean that they will be able to influence the behaviour of others. Hickson, Hinings, Lee, Schneck and Pennings (1971) argue that the effective exercise of power is influenced by external factors, or contingencies, which can advance or impede the use of power by an individual or a department. Hickson and his colleagues identify uncertainty, substitutability and centrality as the main contingencies of power.

Uncertainty

Uncertainty refers to a lack of information about events that may affect an organisation in the future. This may include scarcity of information about the availability of resources, changes to government regulations or laws, actions of competitors or viability of existing markets. Where there is uncertainty in the business environment, organisational planning becomes more difficult, as contingency plans must be made to address all possible eventualities. Pfeffer (1981) argues that the most valued skill within an organisation is the ability to protect organisational members from uncertainty.

Hickson and colleagues (1971) suggest, however, that it is the ability to cope with sources of uncertainty that generates power, rather than uncertainty itself. Pfeffer and Salancik (1978) build on this idea by explaining the link between an organisation's environment and its political processes. They argue that the environment poses uncertainty for an organisation in terms of constraints, contingencies and resources. This, in turn, produces a need for someone to cope with this uncertainty on behalf of the organisation. The ability to cope is translated into power within the organisation.

Therefore, Pfeffer and Salancik (1978) argue, there is a direct relationship between the distribution of environmental uncertainty and the distribution of power within an organisation. Those individuals or departments that can cope with such uncertainty garner power and influence within the organisation. The ability to manage uncertainty, in turn, creates certainty for others and creates power through the dependencies created.

> **Uncertainty:** Limited or no understanding of knowledge or information regarding a given state or situation

SHIFTING POWER BASES IN MODERN HEALTH CARE

Being in a hospital can evoke a profound sense of vulnerability in patients. They often feel exposed and dependent, as their health and wellbeing are in the hands of healthcare professionals. The unfamiliar environment, coupled with the stress of illness or injury, amplifies this reliance. Each interaction with doctors, nurses and other staff becomes crucial, as patients look to these professionals not just for medical care, but also for reassurance and support. Exploring this dynamic through a power lens, the healthcare providers' specialised medical knowledge (expert power), their authority within the healthcare system (legitimate power) and their control over access to treatment and information (informational power) can lead to a dramatic power imbalance between healthcare providers and their patients. To address this imbalance, the Australian government has introduced the Australian Charter of Healthcare Rights, which aims to create a more balanced relationship between patients and their healthcare professionals, by emphasising key principles that promote patient empowerment and involvement in healthcare decisions. The Charter enshrines patient rights, including the right to access health care safely, respectful interactions, participate in decision-making about their health, have privacy, comment on issues regarding their health care and be informed about treatment options, services and costs in a way that can be easily understood. This is an example of an important policy intervention by government to address the perceived power imbalance between healthcare professionals and those they serve. For further information, refer to the website of the Australian Commission on Safety and Quality in Health Care (2024).

Substitutability

Drawing on the work of Hickson and colleagues (1971), Fried (1988) argues that the degree of control an individual or department has over valuable resources can also affect their power in a healthcare organisation. If they have complete control over a highly valued resource – whether it is an expensive piece of medical equipment, money or information – their power over others is heightened. However, if there are alternatives available to replace this important resource, or to access it from a different source, the power of the individual or department that holds the asset is diminished. This is referred to as **substitutability**. The dependence on the holder of the asset is reduced because a substitute asset can be found.

Substitutability: The capability of being replaced

Often, once an individual or department controls a critical resource within the organisation, it is unlikely that they will relinquish this control and thereby dilute their power. For example, a medical college is unlikely to devolve control over the accreditation of hospitals or the training of specialists to third parties, because that would effectively reduce its power and standing.

Centrality

The final contingency noted by Hickson and colleagues (1971) that can affect the exercise of power is **centrality**. This concerns the association between the holder of power and the important activities of the organisation. For example, nursing staff are essential to the functioning of a hospital: without nursing staff, the hospital cannot admit, treat or discharge patients. Hospital management depends on nursing staff to deliver these key functions; therefore, nurses collectively hold a significant degree of power. However, maintenance staff may not hold the same degree of power over hospital management, because their role is not as central to the operation of a hospital. Moreover, some would argue that maintenance workers are more easily substituted compared to highly skilled nursing staff.

Centrality: The position of the power-holder in relation to the important activities of the organisation

Influence tactics

Influence: Deliberate conduct (either positive or negative) that causes measurable results or effects, which may or may not have been intended, in respect to character, aims, processes

Merely possessing the ability to alter people's behaviour is different from influencing their actions. The question of how the sources of power can be utilised to change behaviour brings us to a discussion of the notion of **influence**: conduct that attempts to modify someone else's attitudes or actions.

Over the past 30 years, studies have identified various tactics that people may use to influence others. A summary of the most-frequently identified tactics is presented in Table 14.1, drawing on the work of Kipnis, Schmidt and Wilkinson (1980). Tactics used to influence people can be classified in two broad categories: hard tactics and soft tactics (Kipnis & Schmidt, 1985). Hard tactics rely upon positional sources of power (legitimate, coercion and reward power) to change attitudes and behaviours. Conversely, soft tactics draw on personal power. While hard tactics focus on ways to compel others to behave in a certain way, soft tactics aim for gentler means of persuasion.

Table 14.1 Hard and soft influence tactics

Tactic	Description
Hard tactics	
Authority or sanctions	Using legitimate power to direct others' activities
Assertiveness	Placing pressure on others or making threats to shape their behaviour
Coalitions or networks	Developing an alliance and using the combined power of members to influence others
Upward appeal	Garnering the support and favour of others with position and personal power, and using these to influence others
Soft tactics	
Exchange	Pledging something that is valued in exchange for desired behaviours
Ingratiation	Deliberately establishing oneself in the favour or good graces of others
Rationality	Persuading others by using logic, clear evidence and reasoning

Source: Adapted from Kipnis et al. (1980).

A qualitative study by Rogers, De Brun, Birkin, Davies and McAuliffe (2020) explored how healthcare staff navigate the use of power, authority and influence on goals and decision-making processes in multidisciplinary healthcare teams. They report that introducing changes in healthcare teams is a political process shaped by existing power structures. While influence is used to drive the implementation efforts, the traditional power structures also work to actively constrain the change process. Support from leaders across multiple levels of the hierarchy is crucial for successful implementation because their influence encourages team members to engage with the changes. However, the ways in which this influence is applied, and how it is perceived, are deeply influenced by the historical dynamics within each team. In some cases, these dynamics lead to negative experiences for participants, highlighting the complex interplay between power, perception and implementation outcomes. Another study, by Falbe and Yukl (1992), examined the effectiveness of using one of multiple tactics to influence others. The researchers conclude that combinations of tactics are generally more effective than using a single tactic, and that combinations of hard and soft tactics are more influential than combinations of only hard or only soft tactics.

Authority or sanctions

Authority or sanctions concerns the exercise of legitimate power to generate direct compliance with a request or instruction. The success of this tactic depends largely on the degree of deference shown to this authority (Cialdini & Goldstein, 2004). Some individuals willingly accept a higher degree of unequally distributed power throughout an organisation and will follow the instructions of those in power without question. Others may not be prepared to blindly follow the directions of those in power, and thus other tactics may have to be employed to influence their behaviour.

Assertiveness

Assertiveness involves the application of overt forms of legitimate and coercive power to shape behaviour. This can involve applying pressure upon or coercing workers to comply, or using reward power to modify the actions of others. This may include threatening an individual's job security or withholding rewards such as promotions and salary increases.

Assertiveness: The application of overt forms of legitimate and coercive power to shape behaviour

Coalitions or networks

Another tactic that can be employed to influence others is the formation of **coalitions** or networks. A coalition involves assembling an informal group of individuals with a view to using the collective resources of the group to influence people. These coalitions are likely to exert greater influence than an individual acting alone (Cobb, 1991; Hogg & White, 1999; Mannix, 1993).

Coalition: An informal group of individuals who use the collective resources of the group members to influence people

Collective action tends to lend significance to an issue, as it indicates that many employees believe the issue is legitimate or support a particular course of action. Also, if people can identify with members of the group, they are more likely to accept the decisions or advice of the group. A study by Douglas and Ammeter (2004) found that belonging to a coalition increased employees' perceptions of the effectiveness of their manager and increased the influence of the manager over their subordinates.

Upward appeal

The final hard tactic is **upward appeal**, which is calling on people with significant positional or personal power for assistance in influencing others. This may involve engaging senior people within the organisational hierarchy or those with high levels of expertise both within and outside the organisation.

Upward appeal: A call on people with significant positional or personal power for assistance in influencing others

Ingratiation

One soft tactic is **ingratiation**, which suggests that influence can be heightened by an individual's being amiable or creating the perception that they have much in common with the person they are trying to influence. Typical examples of ingratiation include expressions of admiration or vigorous support for the views of others. However, some studies show that

Ingratiation: The deliberate act of trying to gain benefit from attempting to please or flatter another person

influence can be diminished when individuals exhibit high levels of ingratiation, as they may be perceived to be disingenuous and manipulative (Strutton, Pelton & Tanner, 1996).

Rationality

Rationality: The use of logic, reliable evidence and reasoned arguments to sway the opinions, attitudes and behaviours of others

Another soft influence tactic is **rationality**, which relies on one's ability to use logic, reliable evidence and reasoned arguments to sway the opinions, attitudes and behaviours of others.

Exchange

Exchange: The notion that people feel obligated to 'return the favour', or give something back, when they have received a benefit or advantage (Cialdini, 2001)

Exchange may also be an effective tactic to influence others. It is based on the idea of reciprocity – the notion that people feel obligated to 'return the favour', or to give something back, when they have received a benefit or advantage (Cialdini, 2001). Influence can be exerted through building these exchange relationships and relying on the norm of reciprocity to shape behaviours.

Nurse A could use the exchange tactic to influence Nurse B to cover her shift by reminding Nurse B that she has covered Nurse B's shifts on three previous occasions. Nurse A is relying upon Nurse B to experience some obligation to return the favour and thus agree to cover the shift. Exchange tactics can also be used in senior management negotiations when deciding budget allocations or sharing information.

Increasing power

Political tactics are often used to achieve desired outcomes. However, as noted earlier, these tactics generally rely on individuals possessing some form of power over others. Therefore, the ability to influence the behaviour or attitudes of others is inherently linked to the size of the power base.

How can a person increase their power base? One approach is to create and foster dependencies. If an individual or a department possesses and controls important skills, knowledge, information or materials that are vital to the operation of the organisation, their power is augmented (Pfeffer, 1981). It is likely that those who need access to the resources are likely to acquiesce to any requests or demands made by their holders. Power would be further increased if the resources were scarce, or not substitutable. Another method of increasing power is to work to reduce any areas of uncertainty that the organisation may face. An individual can also increase their importance and power in an organisation by moving into the organisation's critical areas and addressing any problems that may exist therein (Hickson et al., 1971).

Summary

- Political activity is an increasingly important feature of organisational life.
- Political activity in organisations is the process by which individuals debate ideas, challenge assumptions and attempt to ensure that their interests are heard and protected. The ability to influence the behaviours, attitudes and opinions of others is critical to safeguarding such interests.

- The ability to influence others depends on the nature of the power held by an individual. Developing an appreciation of the nature of power and how individuals garner power is vital to understanding political activities within organisations.
- Implementing both hard and soft influence tactics, while being cognisant of the factors that may encumber the use of power, and building a strong power base will contribute to the success of any political activities.

Reflective questions

1. What is power?
2. Discuss the claim that 'power is inherently tied to position in the hierarchy; only managers have power in organisations'.
3. What are the key contingencies that influence the exercise of power? Drawing on your experiences of work or being a student, provide an example of each contingency.
4. How can an individual increase their power within an organisation?
5. Many theorists argue that the basis of all influence can be traced to the notion of reciprocity – that is, an obligation to return a favour. Can you think of a time when someone did something for you? Did you feel obligated to reciprocate? If that person asked you to do something for them, would you feel compelled to do it?

Self-analysis questions

Consider the following scenario. You are a graduate nurse starting your first position at a suburban aged-care facility. Your nurse manager has asked you to dispense to some residents' medication that is not listed on their medication charts. When you question the nurse manager, she instructs you to 'do as she says'. What would you do in this situation? If you refuse to follow the order, what does this suggest about your deference to authority?

References

Astley, W. G. & Sachdeva, P. S. (1984). Structural sources of intra-organisational power: A theoretical synthesis. *Academy of Management Review*, *9*(1), 104–113.

Australian Commission on Safety and Quality in Health Care. (2024). *Charter of healthcare rights*. Retrieved from: https://www.safetyandquality.gov.au/our-work/partnering-consumers/australian-charter-healthcare-rights

Bourdieu, P. (1977). *Outline of a theory of practice*. Cambridge University Press.

Cialdini, R. B. (2001). Harnessing the science of persuasion. *Harvard Business Review*, (October), 72–79.

Cialdini, R. B. & Goldstein, N. J. (2004). Social influence: Compliance and conformity, *Annual Review of Psychology*, *55*, 591–621. https://doi.org/10.1146/annurev.psych.55.090902.142015

Cobb, A. T. (1991). Towards a study of organisational coalitions: Participant concerns and activities in a simulated organisational setting. *Human Relations*, *44*(10), 1057–1079. https://doi.org/10.1177/001872679104401003

Dahl, R. A. (1957). The concept of power. *Behavioral Science*, *2*(3), 201–215. https://doi.org/10.1002/bs.3830020303

Douglas, C. & Ammeter, A. P. (2004). An examination of leader political skill and its effect on ratings of leader effectiveness. *Leadership Quarterly*, *15*(4), 537–550. https://doi.org/10.1002/bs.3830020303

Falbe, C. M. & Yukl, G. (1992). Consequences for managers of using single influence tactics and combinations of tactics. *Academy of Management Journal*, *35*(3), 638–652. https://doi.org/10.2307/256490

Ferris, G. R. & Kacmar, M. K. (1992). Perceptions of organisational politics. *Journal of Management*, *18*(1), 93–116. https://doi.org/10.1177/014920639201800107

French, J. R. P. & Raven, B. H. (1959). The bases of social power. In D. Cartwright (ed.), *Studies in social power* (pp.150–167). Institute for Social Research.

Fried, B. J. (1988). Power acquisition in a health care setting: An application of the strategic contingencies theory. *Human Relations*, *41*(12), 915–927.

Giddens, A. (1997). *Sociology* (3rd ed.). Polity.

Hardy, C. & Clegg, S. R. (1996). Some dare call it power. In S. R. Clegg, C. Hardy & W. R. Nord (eds), *Handbook of organisational studies* (pp. 622–641). Sage.

Hickson, D. J., Hinings, C. R., Lee, C. A., Schneck, R. E. & Pennings, J. M. (1971). A strategic contingencies theory of intra-organisational power. *Administrative Science Quarterly*, *16*(2), 216–229. https://doi.org/10.2307/2391831

Hogg, M. A. & White, K. M. (1999). The theory of planned behaviour: Self-identity, social identity and group norms. *British Journal of Social Psychology*, *38*(3), 225–244. https://doi.org/10.1348/014466699164149

Kipnis, D. & Schmidt, S. M. (1985). The language of persuasion. *Psychology Today* (April), 40–46.

Kipnis, D., Schmidt, S. M. & Wilkinson, I. (1980). Intraorganizational influence tactics: Explorations in getting one's way. *Journal of Applied Psychology*, *65*(4), 440–452. https://doi.org/10.1037/0021-9010.65.4.440

Kumar, P. & Ghadially, R. (1989). Organizational politics and its effects on members of organizations. *Human Relations*, *42*(4), 305–314. https://doi.org/10.1177/001872678904200402

Lewer, K. (2023). Depicting Bourdieu's concepts as a set of stackable and transparent lenses. *Sociology Lens*, *36*(4), 468–473.

Mannix, E. A. (1993). Organizations as resource dilemmas: The effects of power balance on coalition formation in small groups. *Organizational Behavior and Human Decision Processes*, *55*(1), 1–22. https://doi.org/10.1006/obhd.1993.1021

Marie Curie – Biographical. (2015). Retrieved from: http://www.nobelprize.org/

Pfeffer, J. (1981). *Power in organisations*. Pitman.

——— (1978). The micropolitics of organisations. In M. W. Meyer (ed.), *Environments and organisations* (pp. 29–50). Jossey-Bass.

Pfeffer, J. & Salancik, G. R. (1978). *The external control of organisations: A resource dependency perspective*. Harper & Row.

Rogers, L., De Brun, A., Birken, S. A., Davies, C & McAuliffe, E. (2020). The micropolitics of implementation: A qualitative study exploring the impact of power, authority and influence when implementing change in healthcare teams. *BMC Health Services Research*, *20*(1059). https://doi.org/10.1186/s12913-020-05905-z

Runde, C. E. & Flanagan, T. A. (2007). *Becoming a competent leader: How you and your organisation can manage conflict effectively*. Wiley.

Strutton, D., Pelton, L. E. & Tanner, J. (1996). Shall we gather together in the garden: The effect of ingratiatory behaviours on buyer trust in sales people. *Industrial Marketing Management*, *25*(2), 151–162. https://doi.org/10.1006/obhd.1993.1021

Influencing strategically

Mark Avery

15

Learning objectives

How do I:

- develop my skills in respect to influencing tactics and strategies?
- choose key influencing tactics and strategies that might be used in engaging internally in my organisation, as well as outside the organisation?
- understand the importance of influencing strategically as a leader?
- help my department and organisation achieve strategic goals through influencing tactics and strategies?

Introduction

Everyone creates influence during their lives. This may be consciously or unconsciously, through communication, actions or behaviours. A person can be influential through who they are or what they do, such as through their creativity, dependency, vulnerability, position and example.

In complex health organisations, we need effective leadership that articulates vision, inspires, provides guidance and influences, and strong management to plan, organise, direct and control. Leaders and managers have different roles, functions and skill sets. These actions may be visionary, inspirational, task-focused, long or short term, through empowerment and supervision. These roles and responsibilities may be different but need to achieve impact in influencing.

A critically important element of creating change, growth and renewal in health-service organisations is the need for strong and effective leadership, of which influencing skills are an integral part. Healthcare organisations are complex entities with large numbers of internal and external stakeholders. Strategic influence is an important aspect of the leadership and management of these organisations, as leaders and managers rely on their ability to enhance the effectiveness of those working in all parts and levels of the organisations as well as those outside the organisation in the broader system. Healthcare managers can increase their impact and achievements through understanding and applying influence, and key aspects of healthcare leadership relate to the processes of influence.

When they influence to achieve strategic outcomes, leaders and managers work within and across two important areas: transformational change and negotiation. Links between these are important in healthcare leadership and management, as organisational power and personal influence are seen to influence outcomes (Lankshear, Kerr, Spence Laschinger & Wong, 2013).

This chapter explores the issues surrounding influence, particularly as they relate to leadership, management and organisations, as well as how a manager and leader can construct and develop influence to strategically affect projects, initiatives, teams, departments, facilities and organisations.

Influence: Deliberate conduct (either positive or negative) that causes measurable results or effects, which may or may not have been intended, in respect to character, aims, processes and outcomes

Strategic influence: Influence tactics and techniques used to persuade the thinking, reasoning, decisions and outcomes of others with key points, arguments and perspectives to achieve desired results

Definitions

Influence can relate to actions taken but can also be created through individuals or groups as well as in the presence of objects and environments. For example, in negotiating a contract for acquisition of biomedical equipment, the health service procurement manager might undertake a competitive tender so as to apply pressure in the marketplace to maximise the benefit of price. Another example might be found in the existence of an extensive training program for new health graduates in a community health service, which may be a key reward factor creating interest in employment in the service.

Strategic influence supports healthcare leaders in influencing others as part of achieving specific and wider goals, objectives and plans for healthcare delivery. Influence is imparted to persuade others in order to share ideas, concepts, opinions and actions.

Using influence

Healthcare organisations and systems are intricate networks, involving significant complexities and interconnections. Within this dynamic environment, the roles and capabilities of leaders and managers hold paramount importance. Their effectiveness directly affects the growth, development, efficiency, effectiveness, quality and safety of the healthcare sector. Given the collaborative and interconnected nature inherent in healthcare, both within organisations and externally to them, health managers must adeptly navigate and authentically influence various stakeholders to achieve organisational objectives with precision and breadth.

Effective use of influence can affect the behaviours of staff and others in the health system so as to achieve goals and objectives. It aids leaders and managers to engage with and make effective contributions to decision-making processes, as well as enabling them to harness and use their power to maximise engagement and involvement in strategic management processes. Leaders need to understand and work with the situations they find themselves in, and through their relationships with those they seek to influence (Haslam, Reicher & Platow, 2020). Finally, effective use of influence helps leaders to be effective in health-related management, as it enables them to understand and manage the resources and constraints of clinical backgrounds experienced by healthcare managers (Spehar, Frich & Kjekshus, 2014).

The ability to combine influence, strategy and leadership-enabling activities forms a critical pathway towards strategic direction and achievement of outcomes. In health care, leaders seek to move teams, departments, units and organisations towards outcomes, and seek to change them in relation to the environments in which they work. Key strategic activities for managing organisations include identifying problems and goals, decision-making, planning, positioning, learning and reviewing. These activities are framed and managed through effective strategic leadership and management. Vital in these environments is the translation of ideas, directions and activities through internal and external strategic influence. This framing is particularly important in relation to clinical leadership, power and influencing (Saxena et al, 2019).

Targets

The agent of influence is the individual or group of people attempting to exert influence. In considering the strategic use of influence, the targets of the agent need particular consideration. The targets of influence are the people or groups that the agent is trying to influence. Targets can be people who are experiencing a problem, are engaged in the work of the organisation, are at risk or are in a position to make decisions and act. They can also be people and groups who are contributors to specific issues, either through their actions or through their lack of actions.

Healthcare leaders and managers can influence staff by fostering a collaborative environment, setting clear goals, providing feedback, encouraging professional growth and modelling empathy.

It is important to remember that a manager's or leader's influence is not limited to their own direct areas of responsibility. Depending on the effect and outcomes that they are trying to achieve, they may need to influence downwards, influencing those who work for them (subordinates) and over whom they have direct control and responsibility; upwards, seeking to influence those in higher positions of authority, power and responsibility; and laterally, to their peers – those with similar roles and responsibilities, powers and resources. Healthcare managers and leaders may also need to exert influence externally, in other organisations, in the community and with decision-makers in the healthcare system.

Negotiation

Positional authority or power is insufficient to sustain change in complex organisations with large numbers of internal and external stakeholders. Manning and Robertson (2003) report on two areas of influence tactics: strategist-opportunist and collaborator-battler. Strategist and opportunist tactics include those that use reasoning and partnership to effect change, with opportunistic leaders and managers capitalising on favour and exchange for influence. Collaboration tactics use partnering, and battler tactics use coercive and assertive tactics. Framing one's strategic influence style within one of these areas can be useful, because the outcome of one's negotiations is supported by the types of influence strategies used. Consideration of the types of influencing tactics to be used when entering a negotiation can maximise outcomes. In healthcare negotiations, collaboration tactics include active listening, understanding each person's or group's needs, finding shared goals, building trust and proposing win–win solutions.

Frameworks for influencing strategically

Tactics

Research and development of influence tactics, approaches and objectives were carried out between 1990 and 2000 by Gary Yukl from the University of Albany, New York. Yukl's formative work provides a sound understanding and expression of key knowledge about leaders' and managers' abilities to influence. Since this original work, other authors have extended Yukl's list of influencing tactics (Sampson, 2012). However, the influencing tactics reported in the original research offer a useful method for considering how managers might develop their use of influence (Yukl & Chavez, 2002; Yukl & Falbe, 1990). This includes how they might influence others, identification of tactics being used on them and the framing of complex responses when two or more approaches are necessary to achieve a strong influential effect.

Complex problems, situations and operations require a range of responses. In healthcare organisations, it is most likely that influence and influence strategy are not linear in nature or are not confined to a single approach, as different situations may require targeted approaches and strategies to bring about the desired outcomes. Over time, recognition of attributes and changes in personnel, or a change in the direction of goals and outcomes, may also require changes in influencing tactics. The following framework of 11 influencing tactics provides a guide for mapping individual approaches to influential leadership and management as well as tactics to support projects and operations (Yukl & Chavez, 2002; Yukl & Falbe, 1990).

Pressure

Pressure tactics support proposals or requests for help. Alignment is achieved through demands, intimidation, frequent requests or regular returning to the issue. Influence can be direct (such as sending emails or other communication requesting support and outlining consequences) or indirect (such as putting a project or service out to a public procurement tender to force competition).

Upward appeal

This approach is designed to leverage seniority in attaining compliance: senior management or a higher authority is invoked to persuade involvement or agreement from targets. To create such influence, the agent may only have to imply that senior managers would prefer the options being proposed.

Exchange

Exchange tactics involve offering rewards for compliance to a proposal. They can also involve connecting the current proposal to a past favour to be reciprocated.

Coalition

These tactics involve seeking the support or involvement of targets to work on an issue in partnership so as to persuade more targets to give support to the proposal.

Ingratiation

The agent causes the target to think favourably of them or creates an atmosphere of goodwill and connectivity as a prelude to asking for support for a proposal. The agent may activate a relationship or remind the target of a previous relationship or assistance as a mechanism for building connections in order to place the new proposal within that positive relationship.

Rational persuasion

With this approach, the agent provides a factual or evidence-based argument to highlight as the main focus the viability of the proposal to garner support.

Inspirational appeals

The agent appeals to values or ideals to increase the target's confidence in a proposal through emotion, enthusiasm or excitement.

Consultation

The agent gains the target's involvement in the decision-making and planning for a project and thereby creates a situation of target engagement, through which they can work to ensure the target's further involvement.

Legitimation

This approach secures trust in a proposal by connecting it to policies, procedures, rules or other dependable sources inside and outside the organisation.

Apprisement

The agent explains the proposal in a way that shows how it will benefit the target: personal gain and value are highlighted as the results of the target's acceptance of the proposal.

Collaboration

Assistance is offered to the target in return for their acceptance of the proposal, and value alignments between the agent and the target are proposed in return for the distribution of influence to other targets.

> **POPULATION HEALTH MANAGEMENT: ENHANCING HEALTH OUTCOMES AND REDUCING COSTS THROUGH COORDINATED AND INTEGRATED CARE AND PROACTIVE INTERVENTIONS**
>
> In a busy urban community health system, MapleLeaf Health Alliance faced the significant task of improving health outcomes and reducing costs for its diverse client and patient populations. In recognising the imperative for strategic influence, the management team embarked on a comprehensive population health management initiative.
>
> MapleLeaf conducted an in-depth analysis of population health data to identify high-risk client and consumer cohorts, and prevalent health disparities. With these insights, they developed a multifaceted strategy focused on preventative care, care coordination and social determinants of health interventions.
>
> Strategic influencing began by fostering partnerships with community organisations, local government agencies, health and aged-care providers to create a holistic ecosystem of care. Through collaborative efforts, MapleLeaf implemented initiatives such as community health screenings, chronic disease management programs and affordable housing initiatives to address the root causes of poor health outcomes.
>
> The management team championed value-based care models, incentivising providers to prioritise preventative care and proactive population health management. By aligning financial incentives with quality outcomes, MapleLeaf motivated providers to adopt evidence-based practices and embrace care-coordination strategies.
>
> Through continuous monitoring and evaluation, MapleLeaf refined its population health management strategies, demonstrating measurable improvements in health outcomes and cost savings. By strategically influencing stakeholders and fostering a culture of collaboration, MapleLeaf transformed its approach as well as the approach of partner stakeholders to healthcare delivery, ultimately enhancing the wellbeing of its patient population.

Strategies

There are extensive studies and lessons on different types of leadership approaches and their effectiveness. Key to effective and sustained futures for organisations is the use of transformational leadership (Northouse, 2007; Robbins & Davidhizar, 2020) whereby leaders engage in significant influence strategies and actions so as to move followers in organisations to accomplish more than what might usually be expected of them. A transformational leadership style or approach to leading with influence fosters vision, inspires change, empowers teams and drives alignment, which are essential for strategic influence. This style focuses on authentic engagement with stakeholders for involvement and strong ownership of strategic objectives.

In transformational leadership, leaders engage with followers and develop important and new connections that increase motivation for work to be done and achieved. To achieve these relationships within teams, units, departments and organisations, leaders need significant connection to staff, and they make this connection through influencing strategies.

Strategic influence through leadership involves inspiring a shared vision, fostering innovation and aligning team goals with organisational objectives that empower people. Strategic influence and engagement are important within teams, groups and organisations but also in the external environment relating to reputation and community contributions (Yukl & Gardner, 2020).

In considering influential strategy, managers and leaders can discover how they can harness their understanding and knowledge of the various influencing tactics and apply those systematically to support ideas and plans with stakeholders, decision-makers, colleagues and others in key roles or positions.

To achieve consistency and impact in strategic influencing in health organisations, several key actions and activities need to be deployed and coordinated:

- **leadership** – to articulate a shared vision and inspire individuals, teams and organisations to work towards the shared vision
- **stakeholder engagement** – to gain diverse perspectives and build coalition and support, including community outreach and engagement
- **partnerships** – to align goals and objectives so as to capitalise on expertise, resources and innovation opportunities
- **data, analytics and technology** – to develop granular evidence of problems, to develop solutions
- **quality improvement and risk management** – to adapt to changing needs and identify and mitigate program risks
- **financial sustainability** – to achieve sound financial strategy and long-term sustainability based on revenue diversification, cost management and resource allocation.

Important behaviours that managers utilise to strategically communicate with, and to influence the opinions and decisions of others, are found across three areas: the environment in which they are working, individuals and groups with whom they want to align their ideas and thoughts, and individuals and groups with whom they require engagement or connection. Within these three key action areas there are several approaches and behaviours that support successful influence.

Environment

The main vehicle for the use of influence strategies is recognition of an environment in which the manager wants to achieve impact. Healthcare services, systems and organisations are specialised, with their own languages, cultures, priorities, complexities and ways of working. Healthcare organisations tend to have strong cultures, and it requires considerable time and effort to bring about change within them. Similarly, influence strategies need to be proportional, with size and resources aligned to the nature of the issue and targeted to the key levels or parts of the organisation.

Health services operate in a wide range of environments – economic, political, community, scientific and academic – which means that the most effective influence strategies are those that recognise and work in the environment of the setting. It is important to place the influencing strategy in its environmental context.

Alignment

Alignment-influencing strategies focus on the connection and appeal to targets that will maximise the chance of engagement and support. Relationship-building (coalition, ingratiation and collaboration approaches) is an important part of influential strategy. The main strategic goal is to make sound and strong connections with individuals and groups regarding the issues being addressed. Alignment-influencing strategies involve creating a shared vision, clearly communicating goals, linking team objectives with the organisation's mission and consistently reinforcing values through actions and recognition. There are positive effects for organisational performance when alignment to an organisation's strategy is achieved (Kuipers & Giurge, 2016).

This approach is also important when agents are working with large groups or whole organisations. The development of a common vision and achieving agreement on that vision are critical steps in moving organisations in terms of goals, objectives and cultural change. Engendering reciprocal agreement and support for projects and initiatives in organisations is vital to sustained support and the unification of staff and other stakeholders in health organisations.

Engagement

The use of rational persuasion, ingratiation tactics or pressure tactics needs to be managed in the context of dialogue with individuals and groups, and bargaining and empowerment approaches should be presented and managed so that they are constructive in outcome. While it may be necessary to use coercive or pressure tactics to achieve goals, to ensure ongoing working relationships and sustained working environments, these must be managed so as to focus on problem-solving. An example might be the need to create a sense of urgency or understanding of threat in order to drive a change initiative. The object is to present threats, problems or poor outcomes that might occur if advice and suggestions (influence) are not followed, as opposed to creating destructive scenarios or environments that may inhibit further engagement and work between agents and targets.

Engagement-influencing strategies in health care include fostering open communication, recognising achievements of individuals and groups, encouraging team effort, offering growth opportunities and supporting elements of collaborative and inclusive culture (Wittenberg, Eweje, Taskin & Forsyth, 2024).

Summary

- Influence can be exerted in any direction within an organisation: downwards, upwards and laterally.
- Managers and leaders may have influence that is internal and external to their own work unit.

- Knowledge of influence tactics can be useful in understanding how to create influence, how to identify when one is being influenced and how to use separate tactics to achieve the desired effect.
- Managers and leaders need to develop strategies for influence tactics to work effectively.

Reflective questions

1. When considering approaches to influencing strategically to gain support for a proposal, how could you set out a strategy plan for influence?
2. What factors would you consider when deciding whether your influence strategies needed to be aimed downwards, upwards or laterally?
3. Differentiate between influence and strategic influence.
4. When planning to influence someone strategically, what criteria would you use to decide whether to create a formal strategic plan or to implement the tactics in an ad hoc manner?
5. Differentiate between coalition and collaboration-influencing tactics.

Self-analysis questions

Consider the 11 influencing tactics discussed in this chapter. In your experience, which two do you most align with or use? What new skills or experience would you need to improve your use of those tactics? Which two tactics are your least-preferred or used? What new skills or experience would you need to improve your use of those tactics?

References

Haslam, S.A., Reicher, S.D. & Platow, M.J. (2020). *The new psychology of leadership: Identity, influence and power* (2nd ed.). Routledge.

Kuipers, B. S. & Giurge, L. M. (2016). Does alignment matter? The performance implications of HR roles connected to organizational strategy. *The International Journal of Human Resource Management, 28*(22), 3179–3201. https://doi.org/10.1080/09585192.2016.1155162

Lankshear, S., Kerr, M. S., Spence Laschinger, H. K. & Wong, C. A. (2013). Professional practice leadership roles: The role of organizational power and personal influence in creating a professional practice environment for nurses. *Health Care Management Review, 38*(4), 349–360. https://doi.org/10.1097/HMR.0b013e31826fd517

Manning, T. & Robertson, B. (2003). Influencing and negotiating skills: Some research and reflections – part I: Influencing strategies and styles. *Industrial and Commercial Training, 35*(1), 11–15. https://doi.org/10.1108/00197850310458180

Northouse, P. G. (2007). *Leadership: Theory and practice* (4th ed.). Sage.

Robbins, B. & Davidhizar, R. (2020). Transformational leadership in health care today. *The Health Care Manager, 39*(3), 117–121. https://doi.org/10.1097/hcm.0000000000000296

Sampson, S. (2012). Influence tactics and leader effectiveness: How effective, contemporary leaders influence subordinates. [Master of Business (Research) thesis]. School of Management, Queensland University of Technology. Retrieved from: https://eprints.qut.edu.au/52770/1/Susan_Sampson_Thesis.pdf

Saxena, A., Mecchino, D., Hazelton, L., Chan, M-K., Benrimoh, D. A., Matlow, A. & Busari, J. (2019). Power and physician leadership. *BMJ Leader 3*, 92–98.

Spehar, I., Frich, J. C. & Kjekshus, L. E. (2014). Clinicians in management: A qualitative study of managers' use of influence strategies in hospitals. *Health Services Research*, *14*(251). https://doi.org/10.1186/1472-6963-14-251

Wittenberg, H., Eweje, G., Taskin, N. & Forsyth, D. (2024). Different perspectives on engagement, where to from here? A systematic literature review. *International Journal of Management Reviews*, *26*(3), 410–434. https://doi.org/10.1111/ijmr.12361

Yukl, G. & Chavez, C. (2002). Influence tactics and leader effectiveness. In L. L. Neider & C. A. Schiresheim (eds), *Leadership* (pp. 139–165). Information Age.

Yukl, G. & Falbe, C. M. (1990). Influence tactics and objectives in upward, downward, and lateral influence attempts. *Journal of Applied Psychology*, *75*(2), 132–140.

Yukl, G. & Gardner, W. (2020). *Leadership in organizations* (9th ed.). Pearson.

Networking

John Rasa

16

Learning objectives

How do I:

- understand the purpose of networking and where it sits on the partnership continuum?
- use the three levels of networking?
- learn to appreciate the personal and organisational benefits of networking for leadership development?
- enhance my skills in networking?
- overcome the challenges to achieve the potential of intraorganisational and interorganisational networking?

Introduction

Networks, which are defined as groups or systems of interconnected people or things, can be formal and informal in nature and can be applied for different purposes. The capability to network can build influence in groups and organisations to support change or generate new ideas. The process of networking can be seen as a supportive system of sharing information and services among individuals, groups and organisations with a common interest. Networking can be applied at a personal level for career and leadership development, at an intraorganisational level for organisational development and at an interorganisational level for research, knowledge management, process improvement and relationship development.

Definitions

Networking: The practice of establishing or maintaining connections with others for mutual benefit

Networking is a key leadership capability. Besides being a supportive system of sharing information, it can develop trust and a shared understanding of expectations between potential partners, thereby providing a foundation for future connection between individuals and organisations in the initial stages of their working relationship. It is a useful skill in environmental scanning and in managing change.

Advances in technology and the proliferation of mobile devices have changed the way we communicate with each other, and social networks challenge our notions of the flow of hierarchically ordered organisation and information. Social networks such as those created on social media applications are usurping the power of formal, hierarchical networks, and technology is disrupting structural boundaries within organisations (Baker, 2014).

The terms networking, collaborating, partnering and forming an alliance or coalition all involve working with someone else, or with others, in some kind of formal or informal relationship to perform a task and achieve a shared goal. However, networking is positioned on a partnership continuum that moves from networking to coordinating to cooperating and finally to collaborating. Most partnerships or coalitions are built on a clear purpose and value. They move up and down this continuum, which shows progression based on degree of commitment, change required, risk involved, levels of interdependence, power, trust and a willingness to share ground (Himmelman, 2001, p. 277).

Coordination: Exchanging information and resources to achieve mutual benefit, and altering activities for a common purpose

Cooperation: Working together to achieve a shared goal

Collaboration: Working together on a project or activity

Coordination is one step up from networking on the partnership continuum; it involves exchanging information for mutual benefit and altering activities for a common purpose. It requires more time and trust than networking as there is a requirement for action around a common activity that does not include giving ground. **Cooperation**, which means working together to achieve a shared goal, is similar to coordination and also requires significant amounts of time, high levels of trust and concessions to be made. It may require complex organisational processes and agreements, perhaps a memorandum of understanding, in order to achieve the expanded benefits of mutual action. Finally, **collaboration** involves networking, coordination and cooperation, plus a willingness to increase the capacity of another organisation for mutual benefit and a common purpose. Collaboration is defined as working together on a project or activity. It requires the highest levels of trust, considerable amounts of time and widespread territorial exchange. It involves sharing risks and rewards, and can produce the greatest overall benefits.

According to Marinez-Moyano (2006), networking is a recursive process, in which two or more organisations work together to realise shared goals. This is more than the intersection of common goals seen in cooperative ventures; instead, it is a collective determination to reach an identical objective. This may be an endeavour that builds new understanding by sharing knowledge or learnings and achieving consensus. It could be the result of a collaborative trial of a new protocol to reduce variation in clinical practice, or of changing the process of patient referral to improve access to care while enhancing cost performance.

NETWORKING FOR IMPROVED SERVICES

Don Adams, the chief executive officer (CEO) of Murray Regional Health Service, is encouraging clinicians to collaborate and innovate to improve waiting times for patients and reduce operating costs. Dr. Lorraine Thompson, the Chief Medical Officer, suggests that strategic networking could produce the transformative effect the CEO is seeking to enhance health services.

Lorraine believes that by fostering collaboration, the health service can improve the quality and efficiency of its services. Don agrees that the fragmented health system leads to inefficiencies and missed opportunities for patients but is unclear about how to implement strategic networking.

Lorraine argues that they need to invest some funding into a digital platform to connect hospitals, clinics and specialists across the region. Through this network, they can share resources, knowledge and best practices, thereby ensuring patients receive the most comprehensive care possible. She urges Don to imagine the impact if, through this network, primary care providers could gain direct access to specialists, wait times could be reduced and patient outcomes improved.

Lorraine's plan includes the transition of patients from hospital to rehabilitation centres or home care. A connected network will facilitate seamless transitions, eliminate information gaps and ensure continuity of care.

Don asks Lorraine to further explain how the strategic network would operate. Lorraine clarifies that by integrating electronic health records and real-time data exchange, healthcare providers can make informed, timely decisions, which in turn can lead to improved accuracy of the diagnosis and personalised treatments. She points to the power of data analytics within this network, which will enable the health service to identify healthcare trends, predict disease outbreaks and target preventative measures for high-risk populations.

Furthermore, this network has the potential to foster partnerships between academic institutions and healthcare providers, thereby encouraging research, knowledge-sharing and continuous professional development. This can lead to breakthrough innovations that elevate the quality of health care being delivered and position their community as a centre of excellence.

Encouraged by their shared vision, Don and Lorraine embark on mobilising stakeholders, rallying support, seeking innovation funding and translating this vision of strategic networking into a reality to improve healthcare delivery.

Networking is widely seen by the health sector as a crucial way of sharing risk, boosting research productivity, discovering new therapies and ultimately reinventing the way in which health care is delivered. Public and private sector healthcare providers and academia are forming partnerships and strategic networks to drive innovation. These require trust and openness in sharing resources and data, which at times can be challenging. In fact, the level of trust that exists in an organisation greatly influences the volume of knowledge that flows both between individuals and, subsequently, from individuals into the organisation's databases and records (De Long & Fahey, 2000, p. 19).

An important development in strategic networking is the activity of co-creation. An example of this is the development of Melbourne HealthPathways, in which four Victorian Medicare Locals and four Victorian health services (hospital networks) collaborated to develop web-based clinical pathways using evidence-based practice and the latest research to guide general practitioners in making appropriate clinical decisions when referring their patients to hospitals. The framework they used was based on the health pathways model stemming from the Canterbury Initiative in Aotearoa New Zealand (Timmins & Ham, 2013). The benefits of this co-creation, collaboration and networking approach included identification of new opportunities and added credibility to the quality frameworks already in place. The networking partners wanted research that was practical, with commonsense outcomes that people could understand, and the research team was largely able to meet these requirements (Janamian, Jackson & Dunbar, 2014).

A further example of strategic networking is the NHMRC Prevention Partnerships Centre, created to foster partnerships that improve the availability and quality of research evidence for clinicians, managers and policy-makers. Funded in two rounds from 2013 to 2023, the Centre helped build Australia's capacity to produce and use high-quality applied research to find answers to the complex questions that decision-makers face when trying to improve Australians' health and health care (https://www.nhmrc.gov.au/research-policy/research-translation-and-impact/partnership-centres-better-health).

As indicated earlier in this chapter, networking often involves only the sharing of information or only keeping up to date in an area of common interest. It can have a narrow focus on information related to the introduction of a new procedure for handling patient feedback in a health service, or it can have a broader focus such as sharing updates on the introduction of major health reforms, such as the reforms to primary health care in Australia and the introduction of casemix funding to Australian hospitals.

Networking can be 'a powerful way of sharing learning and ideas, building a sense of community and purpose, shaping new solutions to entrenched problems, tapping into hidden talent and knowledge, and providing space to innovate and embed change' (Randall, 2013, p 3). On the other hand, networking can have a more active meaning, of engaging with colleagues attending a college professional development seminar or holding a cross-sectoral health-planning meeting to facilitate better coordination of services, or engaging online when updating profiles on LinkedIn or adding to a professional interest group's blog. All of these activities can be described as different forms of active networking, with varying levels of engagement.

Leadership and networking

Networking is primarily about relationship building. It is, in fact, a leadership capability that involves building and maintaining genuinely helpful relationships with other people for mutual benefit. It is about creating a diversity of connections and win–win alliances with others through nurturing relationships that require some degree of trust. As a leadership capability, networking can be learned and also nurtured with practice.

The ability of health managers or aspiring health leaders to develop networks, coalitions and partnerships is recognised as something worth developing, as evidenced in the leadership frameworks of the Australasian College of Health Service Management, Health Workforce Australia, the American College of Health Executives and the Canadian College of Health Leaders. Hence, conference and professional development events are likely to be structured to enable reasonable networking time.

Ibarra and Hunter (2007), in their work with emerging managers, discovered that there are three distinct but interdependent levels of networking, which are personal, operational and strategic. All three levels play an important role in developing managers to become leaders. Personal networking boosts personal leadership development, operational networking assists managers to meet internal organisational responsibilities and strategic networking opens managers' 'eyes to new organisational directions and the stakeholders they need to enlist' to achieve their goals (Ibarra & Hunter, 2007, n.p.). 'While managers [differ] in how well they [pursue] operational and personal networking, almost all of them underutilise strategic networking' (Ibarra & Hunter, 2007, n.p.). It appears the reasons are both attitudinal and behavioural. Managers often describe networking as somehow manipulative or insincere rather than part of the role of a leader.

Often, the attitude of managers is that their comfort zone and interests lie in the strong command of the technical components or tasks of their jobs and in accomplishing their personal or their team's objectives.

> When challenged to move beyond their functional specialties and address strategic issues facing the organisation, many managers do not immediately grasp that this will involve relational [activity], not analytical tasks. Nor do they easily understand that [meetings] and interactions with a diverse [range] of stakeholders are not distractions from their "real work" but are actually part of what it is to be a leader (Ibarra & Hunter, 2007, n.p.).

Personal networking

While effective personal networking can be more narrowly defined as based on a genuine interest in assisting professional colleagues or significant others, networking is rapidly being recognised as a critical leadership skill that influences a manager's career and organisational effectiveness. Research indicates that as high-performing organisations seek to develop their future leaders and assess the leaders they currently have, they explicitly indicate that the abilities to manage relationships across boundaries and to sell ideas are critical leadership competencies (Ibarra & Hunter, 2007).

Personal networking is a technique for broadening a manager's professional knowledge beyond their usual work setting of acute, subacute, primary healthcare or aged-care services. It enables managers to understand issues confronting other managers in allied organisations, both public and private, and to perhaps find common ground with managers outside their usual professional circles.

There are several avenues through which personal networking can be facilitated. At the one-to-one level, professional mentoring or coaching can play an important developmental role in establishing personal networks by the person firstly gaining a broader understanding and secondly receiving important referrals to key individuals. Mentoring and personal networking can provide a safe space within which a manager can undertake personal development and lay the foundation for strategic networking.

Personal networking is mainly external, often consisting of discretionary links to people who share a common interest or provide possible career opportunities. Personal networks can represent useful referral potential and are an important first step for a manager in transitioning from being operational to strategic. It is part of the development of personal leadership to better understand the inner self and open further avenues for communication.

However, to avoid the possibility of feeling that personal networking is ultimately time-wasting, a health manager needs to link their personal connections to organisational goals as part of a broader strategy. Leveraging a personal network through, say, a professional college relationship could assist a health manager interested in hospital performance and who shares a common interest with a senior colleague who could facilitate a move from a private-sector role with a health insurer to a health department role overseeing public hospital performance. Linking the activity of personal network-building to career advancement, to developing knowledge of what constitutes efficient hospital performance, can benefit a health insurer to manage risk in hospital cost claims experience. The benefit of becoming a strategic networker within a health insurance company becomes clearer.

Personal networking can be either face-to-face or virtual. Increasingly, personal networking is facilitated by electronic means through email, professional networking applications such as LinkedIn, blogs or groups, sometimes enabling personal networks to extend globally to colleagues in other countries. However, while networking on social media is a way to build a personal brand for a professional's career, Baedke & Lamberton (2018) highlight some of the challenges. This is useful for health managers wishing to extend their reach into other health systems, facilitate study tours or undertake international visits. International networking can also cast light on how other health systems have tackled health issues. At the group level of personal networking, membership of professional associations, attendance at continuing professional development activities and keeping in touch with university alumni all assist health managers to gain new perspectives that enable them to advance in their careers.

However, quite often constraints for managers engaging in personal networking are time limitations and pressures of completing immediate work commitments. It is important that managers commit time to ensure personal networking opens future career opportunities.

Reid Hoffman, the co-founder of LinkedIn, maintains that some 'leaders have difficulty with alliances, either because they do not understand the importance of alliances in a networked world, or because they do not understand the types of alliances that are possible with different people. Still others struggle because they fail to see that true alliances are not just a means to an end; they are authentic relationships built upon mutual respect and trust' (Hoffman, 2012, n.p.). He argues that the more valuable and perhaps the more strategic relationships expect commensurate investment of time and energy over time by both parties (Hoffman, 2012).

Operational networking

Operational networking becomes important when a health manager needs to build good working relationships with the senior managers, work colleagues and staff who can help them get their job done effectively. The purpose of operational networking is to 'ensure coordination and cooperation among people who have to know and trust one another in order to accomplish their immediate tasks. That isn't always easy, but it is relatively straightforward, because the task provides focus and a clear criterion for membership to the network' (Ibarra & Hunter, 2007, p. 43). Either someone is integral to getting the job done, or they are not.

In general, operational networking is internally focused and more concerned with sustaining cooperation within the existing network in the organisation than with building relationships to face unforeseen challenges outside the organisation. Operational networking can function within the work team, between departments or divisions in a larger organisation or even interprofessionally, in the case of multidisciplinary care teams delivering acute care or rehabilitation, or managing chronic disease in the primary healthcare setting. But, as managers move into leadership roles, their network must become more externally focused and future-oriented.

Strategic networking

When health service managers begin 'the delicate transition from functional manager to [organisational] leader, they start to concern themselves with broad strategic [and organisational] issues' (Ibarra & Hunter, 2007, p. 47). Lateral and vertical relationships with other functional or business unit managers outside the immediate control of the health service manager become important links, indicating how their own contribution fits into the organisational picture. Thus, strategic networking links 'the aspiring leader into a set of relationships and information sources that collectively embody the power to achieve personal and organisational goals' (Ibarra & Hunter, 2007, p. 43).

As an example, clinical directors, nurse unit managers and allied health department heads may be thrust into a clinical leadership role due to their organisational skills or because of seniority. The rise in managerialism in healthcare reflects organisational demand for efficiency and effectiveness in the delivery of healthcare services. The demand for innovation and continuous improvement in quality of health-service delivery and the relentless push to improve productivity in the model of service delivery are about changing the behaviour of clinicians and patients. The clinical manager is well placed to influence these outcomes.

Leadership for successful innovation for the clinical manager often involves leadership skills such as the 'exercise of political astuteness and [the development of] alignment and sometimes coalitions across different interests implicated by the innovation, in both formal and informal alliances. It involves mobilising existing relationships and developing new ones to encompass the range of practices involved in innovation, as well as seeking funding from [the board or department of health]' (Storey & Holti, 2013, p. 20).

It is important that the healthcare organisation provides the right environment for the clinical leader or manager to develop properly (Leggat & Balding, 2013). The health service organisation should facilitate networking training in areas such as communications, leadership and organisation, human resources and financial systems, and policies and procedures. Networking skills are a capability that can be learned by the transitioning clinician.

The shift from clinician to clinical manager also involves a shift in mindset. 'Many managers need to change their attitudes about the necessity [for] networking' (Ibarra & Hunter, 2007, n.p.). For the clinician, the mindset must shift from the highly valued individual patient focus to organisational objectives, from a narrower clinical focus to a broader organisational and strategic focus. This can often result in a challenge to their identity, from having personal clinical credibility to having a role in the management of people and resources, in which they are less confident. The clinical manager will need organisational support to gain the required management credibility in this new role. At the personal leadership level, unless clinical managers shift their mindset about valuing their management role, they will not allocate sufficient time or effort to getting the job done.

The transition from clinician to manager can be greatly assisted by maintaining clinical networks and leveraging these to develop and support the building of necessary management skills. By encouraging the sharing of ideas regarding intractable clinical process problems, a clinical manager's management challenges can be more effectively addressed.

Organisations can support clinician managers by providing opportunities for internal networking with other managers and encouraging attendance at suitable external events. Developing clinical managers might accompany senior managers to networking events, so as to enable role-modelling of appropriate networking behaviours, or organisations might suggest relevant external websites (for example, ResearchGate, Meetup, LinkedIn) that can assist in further developing personal networks. Organisations can also incorporate networking performance measures into assessment processes and appraise the clinical manager's skill in engaging with others. In these ways, the organisation sends a strong signal that it values networking capabilities.

The Australian Primary Care Collaboratives Program is an example of strategic networking. It used the Breakthrough Series collaborative methodology, which is designed to 'help organisations close [the] gap [in performance] by creating a structure in which teams can easily learn from each other [as well as] from recognised experts in selected topic areas' (Knight, Ford, Audehm, Colagiuri & Best, 2012, p. 956). Staff from general practices that participated in the program attended a series of learning workshops, undertook improvement and change activities in their health service and collected monthly data to track their progress. 'Learning workshops [allowed] participants to [network], hear from topic area and quality improvement experts and actively share knowledge and experiences with their peers' (Knight et al., 2012, p. 956). The workshops enabled practice teams to test ideas and carry out change activities.

Interorganisational networking

Interorganisational Relations Theory, originating from the work of Pfeffer and Salancik (1978), is based on the premise that collaboration among community organisations leads to a more comprehensive, coordinated approach to a complex issue than can be achieved by one organisation alone. In fact, Mena, Humphries and Wilding (2009) found interorganisational relationships promoted stronger collaboration than intraorganisational networking.

Operating beside organisational members with diverse backgrounds, objectives and incentives requires a manager to work through networks that they require in order to compete for resources. Internally, the clinical manager will need to work closely with the health-service management team, comprising the directors of nursing, medicine, finance and allied health services. They form part of a community of practice network, with expertise in leading and organising health professionals, managing finances and assessing operational performance within the organisation.

Externally, clinical managers may be part of an interorganisational community of practice network, in which groups of managers come together to learn, address organisational issues and, where possible, drive innovative practices or design alternative service models. These types of knowledge alliances are important ways for organisations to increase their learning, in order to innovate and remain competitive (Ropes, 2009). Knowledge management in health care is emphasised in evidence-based medicine approaches and through collaborative efforts leading to the development of clinical pathways in which context knowledge is essential (Yamazaki & Umemoto, 2010).

There are many examples of alliances or collaboratives that have formed to facilitate interorganisational learning driven by a strong sense of purpose. The Mental Health Professionals Network (MHPN) in Australia operates a national, multifaceted networking and professional development program tasked with promoting interdisciplinary practice and collaboration to mental health practitioners and general practitioners working in primary care.

In 2022/23, MHPN attracted participation by more than 35,000 mental health practitioners through the National Networks Program and the Online Professional Development Program.

MHPN relies on volunteer practitioners to coordinate local and online network meetings of which there are over 800 meetings per year, with over 10 000 practitioners attending in communities across Australia. MHPN, through its colleges network, provides guest speakers and expert panellists for the extensive webinar and podcast programs. At the organisational level, MHPN has had to develop and maintain productive relationships with relevant mental health professional colleges and associations, with peak bodies representing diagnostic and special-interest areas of activity, including the national grid of 31 Primary Health Networks.

The MHPN platform primarily relies on organisational and individual engagement through the mediums of phone, email and videoconferencing and works with networks in a highly structured manner. There is a strong sense of common purpose and expected outcomes from online programs and network meetings. Structures and processes are well-documented. Network meetings and attendance data from all programs are collected and used to inform interactions with partner organisations.

External, expert clinical advisors are engaged to assist in ensuring the relevance of topics to be considered in complex clinical areas and the identification of expert presenters, thereby complementing the continuing survey of participants' interests. Throughout the networking process there is a strong personal commitment by coordinators to deliver the expected outcomes and achieve shared goals.

Smaller organisations such as MHPN need to learn from each other and can act very rapidly to incorporate new mental health learning and adapt to new approaches to delivery of professional development programs. They also appreciate the need to collaborate, and recognise the respective skills and resources of organisations with which they are networking.

Networking in the 21st century is ably assisted by systems of software, tools and technologies. MHPN has implemented an online platform (portal) that enables members to easily find and join networks, find network meetings of interest and manage their personal information. Members are also able to connect with and refer to each other by using MHPN's network directories, accessible via the portal.

During the COVID-19 pandemic, network meetings were necessarily shifted online. These meetings were hosted on videoconferencing software such as Zoom and Microsoft Teams. The convenience of this delivery format has proven popular, and several networks continue to host hybrid meeting formats since then.

Intraorganisational networking

Research has demonstrated that, at the operational level, an individual's productivity is inextricably linked to their networking capability (Ferreira & Du Plessis, 2009). Effective networkers within organisations reap rewards such as hastened career progression, capitalisation of leadership opportunities, greater job satisfaction and business success.

At the intraorganisational level, studies at Toyota have demonstrated the role of network knowledge resources in influencing an organisation's overall performance. In a sample of United States automotive suppliers selling to both Toyota and United States automakers, Pittaway, Robertson, Munir, Denyer and Neely (2004) found that significant knowledge-sharing in Toyota's supply chain resulted in a more rapid rate of learning within the suppliers' manufacturing operations devoted to Toyota. Indeed, from 1990 to 1996, suppliers reduced defects by 50 per cent for Toyota versus only 26 per cent for their largest United States customer (Dyer & Hatch, 2006).

Recent work on competitiveness has emphasised the importance of business networking for innovation. A systematic review of research by Pittaway and colleagues (2004) linking the networking behaviour of firms with their innovative capacity found that 'the principal benefits of networking ... include risk-sharing, obtaining access to ... new technologies [and external knowledge], speeding products to market and pooling complementary skills' (p. 3). The evidence also shows that:

> those firms which do not cooperate and do not formally or informally exchange knowledge limit their knowledge base [in the] long term and ultimately reduce their ability to enter exchange relationships. At an institutional level, national systems of innovation play an important role in the diffusion of [innovation] in terms of the way in which they shape networking activity. Evidence [suggests] that network relationships with suppliers, customers and intermediaries such as professional associations are important [in] affecting innovation performance and productivity (Pittaway et al., 2004, p. 3).

Summary

- Networking is relationship-building and is a supportive system of sharing information among individuals, groups and organisations with a mutual interest.
- Networking is on a partnership continuum that has its highest form in collaboration, involving high trust, time commitment and risk-sharing.
- Health service managers need to navigate three levels of networking: personal networking, operational networking and strategic networking.
- Networking is an important management capability that can build influence and be applied at the personal level for leadership development or at the intraorganisational level for organisational development and improvement.
- Networking can be applied at the interorganisational level for the purposes of research, knowledge management, process improvement and relationship development.

Reflective questions

1. Why is it important to understand the different forms of networking that are available?
2. Choose one of your organisation's goals or select a personal career goal. Can you map three personal connections you presently have and how, through networking, they might come to assist you in achieving that goal?
3. Reflect on the virtual networks that you currently use and explain why you choose to spend time connecting with other current or aspiring health managers through these media.
4. Based on your personal experience, which form of networking has contributed most to developing your leadership capabilities?
5. If you were given a problem to solve relating to the quality of care in a health organisation, which form of networking do you believe you would use, and why?

Self-analysis questions

List the personal networking activities that you regularly undertake. In what ways have they built your personal influence? What networking activities do you frequently undertake to share information that assists your personal leadership skill development? In what ways have they contributed to you being a better operational manager, a more strategic change agent in your organisation or a more innovative problem-solver? Can you see what you can do differently in the future to become more strategic in your networking? Has your use of social media helped you to build your personal and professional networks?

References

Baker, M. N. (2014). *Peer to peer leadership: Why the network is the leader.* Berrett-Koehler.

Baedke, L. & Lamberton, N. (2018). *The emerging healthcare leader* (2nd ed.). Health Administration Press.

De Long, D. W. & Fahey, L. (2000). Diagnosing cultural barriers to knowledge management, *Academy of Management Executive, 14*(4), 113–119. https://doi.org/10.5465/AME.2000.3979820

Dyer, J. H. & Hatch, N. W. (2006). Relation-specific capabilities and barriers to knowledge transfers: Creating advantage through network relationships. *Strategic Management Journal*, *27*(8), 701–719. https://doi.org/10.1002/smj.543

Ferreira, A. & Du Plessis, T. (2009). Effect of online social networking on employee productivity. *South African Journal of Information Management*, *11*(1), 1–11.

Himmelman, A. (2001). On coalitions and the transformation of power relations: Collaborative betterment and collaborative empowerment. *American Journal of Community Psychology*, *29*(2), 277–284. https://doi.org/10.1023/A:1010334831330

Hoffman, R. (2012). Connections with integrity. *Strategy + Business*, 67. Retrieved from: https://www.strategy-business.com/article/00104

Ibarra, H. & Hunter, M. (2007). How leaders create and use networks. *Harvard Business Review*, *85*(1), 40–47.

Janamian, T., Jackson, C. L. & Dunbar, J. A. (2014). Co-creating value in research: Stakeholders' perspectives. *Medical Journal of Australia*, *201*(3 Suppl), S44–S46. https://doi.org/10.5694/mja14.00273

Knight A. W., Ford D., Audehm R., Colagiuri S. & Best J. (2012). The Australian Primary Care Collaboratives Program: Improving diabetes care *BMJ Quality & Safety*, *21*, 956–963.

Leggat, S. G. & Balding, C. (2013). Achieving organisational competence for clinical leadership: The role of high performance work systems. *Journal of Health Organization and Management*, *27*(3), 312–329. https://doi.org/10.1108/JHOM-Jul-2012-0132

Marinez-Moyano, I. J. (2006). Exploring the dynamics of collaboration in interorganizational settings. In S. Schuman (ed.), *Creating a culture of collaboration* (pp. 69–85). Jossey-Bass.

Mena, C., Humphries, A. & Wilding, R. (2009). A comparison of inter- and intra-organisational relationships *International Journal of Physical Distribution & Logistics Management*, *39*(9) 762–784.

Pfeffer, J. & Salancik, G. R. (1978). *The external control of organisations: a resource dependence perspective*. Harper.

Pittaway, L., Robertson, M., Munir, K., Denyer, D. & Neely, A. (2004). Networking and innovation: A systematic review of the evidence. *International Journal of Management Reviews*, *5*(3–4), 137–168. https://doi.org/10.1111/j.1460-8545.2004.00101.x

Randall, S. (2013). *Learning Report: Leading networks in healthcare*. Retrieved from: https://www.health.org.uk/sites/default/files/LeadingNetworksInHealthcare.pdf

Ropes, D. (2009). Communities of practice: Powerful environments for interorganizational knowledge alliances? In C. Stam (ed.), *Proceedings of the 1st European Conference on Intellectual Capital* (pp. 400–407). Academic Conferences.

Storey, J. & Holti, R. (2013). *Towards a new model of leadership for the NHS*. Retrieved from: http://www.leadershipacademy.nhs.uk/wp-content/uploads/2013/05/Towards-a-New-Model-of-Leadership-2013.pdf

Timmins, N. & Ham, C. (2013). *The quest for integrated health and social care: A case study in Canterbury, New Zealand*. Retrieved from: https://www.kingsfund.org.uk/insight-and-analysis/reports/quest-integrated-health-and-social-care

Yamazaki, T. & Umemoto, K. (2010). Knowledge management of healthcare by clinical-pathways. In S. Chu, W. Ritter & S. Hawamdeh (eds), *Managing knowledge for global and collaborative innovations* (pp. 141–150). World Scientific Publishing.

Part 4
Achieves Outcomes

17 Holding to account

Ged Williams and Linda Fraser

Learning objectives

How do I:

- understand the relationship between manager and employee and the implicit and explicit expectations of this relationship?
- clarify my manager's performance expectations of me and the broader expectations of managers to obtain the best performance from everyone?
- identify why some staff fall below expectations and determine the appropriate approaches to manage these issues?
- develop skills in using frameworks to guide my behaviour and actions in holding staff to account?
- adopt leadership styles that will be most effective in holding others to account?

Introduction

In contemporary healthcare services, managers are required to create and support environments that are complex in nature and are subject to competing forces that place significant demands on both the system and individuals contributing to productivity.

Often, people assume that being held to account is something negative that usually happens only when things go wrong. However, accountability can be viewed as something that can be utilised to ensure success (Smith, 2014). Holding to account can be difficult if the perceptions and expectations of management and staff differ. We cannot assume that people share the same understanding of what they are accountable for, or the standards expected of them, unless they are made explicit and clear.

Definitions

In business, government and healthcare, **accountabilities** may be legislated or described in high-level policy documents to inform senior leaders of their accountabilities and responsibilities (*National Health Act 1953* (Cth); *Public Governance, Performance and Accountability Act 2013* (Cth); *Public Health and Wellbeing Act 2008* (Vic.); Victorian Public Health and Wellbeing Plan 2023–27 (Department of Health, 2023); *Corporations Act 2001* (Cth)). The chief executive officer may delegate accountabilities in a traditional hierarchical fashion to managers, who in turn will hold subordinates to account for responsibilities that are further delegated or directed.

Accountability: The requirement to account for one's actions and outcomes to a higher authority; cannot be delegated

Strategic accountability

At the strategic level of the health system, ministers and department leaders may have their accountabilities legislated through parliament. These accountabilities are well-documented, and expectations are clear and legally binding. The parliamentary process holds to account those in power for delivering on these accountabilities, and if the community is not satisfied with their performance, those in power may not be re-elected.

Publicly available, external peer review is another way in which hospitals and health services are held to account. Health service accreditation through the Australian Council on Health Care Standards (http://www.achs.org.au) and similar accrediting agencies, the Health Round Table (http://www.healthroundtable.org) benchmarking groups and various medical college auditing procedures (Royal Australasian College of Physicians, n.d.) are some examples. External reviews can motivate chief executive officers and the organisations they administer to be accountable to an external standard set by a third party that acts on behalf of the community's interests.

Operational accountability

At the health service or departmental level, key accountabilities are often framed in an operational plan developed to align activities and priorities with the strategic intent. In the operational plan, a list of priorities is outlined and documented using the SMART and/or SIMPLE format (described later in this chapter) with specific individuals identified as accountable officers.

Policy

To provide clarity of expectations among employees at all levels, most organisations rely on written policies. Time and focus are needed to ensure policies are aligned to legislation and are structured with consistent wording and definitions that direct employees to the specific procedures they are required to follow (Watson, 2019). Engaging employees in the consultation process of policy writing is essential to ensure the policy is feasible, easy to read and understand, and that staff have a sense of ownership over the process and expected outcome.

Individual accountability

Overman and Schillemans (2022) refer to 'felt accountability', whereby the individual employee feels accountability in a timely manner and will acknowledge the need to explain their actions and contributions in line with broader organisational and team expectations. Before the accountable officer proceeds with the task, they should examine the accountability structure, specific expectations, allowable resources, authority to act, ability to negotiate or modify expectations (including timeframes) and the consequences of success or failure.

Leadership and holding to account

Managers often seek to be likeable and will attempt to avoid tension, conflict and continuing performance reviews. Accountability can be particularly difficult if personal friendships cloud the professional relationships required at work. However, it is more important for managers to be *respected* than liked (Mitchell, 2017). When managers take **responsibility** and hold themselves accountable for their own actions, they 'model the way' and their colleagues are more engaged and motivated to perform (Kouzes & Posner, 2017).

Responsibility: The obligation of ensuring the required task is complete; can be delegated and/or shared

Holding an employee to account may require the manager to conduct timely and difficult conversations with the employee, and many managers may be reluctant to approach this. Despite feeling apprehensive, by utilising the SIMPLE and/or SMART frameworks set out later in this chapter to guide discussions (and documentation), the manager can approach such issues with confidence and competence.

Although many leadership styles have been studied and documented, no single leadership style will be suitable in all situations. Behavioural leadership styles include autocratic, bureaucratic, participative and laissez-faire; more contemporary styles include charismatic, connective, servant, transactional, transformational and authentic styles. All styles of leadership have currency in various situations, and a skilled leader can vary their style as required for a given context. In a disaster situation, an autocratic style may be necessary; however, in a budget development process, a bureaucratic style may be useful.

Knowing that leadership is more about behaviour than personality (Kouzes & Posner, 2017), and that a leader–follower relationship characterised by fear and mistrust will not produce positive outcomes, most leaders will endeavour to develop positive relationships characterised by respect and confidence. Feedback delivered by a respected and credible authority holds the most value to the recipient and builds both confidence and competence in the team (Foley-Lewis, 2012).

> ## PROVIDING CLEAR EXPECTATIONS
>
> Sally is a four-year postgraduate registered nurse working in a busy medical inpatient unit. She has worked hard to develop her nursing skills since completing her graduate nurse program and is now well regarded as a senior registered nurse. In her performance appraisal and development (PA&D) discussion with her nurse unit manager (NUM), Sally is given the feedback that she is performing well and that her willingness to be a preceptor and mentor to new and unskilled staff has been noted and appreciated. Sally indicates she would like to work towards becoming a clinical nurse (a promotion to a senior ward nurse role).
>
> The NUM takes this opportunity to discuss with Sally the requirements for clinical nurses. Together, they discuss areas for Sally to focus on developing, and Sally is provided with the clinical nurse role description and the role-specific information. Sally and her NUM develop and document a plan collaboratively for Sally to follow to facilitate her development along this pathway.
>
> Over the next six months, Sally works to complete the development plan as laid out in the PA&D and attends a workshop designed for aspiring clinical nurses. She continues to demonstrate sound clinical judgement in the workplace and fills in as a team leader at need in a competent manner.
>
> At the six-month review, Sally and her NUM analyse the plan and Sally's achievements to date. Sally is then offered the opportunity to backfill in the clinical nurse role to cover a period of leave. Sally is delighted her hard work has paid off and agrees to the position.
>
> The NUM ensures that Sally has all the information regarding code of conduct, role description and portfolio responsibilities, and they have an indepth discussion regarding the leadership aspects of the role. This action is recorded on the PA&D, and Sally is provided with a copy of the document. The expectations are both clear and documented.

Holding to account requires very clear communication and decisive directions so that all participants know what is expected. However, not every employee can meet every expectation all the time, and most reasonable managers will demonstrate some latitude in their expectations. When both parties share the same understanding, a failure to perform according to the manager's reasonable **expectations** may be due to unforeseen barriers such as unrealistic timeframes and inadequate resourcing, resulting in unachievable demands, or the accountable individual may lack the necessary competence to complete the task.

It is often easy to find fault in the **performance** of others and yet fail to see our own part in failures or difficulties encountered. How illuminating would it be to see our own contributions to the outcomes achieved?

Expectation: A belief that something will happen as agreed

Performance: Execution of a set of obligations or expectations, usually measured against certain criteria

Frameworks for holding to account

In management, there are many approaches to framing accountability and holding to account. Some simple frameworks are discussed in this section that can assist managers to approach their responsibilities and those they delegate to enable them to implement accountability processes consistently and predictably.

SMART and/or SIMPLE

Accountabilities and expectations, which are essentially goal-setting activities, should be SMART: Specific, Measurable, Achievable, Relevant and Time-based. They should be documented in clear and understandable language. The more important the accountability or expectation, the more important it is to document clearly. If not documented at the outset, specific expectations can be forgotten or confused, leading to argument, wasted time, renegotiation and ill-will.

Miller (2006) articulates a SIMPLE approach to accountability whereby roles and tasks are easy to remember each time a new accountability is established. This approach helps guide managers and their teams in meeting these accountabilities.

Set expectations

Do not assume that employees know what is supposed to be done, when and to what standard unless these are clearly explained at the outset. The clearer these expectations are, the less time is subsequently spent clarifying or arguing about them. To ensure complete understanding, expectations must be **relevant** and **realistic**.

> **Relevant:** Aligned with overarching business objectives, inclusive of goals, mission, values
>
> **Realistic:** Attainable within known constraints

Invite commitment

Most employees will engage if they know the objective will benefit them personally, help move the organisation forward and be open to their input and influence (ownership). Once employees see the benefits and feel they have some control of the process, they are more likely to welcome being held to account for the results.

Measure progress

Key metrics must be quantified and communicated to inform progress and gauge whether the goals and expectations previously committed to have been met. Goals are measurable only when they are quantified. It is important that the measure is agreed and regularly reported so that all stakeholders can monitor continuing performance objectively.

Provide feedback

Sharing the quantifiable measures and constructively commenting on less-tangible markers (such as effort, cooperation and teamwork) can help to keep employees focused and engaged. Feedback will not solve all problems but can open dialogue for problem-solving and follow-up actions, especially if performance is falling short of expectations or unexpected barriers have arisen.

Link to consequences

Consequences guide and focus behaviour and encourage commitments to be taken seriously. Consequences (positive or negative) must be certain, suitable and commensurate with goal difficulty and must immediately follow the outcome or action. Both managers and employees must know that the agreed consequences will follow the action.

Evaluate effectiveness

Using preset goals, an employer can determine how successful they have been in holding employees accountable. The manager must employ self-reflection to review how processes such as communication, feedback, negotiation, compromise and consequences were managed. Reviewing their own performance and heeding supervisor and staff feedback can help a manager develop effective ways to apply the principles of accountability. Holding oneself accountable for holding others accountable is a critical step in becoming an effective manager and leader.

Feedback

Many employees with performance issues often have a better-than-average opinion of themselves, which can result in an enhanced self-worth and a disbelief in the supervisor's judgement (Brown, 2012). High-performing staff will seek feedback on performance to affirm their self-belief and to self-adjust perceived deficits, while low-performing staff will often resist feedback-seeking behaviour as they seldom see the need to improve their own performance (Kuhnen & Tymula, 2012). It is critical for the manager to find ways to provide feedback to individuals so as to establish a realistic, shared perspective of their performance. The most effective feedback to all staff is delivered in a supportive environment by credible and tactful supervisors (Dahling, Chau & O'Malley, 2010).

Before committing to giving feedback, it is helpful to reflect on the intent for the feedback by considering these questions:

- What outcome is to be achieved by the feedback?
- What specific issue is to be addressed?
- Can we agree on a way forward?
- What effect will this have on the relationship between the parties?

Giving feedback can be a difficult and emotional undertaking. It can generate fear and other negative emotions and can lead to a reluctance to both deliver and accept. Despite this, feedback is not always delivered from a higher authority to a lower level but can be effectively delivered by employees who hold their managers to account despite the obvious power differential. It can also be effective when delivered by colleagues at level.

To be effective, feedback must come from an authentic and sincere desire to help or support the other person. It is not about fixing but helping or coaching. Done well, feedback will be accepted as a gift; however, feedback that cannot help someone improve is simply criticism and can lead to accusations of bullying.

Real-time feedback can be delivered to a peer, subordinate or supervisor if behaviour or practice is not in line with the values, standards, expectations or performance goals of the organisation. Providing dignified, caring and honest feedback or a well-placed question immediately the concerning behaviour or practice is recognised enables a brief pause, reflection and a teachable moment. Any group of people working together can, as a group, determine what is and what is not acceptable behaviour based on the organisation's standards; where there is 'a line'. 'Below the line' behaviour is not tolerated and 'above the line' behaviour is encouraged. 'The line' is set by consensus of the group/team and is explicitly stated and documented. By simply stating that a behaviour is 'below the line', an employee provides instantaneous feedback that the concerning behaviour is not acceptable. Just-in-time feedback is delivered after the fact but within a timeframe that enables meaningful action such as a correction or incorporation of change in future behaviour (Nursing Executive Center, 2011).

Eight 'feedback' behaviours of holding others to account and providing feedback are:

- **F**actual – Do not assume or accuse people of something they did not do.
- **E**xpectations – People need to know what you want/need of them.
- **E**arly – Timely feedback needs to follow the event as early as possible.
- **D**iscreet – Coach people in private, never in public.
- **B**alanced – Holding people accountable does not always need to be negative.
- **A**ppreciative – Acknowledge and thank people for positive attempts to improve.
- **C**onsistent – Treat everyone the same way, to the extent possible.
- **K**ind – How would you like to get this input? Show empathy.

Having the right attitude, being calm, managing emotions and treating others as you would like them to treat you are simple but powerful approaches. It is the method of delivery of such feedback that determines its effectiveness. Feedback delivered in a sensitive and supportive manner is more acceptable to the recipient and much more likely to be effective (Dahling et al., 2010).

Leaders who develop and maintain high-quality relationships with their subordinates have been found to provide feedback that is more readily received (Bezuijen, van Dam, van den Berg & Thierry, 2010). Careful, decisive, fair actions and communication are required.

Appraisal methods

Performance appraisal and development

The development aspect of a PA&D covers not only identification of potential deficits in knowledge, skills and abilities but also areas for future development and career progression. A PA&D aims to guide a conversation between employee and manager to review the employee's performance against predetermined criteria, including aspects that are not so easy to measure, such as attitude, teamwork and communication.

Some employers are moving away from the annual appraisal methodology described and are relying on a more frequent conversational approach to achieving positive performance outcomes without the intensity of a single annual performance appraisal (Chellappa, 2022). As described by Javed and colleagues (2017), managers who develop an inclusive leadership style by demonstrating openness, availability and accessibility aid team members to voice their opinions in a safe environment.

Buddy and mentor systems

A buddy or mentor partnership can be formed to provide support to any employee by a capable and respected peer, or a slightly more experienced colleague, who provides real-time and just-in-time feedback on behaviour. If the buddy or mentor process is formal, regular meetings with the supervisor may be required to discuss performance and provide feedback.

Discipline and performance improvement processes

Should feedback and guidance fail to produce the required standards of performance, a disciplinary procedure may be required. Before heading down this pathway, it is first necessary to determine that less-intense options (such as buddy or mentor systems and PA&D reviews) have not been effective or are deemed inappropriate due to the serious nature of the behaviour. Then, a full investigation must be conducted of the alleged poor performance, whether it is clinical or professional or a code of conduct breach. This can be done by the manager or an external investigator. Employees must be afforded a right of reply (natural justice).

Supportive behaviours by work colleagues as well as supervisors will ameliorate negative perceptions of bullying by staff with poor performance (Blomberg & Rosander, 2020). It is not uncommon for staff who overestimate their capabilities to commence 'bullying and harassment' counterclaims towards their supervisors (Goodhew, Cammock & Hamilton, 2008).

It is wise to use human resources experts to inform the process to be followed in responding to such claims. Inviting the staff member to have a support person in attendance can help all parties involved to feel safe, especially if there are feelings of distrust or animosity. The development and documentation of a formal performance improvement plan may be necessary to address issues not resolved by this stage. It may also be necessary to vary the employee's hours of work so that greater supervision of performance and feedback is possible. For instance, bringing a nurse onto day shifts so that more frequent communication and feedback with their manager and/or buddy are possible, and attendance at education and training sessions is achievable. Regular meetings between the supervisor and employee are important (including support persons if appropriate) to maintain momentum and adjustments as improvements are made.

Confidentiality among those participants in the disciplinary process is of paramount importance. Many team members will be aware of the process and will be watching to see how the manager deals with it. It can be profoundly detrimental to the team for this process to be handled poorly or, worse still, not handled at all.

Reprimands, penalties, demotions, transfers and terminations

In the healthcare sector, formal reprimands, financial penalties, demotions, transfers and terminations are severe, often last-resort responses and are generally associated with illegal or unprofessional behaviour. Such issues are beyond the scope of most supervisors to manage on their own and warrant the involvement of human resources, legal, industrial and/or executive and regulatory authority. The Australian Health Professional Regulatory Agency (http://www.ahpra.gov.au) is a valuable resource regarding such complex matters. They have trained managers who can provide advice and guidance on issues of professional malpractice and misconduct.

Summary

- Being accountable means being able to account for one's actions and outcomes to a higher authority. The relationship between managers and employees has explicit and implicit expectations in terms of performance, productivity and behaviour.
- Evidence suggests that managers and employees do not always have shared views or expectations of performance, and these need to be made clear and transparent prior to embarking on work or projects.
- Performance can fall below expectations when an individual does not have the skill required, the expectation is unreasonable, or an individual does not have the will to complete the task.
- There are many ways by which managers can hold an individual to account. By using SIMPLE and/or SMART frameworks as guides, managers can plan their approach despite feeling apprehensive about the process.

- A manager is like a coach who demands the best of each player for the good of the team and its supporters. Regardless of the leadership style, if clear expectations and feedback are given promptly, holding to account can be achieved effectively.
- Developing an inclusive leadership style by demonstrating openness, availability and accessibility aids team members to voice their opinions in a psychologically safe environment.

Reflective questions

1. Consider the five key accountabilities of your current role (or your next role if you are a student). Rate your performance on a scale of 1 to 10 and then ask a supervisor and two peers to rate your performance on the same scale. What are the similarities and differences in the scores? Can you identify reasons for these?
2. Identify two policies in your area that make you specifically accountable for a certain behaviour or performance standard. How do you compare to your colleagues?
3. Identify two specific accountabilities of your manager that you think could assist them in achieving their targets or departmental goals. What could you do to help them improve current performance in each area?
4. Consider a time when you, or someone you know, was considered a low performer relative to peers. What was done to change the situation? How could it have been managed better?
5. Consider an event when many people were responsible for an important task, but no-one did it. What was the outcome? How would you manage that situation differently next time?

Self-analysis questions

Identify your preferred management style. Imagine you are required to performance manage a staff member who has been verbally undermining your management decisions. Identify the pros and cons of using your preferred management style with this individual in the context of a multidisciplinary healthcare setting.

References

Bezuijen, X. M., van Dam, K., van den Berg, R. & Thierry, H. (2010). How leaders stimulate employee learning: A leader-member exchange approach. *Journal of Occupational and Organizational Psychology*, *83*, 673–693. https://doi.org/10.1348/096317909X468099

Blomberg S. & Rosander, M. (2020). Exposure to bullying behaviours and support from co-workers and supervisors: a three-way interaction and the effect on health and well-being. *International Archives of Occupational and Environmental Health*. *93*(4), 479–490. https://doi.org/10.1007/s00420-019-01503-7.

Brown, J. D. (2012). Understanding the better than average effect: Motives (still) matter. *Personality and Social Psychology Bulletin*, *38*(2), 209–219. https://doi.org/10.1177/0146167211432763

Chellappa, S., (2022). Why These 8 Top Companies Redefined Their Performance Management Systems. Retrieved 6 October 2024 from: https://engagedly.com/blog/8-top-companies-redefined-their-performance-management-systems/

Dahling, J. J., Chau, S. L. & O'Malley, A. (2010). Correlation and consequences of feedback orientation in organisations. *Journal of Management*, *38*(2), 531–546. https://doi.org/10.1177/0149206310375467

Department of Health, State of Victoria. (2023). *Victorian Public Health and Wellbeing Plan 2023–27*. Retrieved 6 February 2024 from: https://www.health.vic.gov.au/victorian-public-health-and-wellbeing-plan-2023-27

Foley-Lewis, S. (2012). *Successful feedback*. Sally Foley-Lewis Publication.

Goodhew, G. W., Cammock, P. A. & Hamilton, R. T. (2008). The management of poor performance by front-line managers. *Journal of Management, 27*(9), 951–962. https://doi.org/10.1108/02621710810901291

Javed, B., Naqvi, S. M. M. R., Khan, A. K., Arjoon, S. & Tayyeb, H. H. (2017). Impact of inclusive leadership on innovative work behaviour: The role of psychological safety. *Journal of Management & Organisation, 25*(1), 117–136. https://doi.org/10.1017/jmo.2017.3

Kouzes, J. M. & Posner, B. Z. (2017). *The leadership challenge* (6th ed.). John Wiley & Sons.

Kuhnen, C. M. & Tymula, A. (2012). Feedback, self-esteem, and performance in organizations. *Management Science, 58*(1), 94–113. https://doi.org/10.1287/mnsc.1110.1379

Miller, B. C. (2006). *Keeping employees accountable for results: Quick tips for busy managers*. American Management Association.

Mitchell, B. (2017). Can a Manager be Both Liked and Respected? *ASAE*. Retrieved 10 March 2024 from: https://www.asaecenter.org/association-careerhq/career/articles/talent-management/can-a-manager-be-both-liked-and-respected

Nursing Executive Center. (2011). *Building peer accountability* [Study]. Retrieved from: http://www.advisory.com

Overman, S. & Schillemans, T. (2022). Toward a public administration theory of felt accountability. *Public Administration Review, 82*(1), 12–22.

Royal Australasian College of Physicians. (n.d.). Training Site Accreditation. Retrieved 10 March 2024 from: https://www.racp.edu.au/about/accreditation

Smith, T. (2014). *Holding others accountable* [Video]. Retrieved from: http://www.ozprinciple.com/others/holding-others-accountable

Watson C. (2019, June 19). Policies help to establish accountability at every level. *Australian Ageing Agenda*. Retrieved 10 March 2024 from: https://www.australianageingagenda.com.au/executive/policies-help-establish-accountability-at-every-level/

18 Critical thinking and decision-making

Richard Baldwin

Learning objectives

How do I:

- increase my understanding of the elements of critical thinking?
- counteract the barriers that might limit my critical thinking?
- use critical thinking to identify fake news and evaluate information on social media?
- improve my skills in decision-making?
- identify common decision-making errors?
- make better use of evidence in healthcare decision-making?

Introduction

Managers and leaders need to critically analyse their own thinking and decision-making processes so they can objectively evaluate the problems and issues they face every day. To do this they need to understand their personal preferences, prejudices, values and cultural beliefs, and their motivations and desires. It is also important for them to understand how these factors shape the biases managers and leaders take to decision-making. To achieve success, they require the ability to analyse, synthesise and evaluate material, and to assemble their thoughts in a logical argument.

Critical thinking

Each day health-service managers are faced with large volumes of information from a variety of sources, including social media. When faced with new or conflicting information, managers must ask the right questions to evaluate the situation. The right questions help them to formulate appropriate responses. This is particularly important when assessing information obtained from social media, including that generated by artificial intelligence (AI), and to determine its accuracy (Orhan, 2023). In a systematic review of the literature, Machete and Turpin (2020) report on the capacity of university students to identify 'fake news' in social media. They concluded that critical-thinking skills are helpful to an individual's ability to identify misleading or inaccurate information. They conclude that 'information literacy' (the ability to access and use information), as well as critical thinking, are essential skills to evaluate the credibility of online information.

Critical thinking is a rational, systematic process that involves the assessment of statements and arguments, and the formulation of questions.

A *statement*, like many made on social media, claims that something is, or is not, the case. But a statement, on its own, is not an *argument*. For example, three different statements that by themselves do not form an argument are: 'Smoking tobacco is bad for your health', 'Clinicians without management education make poor managers' and 'Healthcare is too expensive'. **Critical thinking** helps us decide whether there is sufficient evidence to accept these statements.

To decide whether the first of these statements is true requires further information, such as: 'Tobacco contains several chemicals that are known to be toxic to humans', 'Smoking tobacco releases these chemicals' and 'Epidemiological evidence indicates higher morbidity and mortality in people who regularly smoke tobacco'. Put together, these three statements form an *argument*. The argument is also called 'deductive reasoning' and is distinguished from inductive reasoning, in which specific observations are used to develop broader conclusions.

The development of an argument regarding the other two statements may require more than three statements and may be less well-supported by evidence. Managers need the ability to assess which statements support the argument so as to analyse the arguments of others and to formulate their own conclusions.

Critical thinking: The systematic evaluation or formulation of beliefs or statements, by rational standards, that forms the basis of problem-solving, decision-making and emotional intelligence (Vaughn & MacDonald, 2010, p. 119)

Barriers to critical thinking

According to Vaughn and MacDonald (2010), the two most common hindrances to critical thinking arise because of '*how* we think' and '*what* we think'. Our personal predispositions, such as preferences, values and biases, influence how we think. Impediments to what we think tend to be based on beliefs about the world, our cultural heritage and upbringing. A significant influence on how and what we think can come from group pressure to conform and from our own desire to fit in.

To develop critical-thinking skills, individuals need to assess the extent to which their thinking is influenced by the groups to which they belong. Group pressure can come in the form of peer pressure (the pressure to conform), appeals to popularity (a person is harder to like if they think or act differently) and appeals to common practice (doing something the way it has always been done makes survival easier). However, group-centred thinking can degenerate into narrow-mindedness, resistance to change and stereotyping; and in this way it can limit an individual's critical thinking and problem-solving. One of the best defences against group thinking is to always evaluate a claim according to the strength of its arguments – that is, to assess the statements that are being made, their underlying premises and the assumptions that these make to determine whether there is a reasonable argument to support the conclusions offered. Rudinow and Barry (2007) identify the following barriers to critical thinking:

- a limited frame of reference constructed because of a belief structure about the world and the source of the information – for example, placing unjustified faith in what is learned from the internet
- lack of willingness to accept different views and a tendency to make hasty moral judgements
- reliance on untested assumptions, wishful thinking and self-deception – that is, being convinced that something is true because that is the easiest or least painful option, or avoids difficult consequences
- ethnocentricity and cultural conditioning in thinking – that is, the inability or unwillingness to think differently from the familial, tribal or cultural group
- stereotypes or labels used to judge others – for example, holding a prejudice about someone's judgement based on their profession
- peer pressure and inappropriate reliance on authority – for example, simply believing what others say and avoiding thinking for oneself.

Regarding the final point, critical thinking should not be confused with the need to obey a legitimate instruction, order, rule or policy. Careful judgement is needed before ignoring or disobeying legitimate authority.

Thinking is guided by questions. Carefully constructed questions can define tasks, express problems and delineate issues. Questions are important for assessing the strengths of other people's arguments and formulating one's own arguments.

ASSESSING PREJUDICE AND BIASES

A male hospital employee who works as an administrative assistant and has direct contact with patients of the mental health unit has recently informed you and his other work colleagues that he intends to commence wearing women's clothing to work. Under medical advice, he is also commencing the process of changing his sex, which will take some time. The employee has indicated to you that it is important for his own mental health that he continues to function within society as usual during his sex-change process.

Two members of the mental health team, claiming to represent most of the clinical and non-clinical staff, have come to you, as the manager, to express their concerns about the effect this sex change process will have on the patients of the mental health unit. They argue that many of the patients may find it confronting to have to deal with a man in women's clothing. They also argue that the gender ambiguity will hamper this employee's capacity to engage with patients in a general sense. They insist that the staff member be reassigned to work in a different part of the hospital.

As the manager, you need to consider whether the two staff members' concerns are reasonable or are an exhibition of assumptions and prejudice on their part, and to examine barriers to your own critical thinking that might arise as you consider your response to this situation.

- Are the staff members' concerns reasonable or are they an exhibition of assumptions and prejudice on their part?
- How will you test the accuracy of the claims that the staff member's sex-change process will have a negative effect on the patients in the ward?
- Examine barriers to your own critical thinking that arise as you consider your response to this situation.
- How will you, as the manager, respond to this situation?

Developing critical-thinking skills in decision-making

Here are some steps that can help in the development of critical thinking, based on the work of Elder and Paul (2013) and Boogaard (2024).

Listen actively

When having a conversation, instead of trusting that you can passively absorb the message that someone is sending, it is useful to think about what they are saying both through the words they are using and the underlying messages. Active listening involves the listener reflecting to the speaker what they think they heard to confirm correct understanding. Active listening involves neither agreeing nor disagreeing; it is concerned with clarifying understanding of the speaker's meaning.

Stick to the point

When making a disciplined argument, it is important to avoid information and arguments that are irrelevant to the issue at hand and that jump from one point to another in a manner that is not logical or related. Before making an argument, the following questions should be considered: What is the main issue? What information and arguments relate directly to the main issue? What information and arguments are not relevant? How is the argument best developed to relate the relevant information to the main issue?

Be reasonable

There are two steps here: managers must be able to identify unreasonableness in others and identify their own unreasonableness. It is vital for managers to examine closely what people are saying and to form a view as to the strength of their arguments, regardless of whether they challenge the managers' own understanding, accepted position, deep-seated beliefs or cultural preferences. Thus, managers should be prepared to change a point of view when faced with a well-reasoned argument.

Question questions

Managers need to be skilled questioners. Successful questioners form questions that increase understanding and clarify issues. They avoid questions that can be interpreted as challenging, argumentative or loaded. One approach is to formulate several different questions for the same issue. Then select the one that best addresses the issue and is acceptable to the person being questioned; this is the most likely approach that will elicit the result being sought.

Decision-making

Every day we are faced with a wide variety of decisions, but not all of them relate to a problem or need deep analysis – for example, what to wear, what to eat, where to go after work. Decision-making in the workplace takes on a different dimension because we need to decide whether what we are facing is 'business as usual' or an issue that needs a unique decision. Unlike many personal decisions, decision-making in the workplace affects others, so consideration of how to involve others in the **decision-making process** is important. The following steps guide the process of making decisions in the workplace:

- Identify the problem: Ask, 'Is there a problem?' If there is, ask, 'What is it?' Not every issue is necessarily a problem that needs a solution.
- Gather and analyse information: Identify and weigh the criteria that will define the decision-making priorities. Relatively simple analysis is often all that is necessary.
- Identify options: There are always options, including 'doing nothing', and it is vital to consult with stakeholders (people who are affected by or concerned with the issue) about available options.
- Secure the commitment of stakeholders to the recommended option: In many situations an absence of commitment is likely to result in unsuccessful implementation.
- Implement the solution and evaluate its effectiveness.

Decision-making process: Steps that include identifying a problem, selecting an alternative and evaluating the decision's effectiveness (Bazerman & Moore, 2009; Robbins, Bergman, Stagg & Coulter, 2012).

Biases and errors in decision-making

Table 18.1 lists and summarises some of the factors that have been identified as leading in biases and errors in decision-making.

Table 18.1 Possible biases and errors that occur in decision-making, according to their discussion in specific texts

Biases and errors	Description	Source (1)	(2)	(3)
Anchoring	Influence by others (4)	✓	✓	✓
Availability	Bias from most recent events rather than taking a long-term view		✓	✓
Confirmation	Bias-based evidence	✓	✓	
Framing	Shaping the question (4)	✓	✓	✓
Group failure	Assumption that a group of smart, or famous, people cannot be wrong			✓
Immediate gratification	Desire for a quick decision		✓	
Over-prudence	Excessive caution that limits or delays decision-making	✓		
Overconfidence in forecasting	Unrealistic positive views of personal decision-making	✓	✓	✓
Plunging in	Decisions made too quickly			✓
Randomness	Creation of meaning from unconnected information		✓	
Representation	Bias from other like events		✓	
Rule of thumb	Dependence on custom, practice and past experience	✓	✓	✓
Selective perception	Bias-based perception		✓	✓
Sunk costs	Protection of past mistakes	✓	✓	

Sources: (1) Hammond, Keeney & Raiffa (1998): (2) Robbins et al. (2012); Robbins (2004): (3) Russo & Schoemaker (1989). (4) The concepts of anchoring and framing are explored in the following section.

An *anchoring* effect occurs when a manager (or someone else) has limited information upon which to base a decision about an unfamiliar issue and may rely too heavily on the information provided early in negotiations. For example, the manager of a hospital is required to negotiate the initial purchase of a new imaging machine from the only company that sells them. Although the machine is new to this country, the hospital's clinicians have argued that it is essential in the provision of quality health care and will add to the hospital's prestige. No price has been mentioned, and the manager knows that the company is keen to make the first sale. The manager's first impulse is to ask the company for their price, and it comes in higher than the manager is prepared to pay. In preparing a counteroffer, the manager may be influenced by the vendor's first offer; that is, the response will be anchored by the information provided by the company. Hammond and colleagues (1998) offer the following suggestions to avoid the possible effects of anchoring:

- Use different starting points to view the issue. For example, suggest or ask for information about other imaging machines that may be available to minimise the impression of commitment to purchasing the new machine.
- Determine the boundaries to possible solutions. For example, before commencing negotiations, be clear about the cost-effectiveness of the new machine to the health service and how much it is worth to the health service.
- Undertake comparative research. For example, seek information about the pricing of similar machines, or the price of this machine in other countries.
- Use anchoring proactively. For example, as the buyer, make the first offer.

Strategies to avoid the effects of anchoring will vary with different situations. If a manager wants new ideas from their health team about potential changes to health-service design, it may be a good idea for the manager not to suggest their own ideas first. Making the first suggestion may limit the team's responses. Team members may feel the need to respond to the suggestion, possibly negatively, rather than coming up with their own ideas. That is, going first may anchor the team's responses.

Framing is concerned with how a question is shaped and defined. For example, the introduction of a ban on smoking in the workplace in the 1980s was successful because the problem was defined (framed) as an occupational health and safety issue. This framed the issue as concerning the health effects on co-workers and safety in the workplace rather than on the decision of each individual to make about their own health. Shaping the argument against workplace smoking in this way placed legal obligations on both employers and employees to ensure a healthy workplace and removed the option of personal decisions by employees to smoke or not to smoke, even when they worked alone.

Evidence-based management decision-making

Evidence-based decision management has increased in importance in recent decades for both clinical and non-clinical managers in health organisations (Aloini et al., 2018). One useful example of managers using evidence to guide change is in clinical services redesign projects, completed across health services in Australia and overseas (Ham, Kipping & Mcleod, 2003; Li et al., 2022; Masso, Robert, McCarthy & Eagar, 2010; Scott et al., 2011). Typically, clinical services redesign projects are time-limited, sometimes intensive, initiatives. They involve discrete stages; each stage is heavily based on existing data and uses rigorously collected new data. The use of evidence in this way is crucial to the active and supportive involvement of both clinicians and managers.

In health services, research evidence may not be consistent, and opinions are often widely and strongly held. In addition, the availability of evidence does not guarantee that it will be accepted or used. Two examples are relevant to the use of evidence-based decision-making. The first concerns the discovery of the *Helicobacter pylori* bacillus by Australian scientists Barry Marshall and Robin Warren, who in 2005 were awarded the Nobel Prize for what is considered by many to be a paradigm shift in the way in which gastric ulcers are treated. However, 23 years after the first scientific reports emerged, Ahmed (2005) notes that the clinical community 'met their findings, with scepticism and a lot of criticism', and that despite the existence of solid evidence, it took 'quite a remarkable length of time for their discovery to become widely accepted' (para. 3). The second example concerns the use of evidence regarding public health. Botterill and Hindmoor (2012) examined this in relation to the complex issue of obesity and compared it to the simple, and often incorrect, messages articulated by policy-makers and public health officials. They concluded that advisors to decision-makers are 'boundedly rational' (p. 367); that is, complex situations are often reduced to simple messages for senior managers and policy-makers as they are bound by their capacity to make rational decisions which need to be reduced to relatively simple messages when faced with large volumes of conflicting information. Both examples demonstrate that despite overwhelming scientific evidence, managers (and clinicians) can struggle to convert evidence into practice and may hold onto their beliefs rather than change behaviours.

Summary

- Critical thinking is an essential skill for all health services managers and leaders, students and anyone accessing social media. Techniques such as active listening, sticking to the point, being reasonable and asking thoughtful questions are elements of critical thinking.
- Barriers to critical thinking include a limited frame of reference, lack of willingness to accept different views, relying on untested assumptions, wishful thinking, self-deception, ethnocentric and cultural conditioning in thinking, peer pressure and stereotypes.
- Decision-making steps include identifying the problem, identifying and weighing the criteria that will define the decision-making priorities, and gathering and analysing information.
- There are common errors and biases that may adversely influence decision-making.

Reflective questions

1. Can you recall the last time you practised the technique of active listening in your conversations with a friend or colleague? What happened?
2. Can you identify how your cultural and religious beliefs may influence your critical thinking?
3. The director of nursing has complained to you that waiting times in the emergency department exceeded agreed targets the previous Saturday night. Is this a problem and, if yes, what is the problem? Reflect on whether this is a problem that needs investigation and a decision, and, if yes, define the problem.
4. If most of your workforce is predominantly female and aged over 50 years, is this necessarily a problem that needs investigation? If yes, what is the problem?
5. Is a small number of complaints from patients about cancelled minor day-surgery procedures (but with no serious health consequences) a problem that needs investigation and a decision? If yes, what is the problem?

Self-analysis questions

Values and beliefs are often taken for granted, and we are not regularly asked to think about how they may influence our thinking and decision-making. Being in touch with your own values and beliefs is important, because it enables you to be aware of the biases you may bring to your decision-making.

- Write down up to six values that are important to you and that influence your decision-making at work. (Values can include honesty, punctuality, religious belief, relations between the sexes, the work of others etc.)
- Identify your personal positions concerning up to six everyday issues relevant to your workplace. (Issues might include how promotions are made, the balance between collaboration and individual decision-making, the relative power between different professions etc.)
- Write each of your values and personal positions as a single sentence.

References

Ahmed, N. (2005). 23 years of the discovery of *Helicobacter pylori*: Is the debate over? *Annals of Clinical Microbiology and Antimicrobials*, *4*(17). https://doi.org/10.1186/1476-0711-4-17

Aloini, D., Cannavacciuolo, L., Gitto, S., Lettieri, E., Malighetti, P. & Visintin, F. (2018). Evidence-based management for performance improvement in healthcare. *Management Decision*, *56*(10), 2063–2068. https://doi.org/10.1108/MD-10-2018-004

Bazerman, M. H. & Moore, D. A. (2009). *Judgment in managerial decision making* (7th ed.). John Wiley & Sons.

Boogaard, K. (2024). How to build critical thinking skills for better decision-making. *Productivity*. Retrieved from: https://www.atlassian.com/blog/productivity/critical-thinking-skills

Botterill, L. C. & Hindmoor, A. (2012). Turtles all the way down: Bounded rationality in an evidence-based age. *Policy Studies*, *33*(5), 367–379. https://doi.org/10.1080/01442872.2011.626315

Elder, L. & Paul, R. (2013). Learning the Art of Critical Thinking. Retrieved from: http://www.criticalthinking.org/pages/becoming-a-critic-of-your-thinking/478

Ham, C., Kipping, R. & Mcleod, H. (2003). Redesigning work processes in health care: Lessons from the National Health Service. *Milbank Quarterly Online*, *81*(3).

Hammond, J. S., Keeney, R. L. & Raiffa, H. (1998). The hidden traps in decision making. *Harvard Business Review*, (September–October), 2–11.

Li, L., Davis, M., Kim, N., Lipka, S., Branson, B., Amport, S. … Sussman, S. (2022). Clinical redesign: An innovative approach to leading change at an academic healthcare system. *Journal of Healthcare Management*, *67*(1), 13–24. https://doi.org/10.1097/jhm-d-20-00299

Machete, P. & Turpin, M. (2020). The Use of Critical Thinking to Identify Fake News: A Systematic Literature Review. Paper presented at the Responsible Design, Implementation and Use of Information and Communication Technology.

Masso, M., Robert, G., McCarthy, G. & Eagar, K. (2010). The clinical services redesign program in New South Wales: Perceptions of senior health managers. *Australian Health Review*, *34*, 352–359.

Orhan, A. (2023). Fake news detection on social media: The predictive role of university students' critical thinking dispositions and new media literacy. *Smart Learning Environments*, *10*(1), 29. https://doi.org/10.1186/s40561-023-00248-8

Robbins, S. (2004). *Decide and conquer: Make winning decisions and take control of your life*. Financial Times Prentice Hall.

Robbins, S. P., Bergman, R., Stagg, I. & Coulter, M. (2012). *Management 6*. Pearson.

Rudinow, J. & Barry, V. E. (2007). *Invitation to critical thinking* (6th ed.). Thompson Higher Education.

Russo, J. E. & Schoemaker, P. J. H. (1989). *Decision traps: Ten barriers to brilliant decision-making and how to overcome them*. New Doubleday.

Scott, I. A., Wills, R.-A., Coory, M., Watson, M. J., Butler, F., Waters, M. & Bowler, S. (2011). Impact of hospital-wide process redesign on clinical outcomes: A comparative study of internally versus externally led intervention. *BMJ Quality & Safety, 20*(6), 539–548. https://doi.org/10.1136/bmjqs.2010.042150

Vaughn, L. & MacDonald, C. (2010). *The power of critical thinking* (2nd Canadian ed.). Oxford University Press.

19 Managing and leading staff

Godfrey Isouard
With acknowledgement to David S. Briggs

Learning objectives

How do I:

- develop my skills in leadership of human resources as a critical component of health policy and organisational activity?
- understand the challenging role of the management of human resources in a complex, professionally dominated industry that is affected by constant change?
- determine effective strategies for retention policies and practices that are required to respond to the global maldistributions and shortages within the health professions?
- consider the requirements of human resources for the management of four distinct generations in the substantially female and ageing health workforce?

Introduction

In a text on leadership and management in health services, human resource management requires a strategic approach. Health is dominated by a large, diverse, highly professionalised workforce. Human resource management is complex and focuses on the performance effects of human resource systems rather than individual human resource practices (Boon, Den Hartog & Lepak, 2019). The focus is on systems since employees are exposed to an interrelated set of human resource practices which, in turn, are dependent on other multiple sets of systems within the wider health service.

Human resources

In the changing focus of human resources, it remains a key component of health policy and organisational activity that has an increasingly strategic planning and developmental role (Cailhol et al., 2013). The changing context of health care described in this chapter requires a human-resource strategic approach that:

- understands the nature of the existing workforce
- focuses on maximising skills utilisation in adaptive and flexible ways
- strategically develops the workforce in sustainable ways
- emphasises retention of existing staff while also preparing for succession
- develops a responsive, adaptive and innovative workforce.

The concepts of accountability, trust and stewardship afforded to managers are important.

In particular, there is a strong case for a rethink of 'the fundamental theories of stewardship to frame a new concept for corporate disclosure' (Dumay, La Torre & Farneti, 2019, p. 11). These authors found that 'increasing, renewing or extending the information disclosed is not enough to instill trust in corporations' (Dumay et al., 2019, p. 11). Stewardship over the organisation's resources is required to increase trust. Their findings are that the likely implications of contrary behaviour by managers and senior administrators demand stewardship being viewed as an overarching guide for managerial behaviour and disclosure.

It is extremely difficult to consistently provide high-quality health care to patients. One of the greatest challenges for leadership is that teams are large, team membership is continuously evolving and clinicians are often spread across the entire organisation, which may serve multiple units. This, coupled with the fact that patients and their families are generally poorly informed, can affect important decision-making by the manager and leader, and therefore affects the ultimate quality of care.

In this regard, leadership and quality in clinical microsystems are essential to achieving optimal care (O'Leary et al., 2019). The question is how best to support, develop and increase the leadership of the microsystems at the point at which care is delivered. It is important that leaders possess an understanding of leadership as something more than being concerned with hierarchies and control, and that it goes the core of leadership at the service-delivery level, within and between professions.

Skills utilisation

Over the past few years there has been a shift from a focus on 'staff-mix' to 'skill-mix and beyond'. Skill-mix essentially refers to the group of professional development competencies, skills and experiences of the healthcare staff within the workplace that link with specific outcomes while targeting client needs (Rumisha et al., 2020). Rumisha and colleagues (2020) found that a balance of skill-mix and distribution of core human resources was critical to enhancing decision-making processes and subsequent timely responses.

One critical challenge for the manager is addressing workforce shortages. The current focus on staff-mix is restrictive, with a need to focus on staff skills so as to provide a more dynamic human-resources environment that focuses on the effective utilisation of the available health personnel to their fullest potential.

The emphasis on maximising skills requires a human-resources emphasis on skills and competency assessment, training and development so that the workforce can take on new roles and functions. This occurs through role enhancement and/or role enlargement. Altering roles generally tends to be attractive to employees because it offers opportunities, new competencies and greater achievement, recognition and motivation. Evidence in support of these types of strategies is not conclusive, however, and they may cause increased tension or confusion with traditional professional roles and be considered convenient approaches to workforce rationalisation.

Integrated care in treating chronic conditions requires multiple skills, including management, system planning, care planning, negotiation and teamwork, to bring clinical and management roles into alignment. These skills are also required in direct engagement, supporting patients and clients with the capacity to self-manage their disease or chronic condition.

Mobilising 'skills and capabilities in individuals to the teams they work within is critical to positive organisational development and improved patient care' (Elijiz, Greenfield, Molineux & Sloan, 2018, p 135). Elijiz and colleagues (2018) found that effective healthcare delivery is attained through strategic, integrative care using numerous dispersed service providers. In the area of overlapping organisational boundaries, the study suggests that special skills are necessary. These are referred to as 'deep smarts', found in people who play important integrative and networking roles using clinical, organisational and people skills.

One key way to enhance employee skills utilisation is through targeted employee development. As reported by Watts (2011), this approach not only addresses skills utilisation but also strategises towards retention of key employees. The study reports that employees value the personal recognition and skills development they receive. This, in turn, invariably contributes towards improved organisational performance and enhanced morale and motivation in the workplace.

Organisational behaviour and culture

The organisational environment has now significantly changed to the point that a 'new way of work' has been firmly established (Norman, 2022). This new direction has required managers and leaders working closely with human-resources departments to review priorities and place renewed emphasis on building effective human systems and human-focused organisations.

The previous ways of 'doing human resources' are no longer relevant. It is time for human resources to reinvent itself in a post-COVID-19 world. This new role is seen as demanding a 'new style' of human-resources professional.

Implementing human-resource initiatives in the midst of what has become constant health reform requires an understanding of the effects of culture on staff and organisations. Culture is often described as transforming and empowering people to achieve a variety of objectives.

Organisations are also in need of culturally intelligent managers and leaders (Moua, 2012). Leadership with cultural intelligence is regarded as necessary to drive effective changes. Effective leaders need to hone their cultural intelligence to their professional advantage. Moua argues that cultural intelligence is both a strategy and a tool to build cultural competence and proficiency. When this is appropriately integrated and applied in the leadership process, organisations become far more innovative and adaptable, and able to respond to cultural changes.

Having a consistent and coordinated approach between the organisation and its staff as to purpose, mission, values and behaviours ascribed is an important consideration. How management value staff and how they behave towards them are also important. It is important to consistently practise the agreed values and behaviours so that workers have real meaning within the organisation. According to Dubois and Singh (2009, p. 12), an effective organisational structure for the management of human resources includes:

- a relatively flat hierarchy with few supervisors
- worker autonomy
- participative management
- professional development opportunities
- relatively high organisational status for nursing
- collaboration.

Leadership and management

Health managers and leaders are deployed in large health systems, often distant geographically from the services and localities they manage. They are highly qualified, with the predominate field of study being health, followed by management and commerce qualifications (Martins & Isouard, 2024). Health managers are often seen to be implementing health reform but are also affected by constant reform rather than being in control (Briggs, Smyth & Anderson, 2012).

Some health managers have only clinical qualifications; their management experience, both good and bad, having been learned from others. The reported limitations of clinically qualified health managers include difficulty in balancing clinical world and management identity, and a restricted, profession-specific view (Loh, 2015). There are profession-based differences in approach to management roles and tensions between generalist and clinically qualified managers and their peer groups, where the management role is described as contested. Managers need 'to develop emotional resilience, set boundaries, develop personal support structures and understand the formal and informal sides of the organisation' (Briggs, Cruickshank & Paliadelis, 2012, p. 623). The role has moved to leadership and managing change, with emphases on sense making, motivating and communicating.

It involves engagement, relationship-building, learning, thinking flexibly, being resilient and understanding critical thinking (Briggs, Smyth & Anderson, 2012).

Engagement, empowerment and collaboration

The increase in middle management over the past 20 years has been accompanied by a change in management roles. Increased task complexity and new management direction have resulted in direct supervision being replaced by collaboration-led management (Zhang, 2023). The effects of legislation and standards have ensured and made routine many practices such as industrial relations, remunerative practices, work health and safety, affirmative action and anti-discrimination. The human resources concepts of motivation and supervision have moved towards concepts of **work engagement**, empowerment, and collaboration, and the concept of training per se is moving towards learning, knowledge development, coaching, preceptorships and mentoring.

> **Work engagement:** Psychological and emotional connection of an employee to their work and/or workplace

Work engagement is meant to provide 'positive, fulfilling ... work related well-being ... to provide engaged, high energy work focussed staff', broadening the view about the meaning and effects of work (Bakker, Schaufeli, Leiter & Taris, 2008, p. 187). Coaching is recognised as a supportive but challenging process in developing skills in others (Isouard, Thiessen, Stanton & Hanson, 2006) and has been identified as a key competence for healthcare leadership (Kao, Tsai & Schinke, 2021). Mentoring programs enhance job satisfaction of those mentored and, if planned appropriately, can successfully be used for leadership and managerial development (Williamson, 2021). Mentoring is broad-based and concentrates on influencing career progression, scholarly achievement and personal development over time (Richardson et al. 2022).

Effective strategies for recruitment and retention

The health workforce is globalised and 'not equitably distributed with a 6.5-fold difference in density between high-income and low-income countries' (Boniol et al., 2022, p. 1). The mobilisation and strengthening of human resources are seen as critical in sustainable health systems (Karimi, Cheng, Bartram, Leggat & Sarkeshik, 2014; Suriyankietkaew & Kungwanpongpun, 2022). The health (76%) and health management (64%) workforces in Australia are predominantly female, as compared to females employed in all industries (49%) and female managers in all industries (41%) (Martins & Isouard, 2024). The health workforce is multigenerational, multicultural and substantially female. It requires collaboration across sectors on an interprofessional basis and across organisational boundaries, within multidisciplinary teams and networks of service provision.

> **Recruitment:** The process of finding and hiring the best qualified candidate
>
> **Retention:** The degree to which an organisation is able to keep good employees satisfied so that they want to continue to work for that organisation
>
> **Competency:** A specific skill, knowledge or attribute required of a role

Managers need to focus on **recruitment** and **retention** of staff, the development of the workforce, issues of workforce substitution and the achievement of high-performance organisations that attract and retain the right people and provide a healthy work environment.

Liang, Leggat, Howard and Lee (2013) undertook research to identify core **competencies** that are important in developing the capability of health managers, identify staff development and training needs, and the implementation and conduct of performance management systems. The core competencies described are 'leadership; leading and managing change; operations, administration and resource management; evidence-informed decision-making; knowledge of healthcare environment and the organisation; interpersonal, communication qualities and relationship management' (Liang et al., 2013, p. 569). Competencies reflect specific skills and attributes required of a role, and **capability** is used to describe the capacity of individuals to successfully undertake the role and utilise the competencies. Capability goes to broader concepts of 'knowledge, skills and personal attributes' (Briggs, Smyth & Anderson, 2012, p. 73).

> **Capability:** The capacity of individuals to successfully undertake the role and utilise the competencies

Multiple generations

In order to manage and lead staff effectively, it is critical for managers to develop and implement human-resources strategies that take into consideration the four distinct generations employed in the health workforce.

This consideration is important because over recent times it has been reported that people have more employment changes and movement to new employers than occurred previously. As well, it has been reported that these career movement changes have been accompanied by greater diversity, with significant changes in occupational and career paths (Lyons, Schweitzer, Ng, Kai & Culpin, 2015). The study researched career changes for four generations of Canadian professionals. These groups were defined by the authors as: Matures (born prior to 1946), Baby Boomers (1946–1964), Generation Xers (1965–1979) and Millennials (1980 or later). Overall, the study reports significant differences among each group for employment and employer change. Interestingly, the young group, the Millennials, have the most significant changes in mobility.

These generational differences are often described in terms of values, beliefs, expectations and behaviours. Managers need to develop strategies to engage and retain these groups.

A good understanding of generational differences can often result in improved recruitment, retention, succession management, communication, employee engagement and conflict resolution (Jones, Murray & Tapp, 2018).

It has been reported that Millennial workers alone do not tend to link organisational commitment with workplace culture, whereas the other groups – Matures, Baby Boomers and Generation Xers – have a clear link of commitment with culture. The authors demonstrate that Millennials work differently than the other groups and that these differences can be linked to their focus on qualities such as duty, drive and reward (Stewart, Oliver, Cravens & Oishi, 2017). It was shown that through altering performance-evaluation methods to incorporate a range of measures, managers can influence the worker's sense of duty. By enabling greater transparency in the workplace, employers can increase the worker's motivation and show the reward that workers gain. As well, changes that enable new workers to adjust to the work environment can contribute to greater organisational efficiency and therefore greater benefits to all generations (Stewart et al., 2017).

MANAGING CONFLICT IN THE WORKPLACE

In a perfect situation, the workforce would operate in harmony. However, in the real world, conflict within the workplace is seemingly inevitable. Conflict is regarded as differences in perceived interest, values and behaviour among the individuals involved. The relationship between them may result in differences in behaviour (Martins, Isouard & Freshman, 2019). Workers and management nevertheless are expected to demonstrate sensible social skills and openness when conflict strikes (Schiro, 2021).

> ## MANAGING CONFLICT IN THE WORKPLACE Continued
>
> In most organisations there is someone perceived by management as the 'difficult worker', someone who does their job but does not engage in work activities outside the role, who is a champion of defending the status quo – 'the way we do things around here' – and is hence resistant to change, and who is admired by fellow workers for saying what they think and for standing up to management.
>
> Is such a worker really 'the problem', or is the issue more to do with how that person is managed? Based on experience with similar situations, I would spend informal time with this person in their work surrounds (not my office) and find out a bit more about them on a personal level. The experiences and skills that their life experience has provided may come as a surprise. I would ask them for their view or even advice about a particular problem I am confronting. I would find out if they have ever been away from work on a training course or on a visit to a similar facility or service, and if they have not I would make sure it happens in a purposeful way. I would also tell the staff member that I appreciate that they are well liked and respected by other staff and that I see this as something positive to be built on.
>
> This approach means practising an old but important management skill: engaging by walking and talking to staff, identifying issues and responding. If this is done skilfully, the potential of the staff member is developed, and they are empowered to want to come onside and be an effective contributor. This requires skill and effort but could be easier than performance-managing an underperformer out of the organisation.

Effective health teams

Increasingly, healthcare staff work in teams across sectors, in networks and in interprofessional contexts. The healthcare focus is on teamwork in safety and quality care, with one emphasis that comes from the experience of the aviation industry and its approach to crew resource management. Healthcare organisations draw on this experience to develop individual and team behaviours that alter how members communicate a problem or concern, which is viewed outside traditional approaches of apportioning blame, and how tasks are simplified and stepped (Clay-Williams & Colligan, 2015; Kar, 2019). Knowledge, skills and attitudes are summarised in terms of team effectiveness, as team leadership, mutual performance monitoring, backup behaviour or mutual support, communication and adaptability, shared mental models, collective orientation and mutual trust (Leggat & Balding, 2013).

High-performance work systems

The introduction of 'performance management in the health sector is closely related to the development of the concept of "performance in health"' itself (Vidya & Kothai, 2020, p. 4424). The term 'performance' signifies the ability of an organisation to attain desired outcomes within a defined set of parameters that are usually closely related to both the quality of actions and the quality of achievements (Vainieri, Noto, Ferre & Rosella, 2020). Through this process, new definitions of performance in healthcare are needed which control the activities and resources used to achieve those results.

Most members of the health workforce are regularly evaluated through performance reviews, which are based on key performance indicators, competencies, organisational objectives and the perceptions of peers and consumers, a process often referred to as 360-degree reviews. They may also be routinely involved in service reviews, and in how patients and clients generally perceive the quality of teams and services.

High-performance work systems are said to have a positive influence on employees' attitudes and behaviours (Nadeem, Riaz & Riswan, 2019). Several factors have been identified as critical for achieving high-performance work systems (Rabkin & Frein, 2021). These include clearly defined goals, purpose, mission and vision; a supportive organisational structure; demonstrated outstanding team leadership; appropriate health-worker engagement; and the presence of a psychologically safe environment for team members (Rabkin & Frein, 2021).

High-performance work system: A bundle of human-resource management practices related to better organisational performance

It is reported that there are three aspects linked to personal and organisational performance that can be employed in the development of the health-management workforce. These are personal engagement at work, emotional intelligence and conflict resolution (Martins et al., 2019). These key concepts were found to bind and strengthen the management of organisations.

Healthcare is optimal when delivered by high-performance teams that are supported by a culture of equity, support and inclusivity (Coleman, Dossett & Dimick, 2021). Cognitive diversity has been found to lead to increased performance as a result of shared understanding and optimising high-order problem solving. Diverse teams have been reported to outperform standard teams in organisations, as this diversity creates a positive creative culture (Coleman, Dossett & Dimick, 2021). An important contributing factor here is its grounding in inclusive recruitment practices. On the other hand, standard recruitment processes are acknowledged as being unsatisfactory due to the longstanding inequities and exclusion in health care.

Summary

- Human-resource management occurs in a complex, constantly changing organisational arrangement dominated by highly skilled health professionals.
- The context is dynamic and the workforce is global.
- The supply of the workforce is maldistributed, with shortages and projected inability to meet future demands.
- Human-resource leadership needs to increasingly focus on retention and on development of existing employees' skills bases.
- Critical human resource practices focus on engagement and empowerment of a flexible, adaptive workforce.

Reflective questions

1. If you were able to do so, how might you go about improving the number, distribution and skill-mix of the health workforce?
2. How well do you know your fellow workers or your staff? What generations are present?
3. Do you have an effective performance-management review system in your organisation?

4. Do you understand the need to develop leadership at the clinical, microsystem level?
5. How do you go about building knowledge by emphasising the importance of review and reflection?

Self-analysis questions

Research indicates that health-service managers need a high level of self-awareness of their own abilities, sound emotional stability and personal resilience to be able to effectively lead and manage others. Develop a list of the required characteristics identified in this chapter and self-assess your current status of preparedness in these areas. Discuss with mentors and colleagues where they think you need to focus your personal development.

References

Bakker, A. B., Schaufeli, W. B., Leiter, M. P. & Taris, T. W. (2008). Work engagement: An emerging concept in occupational health psychology, work & stress. *International Journal of Work, Health & Organisations, 22*(3), 187–200. https://doi.org/10.1080/02678370802393649

Boniol, M., Kunjumen, T., Nair, T. S., Siyam, A., Campbell, J. & Diallo, K. (2022). The global health workforce stock and distribution in 2020 and 2030: a threat to equity and universal health coverage?. *BMJ Global Health, 7*(6), e009316. https://doi.org/10.1136/bmjgh-2022-009316

Boon, C., Den Hartog, D. N. & Lepak, D. P. (2019). A systematic review of human resource management systems and their measurement. *Journal of Management, 45*(6), 2498–2537. https://doi.org/10.1177/0149206318818718

Briggs, D. S., Cruickshank, M. & Paliadelis, P. (2012). Health managers and health reform. *Journal of Management & Organisation, 18*(5), 641–658.

Briggs, D. S., Smyth, A. & Anderson, J. A. (2012). In search of capable health managers: What is distinctive about health management and why does it matter? *Asia Pacific Journal of Health Management, 7*(2), 71–78.

Cailhol, J., Craveiro, I., Madede, T., Makoa, E., Mathole, T., Parsons, A. N., Van Leemput, L., Biesma, R., Brugha, R., Chilundo, B., Lehmann, U., Dussault, G., Van Damme, W. & Sanders, D. (2013). Analysis of human resources for health strategies and policies in 5 countries in Sub-Saharan Africa, in response to GFATM and PEPFAR-funded HIV-activities. *Globalization and health, 9*(1), 52.

Clay-Williams, R. & Colligan, L. (2015). Back to basics: checklists in aviation and healthcare. *BMJ Quality & Safety, 24*(7), 428. https://doi.org/10.1136/bmjqs-2015-003957

Coleman, D. M. Dossett, L. A. & Dimick, J. B. (2021). Building high performing teams: Opportunities and challenges of inclusive recruitment practices. *Journal of Vascular Surgery, 74*(2), 86S–92S.

Dubois, C. A. & Singh, D. (2009). From staff-mix to skill-mix and beyond: Towards a systemic approach to health workforce management. *Human Resources for Health, 7*(87). https://doi.org/10.1186/1478-4491-7-87

Dumay, J., La Torre, M. & Farneti, F. (2019). Developing trust through stewardship *Journal of Intellectual Capital, 20*(1), 11–39.

Elijiz, K., Greenfield, D., Molineux, J. & Sloan, T. (2018). How to improve healthcare? Identify, nurture and embed individuals and teams with deep smarts. *Journal of Health Organisation and Management, 32*(1), 135–143.

Isouard, G., Thiessen, V., Stanton, P. & Hanson, S. (2006). Managing people in the health care industry. In M. G. Harris (ed.), *Managing health services: Concepts and practices* (2nd ed., pp. 114–314). Mosby Elsevier.

Jones, J.S., Murray, S.R. & Tapp, S.R. (2018). Generational differences in the workplace. *Journal of Business Diversity, 18*(2), 88–97.

Kao, S.F., Tsai, C.Y. & Schinke, R. (2021). Investigation of the interaction between coach transformational leadership and coaching competency change over time. *International Journal of Sports Science and Coaching, 16*(1), 44–53.

Kar, P. (2019). Applying aviation safety to healthcare – Are we missing the fundamental? *BMJ, 364*, 1735.

Karimi, L., Cheng, C., Bartram, T., Leggat, S. G. & Sarkeshik, S. (2014). The effects of emotional intelligence and stress-related presenteeism on nurses' well being. *Asia Pacific Journal of Human Resources*. https://doi.org/10.1111/1744-7941.12049

Leggat, S. C. & Balding, C. (2013). Achieving organisational competence for clinical leadership: The role of high performance work systems. *Journal of Health Organisation and Management, 27*(3), 312–329. https://doi.org/10.1108/jhom-jul-2012-0132

Liang, Z., Leggat, S. G., Howard, P. E. & Lee, K. (2013). What makes a hospital manager competent at the middle and senior levels? *Australian Health Review, 37*, 566–573. https://doi.org/10.1071/AH12004

Loh, E. (2015). Doctors as health managers: An oxymoron, or a good idea? *Journal of work-applied Management, 7*(1), 52–60.

Lyons, S.T., Schweitzer, L., Ng, E.S.W., Kai Peters, C.M. & Culpin, V. (2015). How have careers changed? An investigation of changing career patterns across four generations. *Journal of Managerial Psychology, 30*(1), 8–21.

Martins, J. M. & Isouard, G. (2024). Growing employment and managers in Australian health services 2006–2021. *Asia Pacific Journal of Health Management, 19*(1). https://doi.org/10.24083/apjhm.v19i1.3343

Martins, J. M., Isouard, G. & Freshman, B.D. (2019). Human dimension of health service management. *Australian Health Review, 43*(1) 103–110. https://doi.org/10.1071/AH17063

Moua, M. (2012). *Leading with cultural intelligence*. Saylor Foundation.

Nadeem, K., Riaz, A. & Riswan, Q. (2019). Influence of high-performance work system on employee service performance and OCB: the mediating role of resilience. *Journal of Global Entrepreneurship Research, 9*(13), 1–13.

Norman, P. (2022). *HR: The new agenda*. Knowledge Resources.

O'Leary, K. J., Johnson, J. K., Manojlovich, M., Goldstein, J. D., Lee, J. & Williams, M. V. (2019). Redesigning systems to improve teamwork and quality for hospitalized patients (RESET): Study protocol evaluating the effect of mentored implementation to redesign clinical microsystems. *BMC Health Services Research, 19*(1), 293.

Rabkin, S. & Frein, M. (2021). Overcoming obstacles to develop high-performance teams involving physician in health care organizations. *Healthcare Basel, 9*(9), 1136.

Richardson, E.L., Oetjen, R., Oetjen, D., Gordon, J., Schroeder, L. H., Conklin, S. & Strawn, N. (2022). Micro-advising and mentoring: Small interactions can have broad career-altering impact on learner career progression. *The Journal of Health Administration Education, 38*(4), 1001–1010.

Rumisha, S. F., Kishimba, R. S., Mohamed, A. A., Urio, L. J., Rusibayamila, N., Bakari, M. & Mghamba, J. (2020). Addressing the workforce capacity for public health surveillance through field epidemiology and laboratory training program: the need for balanced enhanced skill mix and distribution, a case study from Tanzania. *The Pan African Medical Journal, 36*(41), 41.

Schiro, H. (2021). Managing conflict in the workplace: Types and phases of conflict. *Journal of Organizational Culture, Communications and Conflict, 25*(S4), 1–2.

Stewart, J. S., Oliver, E. G., Cravens, K. S. & Oishi, S. (2017). Managing millennials: Embracing generational differences. *Business Horizons, 60*(1), 45–54.

Suriyankietkaew, S. & Kungwanpongpun, P. (2022). Strategic leadership and management factors driving sustainability in health-care organizations in Thailand. *Journal of Health Organisation and Management, 36*(4), 448–468.

Vainieri, M., Noto, G., Ferre, F. & Rosella, L. C. (2020). A performance management system in healthcare for all seasons? *International Journal of Environmental Research and Public Health*, *17*(15), 5590. https://doi.org/10.3390/ijerph17155590

Vidya, D. & Kothai, P. (2020). Factors that determine the effectiveness of performance management system: A review. *International Journal of Management*, *11*(12), 4423–4430.

Watts, T. (2011). A collective approach to skills development. *Strategic HR review*, *10*(1), 51.

Williamson, J. E. (2021). Mentorship builds strong leadership skills, confidence and competence. *Healthcare Purchasing News*, *45*(9), 41.

Zhang, L. (2023). The changing role of managers. *American Journal of Sociology*, *129*(2), 439–484.

Project management

Zhanming Liang

20

Learning objectives

How do I:

- improve my skills in project management?
- appreciate project-planning life cycles and the major characteristics of projects?
- recognise the fundamentals and important concepts in project management?
- identify useful project-management tools and resources?
- measure project success?

Introduction

Project management (PM) is a systematic management tool with techniques to bring people and resources together for a single purpose. Since its emergence in the architectural, engineering and building sectors in the early 1900s (Cleland & Gareis, 2006), PM has been systematically applied to other fields and industries as a common tool in managing work and achieving needed change. The rapidly changing operating environment and the frequent, system-wide and large-scale transformation in the health and community care sectors have inevitably changed the PM landscape. In the past 10 years, PM has experienced significant growth in complexity and scope in health and community care. The significant increases in the number of projects undertaken and the investment in developing PM competencies and tools have contributed to the growing project maturity in healthcare organisations (Gomes, Romão & Carvalho, 2016). PM has been broadly used to implement change, trial new service models, develop new programs and technologies, and improve organisational structure and care processes (Dwyer, Liang & Thiessen, 2019). The inclusion of PM competencies as core competencies for health-service managers, public health practitioners and those who may need to be involved in health-related projects further demonstrates its importance in health and community service provision.

This chapter explores the concepts of projects and PM, how projects should be planned and implemented, how to measure project success and, more importantly, how to use PM as a tool to achieve intended outcomes and generate new knowledge for future learning.

Definitions

Project: 'A unique set of inter-related activities designed to produce a set of deliverables and achieve a defined goal within clearly defined time, cost and quality constraints' (Dwyer et al., 2019, p. 2)

3D objective: Meeting quality performance and expectations within the timeframe and budget

Projects are an essential aspect of management in any organisation. Dwyer and colleagues (2019) state that the unique feature of projects can be defined as the **3D objective**, or project triangle: to meet performance expectations in both the scope and quality and within the planned timeframe and budget (see Figure 20.1).

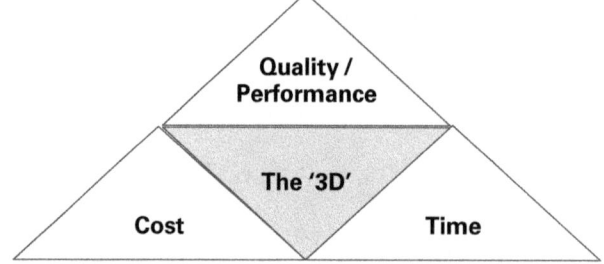

Figure 20.1 The 3D objective of a project

Source: Dwyer et al. (2019).

Project management: A systematic management process with techniques to bring people and resources together for a single purpose

Project management is a one-off effort to achieve a specific purpose; it may not have been done before, or at least not in the particular settings or circumstances, making project design and management challenging. However, projects have some common features and characteristics. For example, all projects have a beginning and end, require resources to support project activities, and move through a life cycle to meet milestones and achieve pre-determined project outcomes (Project Management Institute, 2021). Understanding these common features and factors that influence project progression is important to enable project success.

Frameworks

Although projects are highly varied in focus, size and complexity, they move through four common phases called a project life cycle and including initiation, planning, implementation and closing. This project framework outlines the normal progression of projects from initiation to completion (Kloppenborg, 2009). Figure 20.2 shows the four-phase framework of the project life cycle.

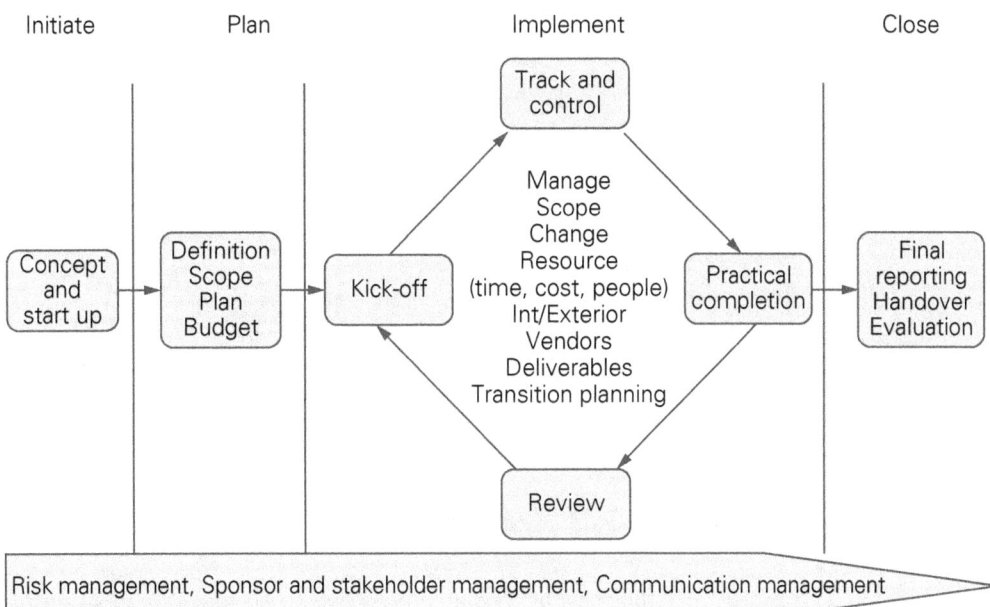

Figure 20.2 Project life cycle

Source: Dwyer et al. (2019).

As the names suggest, project development and management are not usually simple, linear processes but include many cycles of planning, implementation, evaluation and variation (Dwyer et al., 2019). In addition, the development and progression of a project is not clearly divided into phases. The phases included in the basic project framework are part of the joint project process, tend to overlap and often lack clear boundaries. However, having these phases in mind is useful not only for seeing the full picture, but also for better planning and managing each of these four phases. Moreover, projects do not generally proceed exactly as planned and can run backwards; for example, issues identified during project planning may lead to changes in the original design. Therefore, continuous monitoring – identifying problems or variations, modifying the plan and taking action – is a critical role for the project manager. Table 20.1 details possible steps to take during each of the four project phases.

Table 20.1 Key steps in project phases

Project phases	Key steps
Initiate	Identify a problem or opportunity. Develop and scope initial concept. Consider possible solutions and required resources. Identify key stakeholders and potential funders.
Plan	Clarify the goals and define the scope (how big is it?). Determine how, when and by whom the project will be done. Determine resource requirements. Develop stakeholder-engagement strategies. Determine evaluation measures (how project success is judged). Finalise a project plan including all key project components.
Implement	Carry out all tasks as detailed in the project plan. Check work progress regularly. Keep records and collect data necessary for project monitoring and evaluation. Develop interim project reports as per funding requirements. Manage people, stakeholders and risk. Monitor budget (expenses versus income). Meet reporting requirements as per funding/contractual conditions.
Close	Complete evaluation and evaluation report. Develop final project report and seek formal approval for sign-off. Prepare for handover. Maintain final communications to sponsors, funding bodies and key stakeholders. Celebrate with staff for project learning and project success.

Source: Dwyer et al. (2019).

Core components and development

A project has a clear goal to achieve explicitly stated objectives, well-understood strategies to achieve them, well-defined benefits or changes that can be produced and measured, a specified timeline for producing all the benefits or changes, and well-defined resources to implement the strategies and produce the deliverables. Project planning starts with defining problems to be solved, selecting ways of solving the problems and agreeing with the ultimate benefits of solving the problems. In the financially constrained healthcare environment, it is important that an evidence-based process is applied to the identification of problems and relevant solutions to maximise efficiency.

Hence, a rigorous **needs analysis** plays a key role in confirming the health or social problems experienced by a particular group or population, and the types of interventions or strategies that are most appropriate for addressing the problems. A needs analysis guides the design of a project and can ultimately address the proven problems by producing the desired outcomes through successful implementation and completion of the chosen strategies (Royse, Staton-Tindall, Badger & Webster, 2009). It is also worth noting that early consultation of key stakeholders, gaining senior management support and brainstorming among the potential project team are all critical steps in the project-planning phase (Dwyer et al., 2019).

Needs analysis: A comprehensive study or evaluation of the issues and needs of a particular situation

Project goal

A **project goal** is a statement of 'what the project will achieve in response to the problems that the project will address' (Dwyer et al., 2019 p. 65). For example, if an identified problem is high prevalence of type 2 diabetes within the 35–44 years age group in a specified municipal area, a project can be planned with an overall goal of testing the effectiveness of the proposed strategy or intervention in reducing the prevalence of type 2 diabetes within a certain time period among the identified target group. Proven outcomes and learnings from the project will guide the development of a continuing health promotion and intervention program in the municipal area.

Project goal:
A statement of 'what the project will achieve in response to the problems and/or opportunities that the project will address' (Dwyer, Liang & Thiessen, 2019, p. 65)

Project objectives

Project objectives are the immediate outcomes and intermediate benefits that the project needs to produce before achieving the overall project goal (Dwyer et al., 2019).

Ultimately, the achievement of the overarching project goals is the result of achieving the more specific, immediate actions or changes in the course of the project. For example, to achieve a reduction in the prevalence of type 2 diabetes, several changes have to be brought about in the target population, such as adequate daily intake of vegetables and fruit, commitment to daily physical activities, and then reduction in overall body mass index. Sound project objectives should meet the SMART criteria (Doran, 1981): specific, measurable, achievable, realistic and timely.

Project objectives:
Statements of what the project will achieve at a lower level and the intermediate benefits that the project needs to produce

Project strategies

A **project strategy** constitutes a series of related actions designed to achieve the project's objectives, and ultimately contributes to attaining the broader project goal (Eagar, Garrett & Lin, 2001). It describes how the project is going to achieve one or more objectives. A single strategy can contribute to achieving one or more strategies. Using the example of reducing the prevalence of type 2 diabetes, key strategies may be the promotion of good dietary habits through a media campaign and workshops, and organisation of regular physical activities for the target group. Although projects vary in size, achieving the project's goal is normally not a one-step approach. Project teams need to complete many steps, monitoring the results of these steps before the problems can be solved and the project goal is achieved.

It is important to note that a project's goal, objectives and strategies should be closely aligned to the problems that the project is going to solve. The project designer needs to ensure that all intermediate changes that are important in achieving the overarching goal can be produced by implementing all the strategies. Hence, all the intermediate changes that the strategies can produce are captured in the forms of objectives.

Project strategy:
A collection of actions to achieve project goals

Project plan

Once the goal, objectives and strategies for a proposed project are clear, planning the activities, timing and resources needed to achieve them is the next step. There are many tools and methods for this, such as work breakdown structures, Gantt chart and linear responsibility charts, which can make planning easier. To complete this step, the project team needs to carry out the following tasks, identified by Dwyer and colleagues (2019):

- Document all the key activities and associated tasks that must be completed in order to achieve the objectives.
- Break down the activities and tasks into manageable chunks – a mechanism for decomposing the project goals into manageable tasks to enable estimation of project time and costs (Kliem, 2007).
- Identify the resources required to complete each of the tasks.
- Explore the relationships and dependencies between the tasks.
- Put activities and tasks in the right sequence; some my run in parallel.
- Estimate how long the project will take and any deadlines (or critical points) within the project.

These steps can be time-consuming. For large and complex projects, extensive experience and expertise in projects and PM maybe required. Hence, inputs from colleagues with various levels of expertise and experience maybe very helpful in giving inexperienced project designers the required confidence and experience. Project strategies cannot work unless there is a clear action plan, with the necessary staff, resources and equipment at hand. Estimation also needs to take into consideration the additional time and resources required for pretest strategies, when these are considered necessary. For example, a project team developing a training workshop for a large population group could pretest it on a small sample to discover whether the training and materials are relevant and appropriate. Modifications and revisions to the workshop and relevant materials may then be required before rolling it out to the target population group. These activities should be identified in the planning stages and written into the plan.

Deliverables: The products, services or outcomes provided as the result of a project

Work breakdown structure: 'A tool that the project team uses progressively to divide the work of a project into smaller and smaller pieces' (Kloppenborg, 2009, p. 142)

The simplest way to make a project plan is to start with a clear problem statement, the goals, strategies and **deliverables**, simplifying them with subheadings and expanding them into a list format. In PM terms, this is called creating a **work breakdown structure** (WBS): 'a tool that the project team uses progressively to divide the work of a project into smaller and smaller pieces' (Kloppenborg, 2009, p. 142) and a mechanism for decomposing the project goals into manageable tasks to allow estimation of project time and costs to take place (Project Management Institute, 2021).

The process of building a good WBS forces significant issues to arise early rather than late in a project, and also provides the basis for estimating the time and cost of the overall project. WBS is a powerful tool for expressing the scope of a project in a simple graphic format (Dwyer et al., 2019). The two common approaches in developing a WBS are deliverable-based WBS and phase-based WBS.

Evaluation and learning

Project evaluation can be a powerful method of producing evidence required to secure future project or program funding and building cumulative knowledge for later projects. It provides an opportunity to reflect on outcomes, processes, organisation and methods. It assists funders to make informed decisions about whether to support the continuation or extension of a project (South Australian Community Health Research Unit, 2012) and for organisations to learn from their project experience and apply that knowledge to the design and conduct of future projects. Evaluation requires the collection of different types of data throughout the project, hence the consideration and design of evaluation needs to be included in the project's planning process. It does not just magically happen at the project's end (Dwyer et al., 2019).

Regardless of whether the evaluation is simple or complex, it needs to be planned and built into the project at the planning stage to guide the correct collection at the right time of the most appropriate types of information (Dwyer et al., 2019). One of the reasons the benefits of evaluation can be compromised is not planning it early enough to enable important data to be collected on time.

To conduct project evaluation, a range of qualitative and quantitative methods and data collection techniques can be employed. Following are some examples of methods that can be used to collect information for evaluation:

- **analysis of records** – attendance, admission and demographic details
- **surveys** – mail and email
- **interviewing individuals** – face-to-face and by telephone or videoconferencing
- **interviewing groups** – focus group discussions
- **documentation** – journals, diaries, logs and progress reports
- **triangulation** – combining and comparing data from different sources and methods.

Different types of evaluation seek to answer different questions at different stages of the project. To understand project progression, questions include: Is the project going well? Did we do what we set out to do? Is the project likely to produce the benefits as planned? To understand whether the project is achieving the intended immediate benefits or changes as stated in the objectives, evaluation involves asking: Has the project achieved all its intended objectives and are they directly and indirectly relevant to the target population or the goal recipients? A period after the project has been concluded, it is important to ask: Were the benefits achieved at the end of the project sustained over time? Have the long-term benefits been realised as anticipated?

The four basic evaluation types include process, impact, outcome and economic evaluation, which may require different approaches.

Process evaluation

Process evaluation measures the effectiveness of strategies and methods used in the project and assesses and monitors how they are implemented. It gives people real-time feedback on what is happening and whether the planned outputs and deliverables have been produced, which can enhance the project's chance of success. Process evaluation also provides an indication of whether the project team has completed all the required steps essential to producing the intended outcomes.

Process evaluation: A measure of the effectiveness of the strategies and methods used in the project and the extent to which planned outputs and deliverables are produced

Impact evaluation

Impact evaluation measures the achievement of the project's short-term effects as stated in the project's objectives. It should be conducted immediately after the project has been conducted or implemented, but not before all activities and strategies have been executed as planned. However, data collection may commence at the beginning of the project, such as collecting baseline data. For large and complex projects, impact evaluation requires substantial planning, which may include choosing or designing **indicators** to measure the complex changes and the effects of complex changes.

Impact evaluation: A measure of the achievement of the project's short-term effects, normally called 'project objectives'

Indicator: Signals of the success of a project

Outcome evaluation

Outcome evaluation: A measure of the longer-term achievements of the project, which are closely related to the project's goal

Outcome evaluation measures the longer-term achievements of the project, which are closely related to the project's goal. Both impact and outcome evaluations measure effects, benefits or intended changes, focusing on assessing the effects of the completed project over different time periods (Hawe, Degeling & Hall, 1990). Since outcome evaluation takes places after the project has been completed, it is not commonly built into evaluation plans for projects, especially small projects in health and community services (Dwyer et al., 2019).

Economic evaluation

Economic evaluation: An estimate of the relative value of alternative options using a range of economic and financial techniques

When financial constraints are present, economic considerations become paramount: resource allocation decisions should maximise efficient use of those resources. **Economic evaluation** estimates the relative value of alternative options including benefits and costs (Gray & Wilkinson, 2016) and is designed to help decision-makers answer the following questions: Is this project worth doing compared with other projects we could do with the same resources? and 'Are we satisfied that resources should be spent in this way rather than another way?' (Dwyer et al., 2019, p. 135).

Economic evaluation of interventions or services has three main methods: cost-effectiveness analysis, cost–benefit analysis and cost–utility analysis. This type of evaluation requires specific levels of expertise and is generally conducted by an economist. However, it is important to be aware of what it is and when it should be commissioned.

PROJECT GOAL, OBJECTIVES AND STRATEGIES

This case study outlines the specific project-planning features and how goals, objectives and strategies are developed.

Problem statement: There has been an increased number of falls among residents of a high-care nursing home in the past 2 years. Residents' fear of falling has led to their reduced activity, affecting their functioning and further increasing the risk of seriously harmful falls.

Project timeframe: 1 year

Project target population: Residents at the high-care nursing home

Project goal: To reduce falls among elders at the high-care nursing home, improve mobility and reduce mortality

Project objectives:

- To improve residents' commitment to regular physical activities within 6 months
- To increase residents' balance and strength by 20 per cent within 12 months
- To reduce the incidence of falls by 50 per cent within 12 months

Project strategies:

- To develop an exercise program in the high-care nursing home by the end of the second month and to implement the program throughout the project
- To implement a falls monitoring system in the high-care nursing home by the end of the third month

- To develop and implement a regular falls-risk assessment method and procedure by the end of 6 months
- To ensure all staff are competent in applying falls-prevention methods and following the falls-prevention procedure by the end of 8 months
- To identify and remove the falls hazards in the facility by the end of the 8th month.

Management of projects

Achieving good project outcomes depends upon sound PM, which includes having the right person in the role of project manager. Effective project managers can get the job done, keep the project moving, understand what the project must achieve. They are responsive to contingencies, open and flexible, aware of the situation and able to deal with crises. For a small project, all tasks may be completed by the project manager, who takes on all functions that are required for the implementation of the project. However, for larger and more complex projects, many other roles may be involved that will build up a project team. These roles may include a project director, project manager, group leader, team member and technical manager. Having PM skills among health managers has become relatively common in the past decade.

Given the uniqueness of projects, PM requires a balance between strong content knowledge and PM ability. Therefore, as Dwyer and colleagues (2019, pp. 58–59) suggest, general skills and knowledge required for PM may include some or all of the following:

- leadership ability, particularly to create and share the vision for project success and to motivate the team and stakeholders
- discipline and drive, including application to the task, taking responsibility, decisiveness and ability to work effectively at both strategic and detail levels
- excellent communication and interpersonal skills, which involves talking to the right people, influencing others, building consensus, making the project visible, negotiating, lobbying for the project and managing conflict
- initiative and organisation, including working independently, meeting deadlines and ensuring follow-through
- technical PM skills, know-how and experience
- knowledge of the working environment and the ability to adapt tools and methods to suit
- analysis and reflection, which involves monitoring progress, understanding risks, ability to read situations, flexibility and responsiveness.

Structure and stakeholders

Each project is unique; however, it does not stand alone and is part of an organisation's activities. Understanding of how the project fits into the organisational structure is extremely important, as it demonstrates the line of accountability and reporting requirements, and makes managers aware of where and how to seek help in times of doubt and when difficulties are encountered. Since a project is usually a way of trialling new ideas, internal and external expertise and guidance can minimise mistakes in project design and implementation. Such expertise and guidance can be provided formally, by way of establishing an advisory committee.

A project advisory committee consists of representatives from project sponsors, key stakeholders and project staff, usually providing advice and support, and helping the project to succeed as planned. The design of advisory committees, and their ways of working, will depend partly on whether the project is internally or externally focused. It is important that the role of the advisory committee is clarified upon its establishment.

Project sponsors are individuals and/or organisations that provide funding or financial support (including in-kind donations) to a project. Stakeholders are the individuals and/or organisations that are actively involved in the project, whose interests may be affected because of the project or who may exert influence over the project and its results (Project Management Institute, 2021, p. 34). Stakeholders bring positive influence or risk to the project. It is important that they are identified and their interests are understood in the project-planning phase. Increasing evidence has shown that adopting a co-design approach by working closely with key stakeholders in the design and implementation of a project is one of the keys to project success. It ensures that 'ideas' can be turned into workable solutions suitable to the specific context (Bird et al., 2021; Slattery, Saeri & Bragge, 2020).

Methods

PM methodology is an approach that can guide the conceptualisation of project ideas, understanding of the required tasks of managing a project and 'use of project management tools and techniques that enable projects to progress in effective, disciplined and reliable ways' (Dwyer et al., 2019, p. 50). However, the use of PM methods does not guarantee successful project outcomes, and a fixed method may not always work. For example, some government departments have adopted specific PM methods as frameworks, with or without local modifications, thus making them too rigid for project staff to use. If the project involves a tender process or is subject to certain funding requirements, some standardised methods may be stipulated as part of the funding arrangement.

There are several methods of PM in use in the health and community services sector – for example, the Project Management Body of Knowledge (Project Management Institute, 2021); PRINCE2®, which stands for PRojects IN Controlled Environments (Central Computer and Telecommunications Agency, 1997); and the Agile approach (Alexander, 2018). In health and community services, many organisations use their own in-house tools and methods. While certain principles and methods are necessary for project success, in most instances there is no single best approach (Dwyer et al., 2019).

Tools

A project team may use specific PM tools to achieve project tasks. Common tools are Gantt and PERT charts, and computerised scheduling and tracking tools such as Microsoft Project and Mac Project (Dwyer et al., 2019). Organisations may provide project teams with standard tools and templates for project proposals, plans, communications, risk management, and status and variation reporting. Some organisations may use specific software programs to facilitate PM processes. It is useful for project managers to check what resources are available in the workplace.

Project managers require knowledge of when and how to use the available tools and techniques as PM tools may be effective in certain contexts, industries or organisations but not in others. In addition, many tools and techniques may be ineffective unless they are supported by strong management practices such as effective negotiation, communication, leadership, use of alliances and networks, and change-management methods (Dwyer et al., 2019; Ershadi, Jefferies, Davis & Mojtahedi, 2020; Ellahi, Rehman, Javed, Sultan & Rehman, 2022). Organisations in health and community services generally use local adaptations of PM methods and tools to guide project design, implementation and management.

Summary

- Large projects are unique and complex, and vary in scope and need.
- A project is a cycle not a linear process. Project life cycle has four phases: initiation, preparation, implementation and closure.
- Project planning involves the development of achievable goals, objectives and strategies.
- Many frameworks, models and tools can be used to assist in project design and PM; the key is to select the approach that is suitable to the project and its context.
- Understanding the needs of key stakeholders and engaging them in the design and implementation process are key to project success.
- Evaluation is critical for project learning and should be included in the project-planning phase.

Reflective questions

1. What makes projects unique?
2. What are the key phases in a typical project life cycle?
3. Why is project planning not a linear process?
4. What are the purposes of work breakdown structures in project planning?
5. What are reasons for project evaluation and the basic evaluation types?

Self-analysis question

Projects have become a common part of getting work done in health and community services. As a manager in your organisation, how could you improve PM competence among your staff so that PM tools are properly used to implement changes and trial new ideas?

References

Alexander, M. (2018). Agile project management: 12 key principles, 4 big hurdles. *CIO*. Retrieved from: https://www.cio.com/article/3156998/agile-project-management-a-beginners-guide.html

Bird, M., McGillion, M., Chambers, E.M. et al. (2021). A generative co-design framework for healthcare innovation: Development and application of an end-user engagement framework. *Res Involv Engagem 7, 12.* https://doi.org/10.1186/s40900-021-00252-7

Central Computer and Telecommunications Agency. (1997). *PRINCE 2: An outline*. Stationery Office.

Cleland, D. & Gareis, R. (2006). *Global project management handbook.* McGraw-Hill Professional.

Doran, G. T. (1981). There's a S.M.A.R.T. way to write management's goals and objectives (PDF). *Management Review, 70*(11), 35–36.

Dwyer, J., Liang, Z. & Thiessen, V. (2019). *Project management in health and community services: Getting good ideas to work* (4th ed.). Allen & Unwin.

Eagar, K., Garrett, P. & Lin, V. (2001). *Health planning: Australian perspectives.* Allen & Unwin.

Ellahi, A., Rehman, M., Javed, Y., Sultan, F. & Rehman, H. M. (2022). Impact of servant leadership on project success through mediating role of team motivation and effectiveness: A case of software industry. *SAGE Open, 12*(3). https://doi.org/10.1177/21582440221122747

Ershadi M., Jefferies M., Davis P. & Mojtahedi M. (2020). Towards successful establishment of a project portfolio management system: business process management approach. *Journal of Modern Project Management, 23*(8), 1–20.

Gomes, J., Romão, M. & Carvalho, H. (2016). Successful IS/IT projects in healthcare: Pretesting a questionnaire. *Procedia Computer Science, 100*, 375–382. http://dx.doi.org/10.1016/j.procs.2016.09.172

Gray, A. M. & Wilkinson, T. (2016). Economic evaluation of healthcare interventions: Old and new directions, *Oxford Review of Economic Policy, 32*(1), 102–121.

Hawe, P., Degeling, D. & Hall, J. (1990). *Evaluating health promotion: A health worker's guide.* Maclennan & Petty.

Kliem, R. L. (2007). *Effective communications for project management.* Auerbach.

Kloppenborg, T. J. (2009). *Contemporary project management: Organize, plan, perform.* South-Western Cengage Learning.

Project Management Institute (PMI). (2021). *A guide to the project management body of knowledge (The PMBOK guide)* (7th ed.). PMI.

Royse, D., Staton-Tindall, M., Badger, K. & Webster, J.M. (2009). *Needs assessment pocket guide to social work research methods.* Oxford University Press.

Slattery, P., Saeri, A. K. & Bragge, P. (2020). Research co-design in health: A rapid overview of reviews. *Health Research Policy and Systems, 18*(17). https://doi.org/10.1186/s12961-020-0528-9

South Australian Community Health Research Unit. (2012). *Planning and evaluation wizard.* Flinders University.

Financial management 21

Christine Dennis
With acknowledgement to Ian Edwards

Learning objectives

How do I:

- use assets, liabilities, equity, revenues and expenses in the financial management of a service, department or organisation?
- develop an appropriate budget and cashflow?
- enhance my organisation's financial position through a casemix classification and funding system?
- use variance analysis to improve the performance of my service, department or organisation?

Introduction

The financial management of healthcare organisations is a key management responsibility for both public and private facilities. While this responsibility has always been important, it is becoming increasingly so with the rising costs of healthcare provision due to advances in technology and rising rates of chronic disease and ageing populations. The responsible use and management of scarce healthcare resources requires knowledge and information. The accounting process provides the necessary information to develop and monitor a budget. However, it is the financial management of the budget and associated activity levels that provide the necessary framework to ensure budget integrity and financial governance.

Financial accounting is mainly concerned with the transactions of accounting, with the systematic recording of the financial events of the organisation. The main accounting groups are:

- **Assets** are items of value owned or controlled by an organisation, such as cash, inventories or land.
- **Liabilities** are amounts owed by an organisation to external parties, such as loans or wages.
- **Equity** is the funds invested in the organisation by its owner, either as capital investment or as retained earnings.
- **Revenues** (or income) are the flows of resources into an organisation from government, grants, sales or services performed.
- **Expenses** are outflows of resources from the organisation to purchase goods or services, or to carry out its general operations.

These five basic accounting groups represent the essence of how financial information is recorded to provide the means for financial management.

The basic accounting equation is represented in the relationship between the assets, liabilities and owner's equity of a business. It can be expressed as assets equal liabilities plus equity or equity equals assets minus liabilities. Perhaps the easiest way to understand this equation is to relate it to purchasing a house:

$$\text{equity (amount invested or owned)} = \text{asset (value of house)} - \text{liability (mortgage)}$$

Suppose the relationship between the asset, liability and equity in this house purchase is as follows:

$$\text{asset (\$500 000)} = \text{liability (\$200 000)} + \text{equity (\$300 000)}$$

In this example, the equity (or the amount owned by the purchaser) is $300 000. The house is valued at $500 000 minus the loan or mortgage of $200 000.

Types of budgets

Simply put, a budget is written plan of what managers expect to happen in the future in terms of dollar inflows (revenue) and outflows (expenses). Budgets play a pivotal role in the operational decision-making of the organisation.

There are many different types of budgets. However, each budget's use and application depends on its purpose as well as the size and financial maturity of the organisation (King,

Clarkson & Wallace, 2010). There is no single type of budget that fits all circumstances. As organisations mature, they typically move from a historical type of budget to a zero-based or activity-based budget. However, the cost of developing the information required to support construction of a more sophisticated budget needs to be taken into consideration.

Prior to 2011, Australian public hospitals mainly used historical budgeting. Hospitals would develop budgets for the following year based upon the previous financial year's budget allocation or simply based upon the actual expenditure of the previous year. The difficulties inherent in this approach included a lack of flexibility to adjust the budget for increases in volume or activity during the budget period; a lack of emphasis on control mechanisms to ensure that funds are being utilised in the most efficient and effective manner, and an inability to effectively **benchmark** activity, efficiency and health outcomes.

The National Health Reform Agreement, signed by the Australian government and all jurisdictions in August 2011, shifted the funding model for public hospitals to activity-based funding where practicable.

Regardless of the funding model, the development of a budget can drive planned approaches to the allocation of resources and evaluation of performance (Gapenski & Pink, 2007). There are several different approaches available in constructing a budget. The major approaches include those discussed in the following section.

Benchmark: To measure and compare services with an agreed standard (Heslop, 2012)

Global budgets

In a global budget, funds are allocated to an organisation as a bulk amount. It is then the responsibility of the organisation to distribute the funds internally. This type of budgeting is often referred to as 'base budget allocation' and is usually determined on an incremental basis, with the previous year's final budget allocation plus a percentage increase. This method leaves little scope for new services or initiatives other than those funded from efficiency savings; however, it does enable resources to be reallocated and reprioritised within the organisation and within a predetermined amount.

Historical budgets

Historical budgets are also known as static, fixed or forecast budgets. They are developed on the premise that revenue and expenditure will remain relatively constant from one year to the next. Historical budgeting is designed to maintain the status quo. Historical budgets are primarily based on the belief that business operations will continue in the same fashion. At times, it may leave little room for sudden changes, such as adapting to events such as the COVID-19 pandemic (Reed, 2021).

Flexible budgets

This type of budget is adjusted for changes in the unit level of the cost driver. For example, a flexible budget can be based on the previous year's budget but make allowance for adjustments to the budget depending on variable factors such as occupancy rates and planned workload.

Zero-based budgets

Zero-based budgets take an approach that ignores (to some extent) the previous year's budget allocation and expenditure, and uses the assumption that the budget is to be developed from scratch. While zero-based budgeting encourages the supply of detailed and strategic information into the budgetary process, it can be extremely time-consuming in its development (Dionne, Mitton, Smith & Donaldson, 2009).

Activity-based budgets

This is a method of budgeting for activities and services that incur costs in every functional area of the organisation. The budget is developed in terms of the cost of an organisation's products and services – for example, the cost of providing an occupied bed day in an orthopaedic ward. The budget is developed on the basis of the specific activity targets that are planned for each area of the organisation. A critical part of activity-based budgeting is the development of a plan for the level of activity that is likely to be performed by the organisation (Heslop, 2012). The budget that is developed relates to the level of activity that is planned for that area of the organisation and is the composite of the cost associated with each production activity multiplied by the quantity (Zhang & Bohlen, 2023)

Importantly, activity-based funding enables health services to get paid for the number and mix of patients they treat, to measure what they do and what that activity costs compared to an agreed price.

> ### BUDGETING FOR THE FUTURE
>
> Martin is the nurse manager of a busy ward in a large public hospital. He has been in this position for the previous 4 years. During this time, Martin has noticed an increase in both the number and complexity of patients. However, there has been little change in the annual budget other than a notional increase each year that reflects consumer price index. Nursing staff have also noticed the change during this period and have raised this concern in several team meetings, stating that nursing staff in other wards in the hospital 'do not have to work as hard as they do, they seem to have less complex patients and a higher staffing establishment'.
>
> Martin has discussed the situation with senior management and the finance manager. However, the historic budgeting process used by the hospital does not enable an increase in budget without other areas receiving reduced budgets. While this might sound like a simple solution, moving financial resources from one area to another can create problems where there are fixed costs (staffing or utilities) and fixed budget expectations and also assumes that the factors that influenced past financial performance will remain consistent in the future; that is, the ward that appears 'less busy' may see an increase in activity in future.
>
> A new finance manager is appointed to the facility and receives executive management approval to implement activity-based budgets. Martin is sceptical that the new budgeting process will make any difference but acknowledges that better alignment of activity with budget will increase transparency and contribute to a more equitable approach.
>
> The finance manager outlines that this budget approach takes into consideration that care of some patient groups is more complicated and resource-intensive than others. Martin is now able to monitor his budget allocation along with performance against commissioned activity. The data also enables him to benchmark outcomes, identify inefficient practices and reduce unnecessary costs.

Healthcare funding

Healthcare sectors in Australia are funded differently, which can influence both the budgeting process and the ongoing management of funding. The funding for public hospitals is provided from a range of different sources; however, most funding is provided by national (42%) and state/territory (52.5%) governments. The bulk of the funding that is provided by the government is capped. This **capped funding** affects the development and management of the budget and the levels of service. Both must be managed to ensure that the budget revenue and expenses are balanced. In contrast, while private hospitals also receive their funding from different sources, this funding is not capped. This is a significant difference and enables private hospitals to use activity-based budgets that can change during the budget period, based on the levels of clinical activity.

Capped funding: A set amount or level of funding to the healthcare facility to provide services; it does not increase if additional services are provided above the funded levels of activity

About two-thirds of the funding for residential aged care is provided by the Australian federal government. Subsidies are paid directly to aged-care homes on behalf of their residents. The Australian National Aged Care Classification (AN-ACC) funding model confirms the subsidy based on service type and each resident's care needs. Also, residents who can afford to do so contribute to the cost of their care.

Expenditure is contained by capping the number of subsidised aged-care places by approved providers.

Casemix

Casemix is a generic term for the method of classifying the activities that health services deliver.

The origins of casemix can be traced to surgeon Ernest Codman (1869–1940) in the United States, who proposed methods of standardising and comparing outputs and outcomes between different hospitals. Acknowledged as the 'founder of outcomes-based patient care', Codman believed that information on patient outcomes should be made public in order to guide patient choice. Important to note is that casemix was founded in clinical terms, not in financial or economic terms (Heslop, 2012).

Casemix-based hospital funding was introduced in Australia in the early 1990s and in Aotearoa New Zealand in 1998–99. The previous standards of measuring activity, based on occupied bed days and admitted patients, evolved into a system that considers the **acuity** of the patient and the cost of the likely resources to be used.

Acuity: The level of clinical care required by the patient based on their condition

For a casemix classification system to be useful, several design principles must be incorporated (Madden, 2013). Firstly, to be useful, classification systems in health must have clinical meaning. Patients in the same class should be similar from a clinical perspective. Episodes of care in the same class should contain similar diagnoses and treatments. Secondly, homogeneous resource use is required. The cost of the health care provided should be approximately the same for all patients within the same class. Finally, there should be about the right number of classes in the system – that is, not too many classes and not too few.

There are several casemix-based funding instruments being used in Australia – for example, the AN-ACC funding model (previously the Aged Care Funding Instrument) and the Australian Refined Diagnostic Related Groups (sometimes called AR-DRGs). The diagnosis-related groups classification provides a clinically meaningful way to classify acute admitted patient episodes in public and private hospitals. Episodes of care are assigned disease and intervention codes by health-information managers or clinical coders. AR-DRGs are then assigned based on these codes and several other routinely collected variables including age, sex, separation mode, length of stay and, for example, admission birthweight for neonates (https://www.ihacpa.gov.au/health-care/classification/admitted-acute-care/ar-drgs).

Each episode of care is assigned to one of 23 major diagnostic categories. Most of these categories are defined by major organ systems of the body and correspond with a particular medical or surgical specialty – for example, the respiratory system. The classification of patient episodes of care to AR-DRGs enables an accurate method of understanding the type and level of clinical activity within a hospital. In addition, each diagnostic-related group is allocated a weight, which has been calculated to represent the acuity of the service provided and the average use of resources in comparison to other groups.

> A National Weighted Activity Unit (NWAU) is a measure of health service activity expressed as a common unit against which a National Efficient Price (NEP) is paid. It provides a way of comparing and valuing each public hospital service, whether they are emergency department presentations, admissions or outpatient episodes, weighted for clinical complexity. (National Health Funding Body, 2023, n. p.)

> The average hospital service is worth one NWAU – the most intensive and expensive activities are worth multiple NWAU, the simplest and least expensive are worth fractions of an NWAU (National Health Funding Body, 2023, n. p.)

As part of the activity-based funding model, the efficient price of a public hospital service is calculated by multiplying the NWAU allocated to that service by the national efficient price (NEP) for that financial year. For example, in 2022–23 the NEP was $5797 per NWAU:

- A tonsillectomy has a weight of 0.7400 NWAU, which equates to $4290.
- A coronary bypass (minor complexity) has a weight of 5.3925 NWAU, which equates to $31 260.
- A hip replacement (minor complexity) has a weight of 3.4152 NWAU, which equates to $19 798.

The Independent Health and Aged Care Pricing Authority provides a national benchmarking portal that improves health managers' ability to compare differences in cost, activity and efficiency at similar hospitals using the NWAU.

Casemix and other contexts

Increasingly, other sectors are moving to a casemix-based system of allocating funds. In October 2022, the aged-care funding system transitioned from the Australian Aged Care Funding Instrument to the AN-ACC to enable improved capacity to identify the care needs of aged-care residents and provide funds accordingly. The tool considers physical ability, cognitive ability, behaviour and mental health.

The key components of a funding allocation system are shown in Table 21.1. Importantly, any funding allocation system should:

- Ensure equitable allocation of funds.
- Enable sound business decisions about resource allocation.

- Analyse the link between the costs and funding of services, and the care provided.
- Provide a basis for comparison of activity and outcomes.
- Drive the most efficient and effective use of resources.

Table 21.1 Key components of a funding allocation system

Product identification and classification	A system of taxonomies that adequately classifies care across different care types and settings and to a level that enables variation in complexity and care needs.
Product counting	A system that supports accurate, electronic counting of all patient-related services, linking clinical and accounting feeder systems.
Product costing	Product-level costing with as close to full cost absorption as possible, yielding a recognised unit cost per product type.
Data management, analysis and reporting	Data management, analysis and reporting provide a supporting element for counting, costing and benchmarking while supporting flexible local reporting requirements.
Funding	A system of activity-based funding based on accepted activity-based costs and classification of products.
Governance and management	A model of clinical and corporate governance at a jurisdictional and regional or local level. It includes activity-based management systems and processes.

Source: Department for Health and Wellbeing (2022).

Reforms in funding

There has been significant change to Australian public hospital funding arrangements over the past decade. A key feature of this reform was the introduction of national activity-based funding, which commenced in July 2012 following a signed National Health Reform Agreement between the Australian government and all states and territories, committing to the funding of public hospitals using activity-based funding where practicable.

The Independent Hospital Pricing Authority (IHPA) was established as a statutory authority in December 2011 by the *National Health Reform Act 2011* (Cth). In 2022, IHPA commenced a formal transition as its functions expanded to include the provision of costing and pricing advice on aged-care services. The authority subsequently changed its name to the Independent Health and Aged Care Pricing Authority. The authority is responsible for determining the national efficient price for healthcare services provided by public hospitals where the services are funded on an activity basis.

The National Health Reform Agreement 2020 to 2025 continues to drive agendas focused on delivering high-quality care, prioritising prevention, best practice and improving efficiency to ensure financial sustainability.

Additionally, there is increasing interest in complementing activity-based funding models with other approaches such as value-based health care and bundled payments. Pay-for-performance models reward specific, measurable aspects of value. An example of pay-for-performance is the Medicare Practice Incentive Program, which rewards general practices for targeted levels of care in areas such as diabetes and asthma.

Management and financial performance

An organisation's financial performance must be planned and controlled with sound budgeting procedures and as thoroughly as possible if acceptable results are to be achieved. This statement holds true for both public and private organisations. While public organisations do not operate for profit, they are responsible for delivering services to the public within an allocated budget. Both public and private healthcare organisations depend on the development of budgets to plan for the effective use of the available resources (Horngren, Datar & Foster, 2006). The major benefits of budgeting are that:

- It forces management to plan and anticipate the future on a systematic basis.
- It provides management with realistic performance targets against which results can be compared.
- It coordinates the various segments of the organisation.
- It serves as a communication device with which the various managers can exchange information concerning goals, ideas and achievements.

Costs

The development and subsequent monitoring of a budget requires an understanding of the various types of costs and their behaviours. The total costs of an activity or service consist of three types of costs, and their relationship can be expressed as:

$$\text{total costs} = \text{fixed costs} + \text{semi-variable costs} + \text{variable costs}.$$

Fixed costs have to be paid regardless of the level of activity or production – for example, rent, security staff and maintenance contracts. Variable costs change in direct proportion to the level of activity or production. The greater the level of activity, the greater the variable costs – for example, clinical drugs and pathology. Semi-variable costs are fixed in the short term but vary over time or with large changes in activity or production – for example, the availability of an additional CT scanner due to patient demand.

In addition to fixed, semi-variable and variable costs, direct and indirect costs also need to be considered in developing a budget. Direct costs can be directly associated with the activity or production, and they can be either fixed or variable depending on the nature of the costs – for example, nursing services and medical supplies. Indirect costs, also called overheads, are not directly related to producing the activity or service. They can be either fixed or variable depending on the nature of the costs – for example, administrative departments and medical records departments.

It is important to understand the relationship between the revenue received and the costs incurred for delivering the activity.

Variance

Variance analysis is an essential financial-management control function. The difference between a budgeted amount and the amount expended represents a variance. Managers need to investigate variances to determine their cause. Actions taken in response to variances can often dramatically improve the financial outlook of the healthcare organisation (Henderson, 2003b). There are several types of variances, which are discussed following.

Volume variance

This is caused by a change in the total number of services being provided. This can be both higher and lower than expected. There is a cost associated with each product, and the costs will vary according to the number produced. If a day-surgery unit sees an additional 5 per cent of cases in a month, it will be reasonable to expect the variable costs of providing the service to be 5 per cent higher.

Mix variance

Mix variance is caused by a change in the proportion and types of services being provided. While the total volume of patients or services may be as planned, the complexity may increase, and this may result in an increase in nursing care.

Utilisation variance

This is caused by changes in efficiency. Efficiency variances relate to the level of resources used in producing each output and reflect a manager's performance in resource management – for example, the number of hours of nursing care per occupied bed day.

Budget development

The first stage in the development of a budget is identifying the goals and objectives. To illustrate the budget development process, assume that we have to develop a budget for a 30-bed ward with a planned occupancy rate of 90 per cent. As shown in Table 21.2, the level of nursing care will be 5.0 hours per occupied bed day. (An occupied bed day is a hospital inpatient bed occupied at midnight.) The number of full-time equivalents (FTE) required (26.7 FTE) has been calculated as per Table 21.2 and considers fixed nursing costs, consisting of the unit manager and the assistant, and variable nursing costs, which include the remainder of the staff.

Nursing Hours Per Patient Day

Nursing hours per patient day (NHPPD) is a nursing workload measurement that provides a guide to the number of hours needed to care for each patient in a given ward or unit. Unlike an occupied bed day (hospital inpatient bed occupied at midnight), NHPPD takes into consideration patient acuity, direct-care needs and other factors. NHPPD supports healthcare facilities to measure productivity and efficiency. The metric is convertible to a nurse-to-patient ratio through a simple equation:

$$NPR = 24 \div NHPPD$$

Table 21.2 Goals and objectives in a budget development for a hospital ward

Ward details	Required amounts
Number of beds	30
Beds per week[a]	210
Occupancy rate (%)	96.6
Weekly occupied bed days[b]	202.9
Nursing hours per occupied bed day	5.0
Nursing hours per week[c]	1,014.5
Full-time equivalent nursing staff[d]	26.7
Fixed nursing costs	
Unit managers	1.0
Assistant / Associate nursing managers	1.0
Total fixed nursing full-time equivalents	**2.0**
Total nursing full-time equivalents	28.7

Notes: (a) Number of beds × 7; (b) Beds per week × occupancy rate; (c) Occupied bed days × nursing hours per occupied bed day; (d) Nursing hours per week ÷ number of hours per week per full-time equivalent (1 full-time equivalent = 38 hours per week). Clinical nurse managers, nurse unit manager and associate nurse managers are usually excluded from NHPPD calculations.

The second task is the development of the average penalty rates for the different categories of staff. Table 21.3 calculates the average penalty rates (14.6 per cent) for the registered nurses on the ward.

Table 21.3 Calculating average penalty rates for registered nurses in a budget development for a hospital ward*

Shifts	Penalty rate[a]	Frequency[b]	Total[c]
Night duty	15.0	7	105.0
Sunday and public holiday	75.0	1	75.0
Saturday	50.0	1	50.0
Evening	15.0	7	105.0
Day duty		7	0
Total		**23**	**335.0**
Average[d]			**14.6**

Notes: *This is a guide only. Rates will vary between jurisdictions and following award negotiations (a) Percentage of base pay rate; (b) Number of shifts per four-week roster; (c) Penalty rate × frequency; (d) Total ÷ frequency.

The various categories of leave entitlement need to be included in the budget. This can be achieved by constructing information about the various categories. Table 21.4 calculates the leave entitlement for the variable nursing staff.

Table 21.4 Calculating leave entitlement for variable nursing staff in a budget development for a hospital ward

Types of leave	Amount of leave entitlement	Proportion of on-costs (%)
Annual	5 weeks backfill[a]	9.60
Annual loading	17.5% loading for 5 weeks[b]	1.68
Long service	1.3 weeks backfill per year[c]	2.50
Sick	1 week backfill[d]	1.90
Study	2 days (not replaced)	0
Total on-costs		**15.68**

Notes: (a) 5 ÷ 52 × 100; (b) 5 × 17.5 = 87.5; 87.5 ÷ 52 = 1.68; (c) 1.3 ÷ 52 × 100; (d) 1 ÷ 52 × 100

Finally, all the information is used to develop an appropriate nursing budget for the ward given the initial goals and objectives. As calculated in Table 21.5, the final nursing budget requirement for the ward is $2 992 509 for the year. The fixed nursing costs are $274 314, and the variable nursing costs are $2 718 195. Understanding the various costs and how they behave assists in both the development of a budget and the continuing management of the budget. The development of a budget requires knowledge of the staff that are to be employed (classification), award rates, superannuation rates and organisational policy regarding study leave and other allowances. Clearly, an understanding of the casemix profile of a ward or area will ensure the correct allocation of NHPPD.

Table 21.5 Calculating the nursing budget in a budget development for a hospital ward

	Types of nurses					
	NM	ANM	RN	EN	AIN	Total
Number of full-time equivalents	1.00	1.00	9.00	13.7	4.00	28.70
Number of weeks employed	52	52	52	52	52	
Hourly rate of pay ($)	55.00	50.00	45.00	40.00	30.00	
Hours per week employed	38	38	38	38	38	
Annual base pay ($)	**108 680**	**98 800**	**711 360**	**940 576**	**177 840**	**2 037 256**
Superannuation at 11.5% ($)	12 498	11 362	81 806	106 166	20 451	232 283
WorkCover	1030	1482	10 670	14 109	2668	30 559
Professional development ($)	1500	1500	12 000	17 850	4500	37 350
Uniform allowance ($)	250	250	2000	2975	750	6225
Total leave on-costs (%)	**13.78**	**13.78**	**15.68**	**15.68**	**15.68**	
Total cost of leave ($)	**14 976**	**13 615**	**111 541**	**147 482**	**27 885**	**315 500**
Shift allowance (%)	0.0	0.0	14.6	12.4	11.8	
Total cost of shift allowance ($)	**0**	**0**	**103 859**	**116 631**	**20 985**	**241 475**

Table 21.5 (cont.)

	Types of nurses					
	NM	ANM	RN	EN	AIN	Total
Subtotal ($)	139 534	127 009	1 033 236	1 345 789	255 079	2 900 647
Payroll tax at 4.75% ($)	6628	6033	49 079	63 924	12 116	137 437
Total labour costs ($)	**145 819**	**133 042**	**1 082 315**	**1 409 713**	**267 195**	**3 038 083**
Fixed nursing costs ($)	145 819	133 042				274 314
Variable nursing costs ($)			108 231	1 409 713	267 195	278 861

Notes: NM: nurse managers; ANM: assistant nurse managers; RN: registered nurses; EN: enrolled nurses; AIN: assistants in nursing

Few would argue that the development of an accurate budget and knowledge of how it was constructed are important. However, it is equally important that the budget is apportioned to each month (cash flowed), reflecting the planned expenses for that month (Bryans, 2007). This will support management of the budget, as any variances between the budget and expenditure will be meaningful.

Therefore, to continue with the example, the annual nursing budget needs to be apportioned to each month of the year. The fixed nursing costs are not influenced by the number of patients on the ward. Therefore, it would be reasonable to apportion the budget to each month based on the number of days in each month. However, the variable nursing costs have a direct relationship to the number of patients in the ward and the acuity or casemix of the patient population. Analysis of the occupied bed days for the previous 2 years provides a trend over the 12-month period. As shown in Table 21.5, the annual planned occupied bed days are apportioned to each month based on the past trend. The variable nursing budget is then apportioned to each month based on the number of planned occupied bed days for each month (see Table 21.6).

Table 21.6 Calculating the variable nursing budget in a budget development for a hospital ward

Month	No. of days in month	% of annual days	No. of OBD	% of annual OBD	FNC ($)	VNC ($)	Total budget ($)
July	31	8.5	887	9.0	23 298	244 651	267 949
August	31	8.5	900	9.1	23 298	248 237	271 535
September	30	8.2	851	8.6	22 546	234 722	257 268
October	31	8.5	799	8.1	23 298	220 379	243 677
November	30	8.2	821	8.3	22 546	226 447	248 994
December	31	8.5	628	6.4	23 298	173 214	196 512
January	31	8.5	740	7.5	23 298	204 106	227 404
February	28	7.7	792	8.0	21 043	218 449	239 492
March	31	8.5	890	9.0	23 298	245 479	268 777
April	30	8.2	809	8.2	22 546	223 137	245 684

Table 21.6 (cont.)

Month	No. of days in month	% of annual days	No. of OBD	% of annual OBD	FNC ($)	VNC ($)	Total budget ($)
May	31	8.5	858	8.7	23 298	236 653	259 951
June	30	8.2	880	8.9	22 546	242 721	265 267
Total	**365**	**100.0**	**9 855**	**100.0**	**274 314**	**2 718 195**	**2 992 509**

Notes: OBD: occupied bed days; FNC: fixed nursing costs; VNC: variable nursing costs

The heath service-delivery environment has different trends that affect different types of expenditures. For example, during the winter months, medical wards in hospitals typically experience higher occupancy rates, due mainly to respiratory conditions. While all budgets need to be cashflowed, there must be a balance between the annual budget and the level of work undertaken to cashflow it. If the annual budget is small – for example, $5000 – it may be simpler to simply divide it by 12 months rather than understanding what the expenditure driver is for that budget and then allocating it according to anticipated monthly usage.

Controlling and monitoring a budget

The management of a budget should be undertaken in conjunction with other performance information. Accountable managers use strategies to ensure that processes are aligned with activity and financial goals. Monitoring and evaluation enable managers to decide when to implement changes. Short-term and long-term monitoring and evaluation strategies are used to manage expenditure and activity levels to meet budget and, ultimately, strategic plan objectives (King et al., 2010).

Benchmarking is a quality improvement tool that enables organisations to compare their performance with others and learn from processes and systems that obtain better results, and to achieve and sustain best practice (Henderson, 2003a).

As illustrated, many health services use casemix information to benchmark health services in several different ways, in particular to compare the average length of stay for diagnostic-related groups. Differences in clinical practice, the efficiency of the labour and materials utilised, and the type of service delivery are other concepts that may benefit from benchmarking. The challenge in benchmarking is to balance economic outcomes with improvements in quality of care.

Developing an accurate budget and an appropriate cashflow for the accounting period is fundamental to the management of the budget (Gapenski & Pink, 2007). If the budget and cashflow are not prepared with accuracy, the various monthly variances will not be able to be analysed (Zelman, McCue & Glick, 2009). The variances may simply be due to the poor cashflow of the budget; if this is the case, the true position of the budget will not be known until the end of the accounting period.

With accurate budgeting and cashflow, the analysis and management of budgets becomes a manageable task. The objective of the analysis is to understand why variance has occurred. This can be achieved only with an array of performance indicators, the variance between the budget and the expenditure being only one of these. Information regarding the planned activity level and actual activity level also needs to be included, together with quality indicators.

Summary

- The five basic account groups are the essence of how financial information is recorded, which enables the development of budgets and the means of financial management and variance analysis.
- There are many types of budgets, and their application depends on what they are being used for, as well as the level of maturity and the management of the organisation.
- The casemix classification system provides significant levels of information that can be used within health care for clinical outcomes benchmarking and to better manage healthcare resources.
- The development of an accurate budget and cashflow based on the levels of planned outcomes is a critical part of financial governance for all types of healthcare organisations and an essential function of good financial management.
- The development of an appropriate budget and cashflow enables analysis of any variations from the planned expenses.

Reflective questions

1. Why is it important to separate fixed and variable costs in developing a budget?
2. What are the challenges associated with activity-based funding?
3. What factors would you need to consider in benchmarking clinical services?
4. What type of information would you require to undertake a budget-variance analysis?
5. What is the role of the Independent Health and Aged Care Pricing Authority?

Self-analysis questions

Think about how budgets are developed and managed in your current or previous place of employment. What types of budgets do you think are used? How are the budgets developed? What level of transparency exists in the organisation about how budgets are developed? Do the budgets have clear objectives that need to be achieved? How are the budgets monitored? If analysis has been undertaken, did it assist with the development of strategies to maintain a balanced budget? In considering these questions, is there an opportunity for you to do things differently?

References

Bryans, W. (2007). *Practical budget management in health and social care*. Radcliffe.

Department for Health and Wellbeing. (2022). 2022–23 Funding Allocation Methodology for South Australian Public hospitals. Retrieved from: https://www.sahealth.sa.gov.au/wps/wcm/connect/public+content/sa+health+internet/resources/funding+allocation+methodology+for+south+australian+public+hospitals+2022-23.

Dionne, F., Mitton, C., Smith, N. & Donaldson, C. (2009). Evaluation of the impact of program budgeting and marginal analysis in Vancouver Island Health Authority. *Journal of Health Services Research & Policy, 14*(4), 234–242. https://doi.org/10.1258/jhsrp.2009.008182

Gapenski, L. & Pink, G. (2007). *Understanding health care financial management* (5th ed.). Health Administration.

Henderson, E. (2003a). Continuing professional development: Budgeting (Part 1). *Nursing Management*, *10*(1), 33–37. https://doi.org/10.7748/nm2003.04.10.1.33.c1919

——(2003b). Continuing professional development: Budgeting (Part 2). *Nursing Management*, *10*(2), 32–36. https://doi.org/10.7748/nm2003.05.10.2.32.c1926

Heslop, L. (2012). Status of costing hospital nursing work within Australian casemix activity-based funding policy. *International Journal of Nursing Practice*, *18*(1), 2–6. https://doi.org/10.1111/j.1440-172X.2011.01992.x

Horngren, C., Datar, S. & Foster, G. (2006). *Cost accounting: A managerial emphasis* (12th ed.). Pearson.

King, R., Clarkson, P. M. & Wallace, S. (2010). Budgeting practices and performance in small health care businesses. *Management Accounting Research*, *21*(1), 40–55. https://doi.org/10.1016/j.mar.2009.11.002

Madden, R. (2013). ICF and casemix models for health care funding: Use of the WHO family of classifications to improve casemix. *Disability and Rehabilitation*, *35*(13), 1074–1077. https://doi.org/10.3109/09638288.2012.720349

National Health Funding Body. (2023). Calculation of National Weighted Activity unit. Retrieved from: https://www.publichospitalfunding.gov.au/calculation-national-weighted-activity-unit?#:~:text=A%20National%20Weighted%20Activity%20Unit,Price%20 (NEP)%20is%20paid

Reed, C. (2021). Historical Budgeting: How it Works. Retrieved from: https://firewalltimes.com/historical-budgeting/

Zhang R. & Bohlen J. (updated 2023). *Healthcare business budgeting*. StatPearls Publishing.

Zelman, W., McCue, M. & Glick, N. (2009). *Financial management of health care organizations: An introduction to fundamental tools, concepts, and applications* (3rd ed.). Jossey-Bass.

22 Negotiating

Sandra G. Leggat

Learning objectives

How do I:

- improve my skills in negotiating?
- plan a negotiation?
- decide whether I should accept a proposed solution?

Introduction

Negotiation is important for healthcare managers (Higazee & Gab Allah, 2022; Marques, Nogueira, Gonçalves & Rocha, 2023). In the past, negotiation was largely conducted face-to-face but that changed during the COVID-19 pandemic. Many negotiations are now conducted virtually over videoconferencing platforms such as MS Teams (Bjola & Coplen, 2022). This chapter introduces negotiating that can assist readers to develop their skills for use in personal and professional negotiations.

Concepts

Once two or more parties agree to enter into a **negotiation**, they may use either an integrative value-creation approach (win–win) or a distributive value-claiming approach (win–lose). The creation of a preferred health-service provider relationship can be integrative as the provider wins because they have negotiated a steady cashflow, while the organisation wins with the guarantee of quality health services at an agreed price. Integrative approaches involve more than one factor, such as price, volume, availability, quality and mode of delivery. A metaphor used to describe the **integrative approach** to negotiation is that it increases the size of the pie to be shared.

In contrast, the **distributive approach** assumes that the factor (or pie) under negotiation cannot be increased; therefore, if one negotiator gets more, the other gets less (Bazerman & Neale, 1992). This approach to negotiation is recommended when there is a need for a quick outcome that is more important than the relationship of the negotiators. For example, a distributive approach enables swift resolution with a child who is trying to negotiate not wearing a seatbelt. However, 'most negotiations take place in the context of an ongoing relationship where it is important to carry on each negotiation in a way that will help rather than hinder future relations and future negotiations' (Fisher, Ury & Patton, 1991, p. 22). Hart and Schweitzer (2022) developed the **ERRO** to measure the economic value of the relational outcomes of a negotiation. Negotiations dependent on the post-negotiation relationship, such as continuing service delivery, are considered high in ERRO and require a collaborative approach.

Negotiation: 'Back-and-forth communication designed to reach an agreement when you and the other side have some interests that are shared and some that are opposed' (Fisher et al., 2012, p. xxv)

Integrative approach: A negotiation method used when the negotiators believe that both parties can achieve their goals, with neither negotiator feeling like they are losing

Distributive approach: A negotiation method used when the factor under negotiation cannot be increased, and therefore if one negotiator gets more, the other gets less (Bazerman & Neale, 1992)

ERRO: Economic Relevance of Relational Outcomes, which requires consideration of the longer-term relationship

Frameworks for negotiating

De Janasz, Dowd and Schneider (2012) propose five stages of negotiation, each of which is discussed following.

Prepare and plan

Planning is essential to a successful negotiation, as it is important to be clear about what is wanted from the negotiation. Skilled negotiators suggest that this is the stage to identify the **BATNA**.

A BATNA requires identification of the options available if an agreement is not reached. Once these have been outlined, the option that is the best in terms of potential deals with

BATNA: Best Alternative To a Negotiated Agreement, which should be used as the standard against which a proposed agreement is measured (Fisher, Ury & Patton, 1991)

the counterpart is identified (Sebenius, 2017), which enables the terms of a proposed agreement to be evaluated. Never accept an agreement that leaves you worse off than your BATNA.

The BATNA is influenced by the options available for achieving the required result from the negotiation. For example, if a person buying a car would be happy with 10 or 12 different types of cars, their BATNA will be lower than if they want a specific car. It is easier to find a negotiated solution that is better than their BATNA.

At the preparation stage, consider the possible interests and negotiating strategies of the other party. Fisher and colleagues (1991) suggest that writing down both one's own interests and the possible interests of the other party helps to create more options. Consider the other party's BATNA. In the car-buying example, at the end of a slow month dealers may be willing to reduce their profit, as one sale at a lower price is likely to be better than a BATNA of no sales at all.

The area in which negotiating parties' BATNAs overlap is known as the **zone of possible agreement**. If a car dealer will not sell for less than $20 000 and a car buyer has only $18 000 to spend, there is no zone of possible agreement. However, if the car buyer has $25 000 to spend, the zone between $20 000 and $25 000 is open for possible agreement.

> **Zone of possible agreement:** The common ground between two or more parties to a negotiation, where the possible solutions are all at least as good for each negotiator as their BATNA

CALCULATING A BATNA

Sally works in the city, managing a health promotion service at a community health centre. Her organisation has just opened a new site in a regional town and has asked her to move there to complete the planning and development of the service.

Sally calculates her BATNA in preparation for the discussions with her manager about this new role. Her salary is currently $115 000. Not accepting the new position might mean her BATNA is $115 000. If she accepts the new position, Sally will be leaving friends, family and her house in the city, which she loves. She recognises that the regional lifestyle comes with generally lower housing costs and thus will be a benefit. She also considers that a bonus of $5000 to help with the move and to enable regular travel to visit her friends and family in the city might make her happier to move.

Sally feels that she needs to accept the move if she does not want to be disadvantaged in her current organisation. But she has the option of staying in the city and getting a new job. She looks at the jobs available for people with her education, experience and skills, and finds some with salaries of $125 000, for which she would be qualified.

Sally has therefore calculated her BATNA as a salary of $125 000 plus a $5000 incentive payment. She is ready to talk to her manager about her expectations if she were to move to the regional town.

Define ground rules

The ground rules of a negotiation address the following factors:

- who will participate in the negotiation
- who may be present to watch or provide information and support during the negotiation

- the location of the negotiation
- the time that will be allocated to the negotiation
- the parameters for the negotiation process.

Negotiation parameters may include the requirement that parties are polite, procedures for calling time-out, the types of issues that will be discussed and which of these may be set aside for later, and a protocol that will be followed if the negotiation process is not successful. It is more difficult to agree on ground rules for a negotiation if one has not already considered what they may entail. Documenting the ground rules that one considers important before entering the negotiation can assist in subsequent work with the other party to outline a mutually acceptable process.

Negotiation in a virtual venue may require additional ground rules. The limitations of not having face-to-face negotiations have been identified (Akpinar, Alfano, Kersten & Yu, 2017; Bjola & Coplen, 2022), with suggestions to improve the process with use of emoticons (Gettinger & Koeszegi, 2015).

Clarify and justify

During this stage, often referred to as 'principled negotiation', or separating the people from the problem, each party presents their interests and asks questions to clarify the interests of the other party. It is essential to negotiate on interests and not get stuck on the positions of the people involved in a negotiation (Bazerman & Neale, 1992), with the need to understand different cultural contexts (Adair et al., 2013). Negotiations regarding land claims of Indigenous peoples illustrate this concept. If the interests are seen to be solely about ownership of the land, the positions will be adversarial. If, however, the interests are regarding how best to manage, preserve and develop the land, the issue becomes one of management and not property rights, and might therefore be able to end in an agreed plan.

Research has shown that how issues are framed has an effect on how likely people are to accept and to encourage others to accept a proposal. If people perceive that they are getting a good deal, they are more likely to accept a proposal than if they perceive they are being taken advantage of. **Framing** issues in a positive light generally results in less risky choices, while negative framing often results in riskier choices (Tversky & Kahneman, 1981).

Negotiators often become fixated on irrelevant **anchors**, which are the initial offers made by parties to a negotiation. The anchoring effect is the common tendency to rely too heavily on anchors when making the next decision. For example, the initial price offered for the purchase of an item sets the standard for the rest of the negotiation. This means that prices lower than the initial asking price can seem more reasonable to a buyer, even if they are higher than the item's true worth.

There is disagreement among expert negotiators as to who should make the first offer. Some recommend that the other party should be encouraged to make the first offer, as this enables further gathering of information. Others suggest that whoever makes the first offer achieves the best outcome. If the other party makes the first offer, it may be important to follow quickly with a counteroffer to avoid the first offer becoming a strong anchor. Equally, if the other party rejects an offer and asks for a new, better offer, this should be declined. Instead, a counteroffer is worth insisting upon; otherwise, one party ends up negotiating with itself.

Framing: Careful choice of the language used to describe an issue so that it appears more positive or more negative

Anchor: The first offer made by a party to a negotiation

Bargain and problem-solve

In this stage, the parties to the negotiation should be actively exploring the solutions that will enable each to address their interests. A recent study suggested that nurse managers tended to compromise when there were opportunities for collaboration to ensure a better outcome for all (Higazee & Gab Allah, 2022). This is a skill to be developed – keep an open mind and determine whether there are ways to increase the size of the pie and a win–win agreement.

During this stage, it may be useful to check that one's style of negotiation is sensitive to the values, perceptions, norms of behaviour and mood of the other party (Ardianto & Hermawan, 2022). Varying the pace and level of formality of communications, and even the location, as the negotiation progresses can be useful.

If the parties are not able to come to an agreement but want to continue bargaining, it may be useful to include an independent third party. De Janasz and colleagues (2012) suggest allowing the third party to draft a plan that considers the interests of all negotiators and then giving the negotiators the opportunity to revise the plan. This process can continue until there is agreement. A third-party **mediator** can often establish a constructive environment that requires all parties to continue to discuss issues cooperatively and objectively. Sometimes, however, unresolvable issues are sent to an **arbitrator.**

> **Mediator:** Someone who attempts to help people involved in a conflict come to an agreement
>
> **Arbitrator:** Someone who is independent from either party in a conflict and is given the power to impose a settlement to the dispute

Close and implement

At this stage, either an agreement has been reached or the parties walk away from the negotiation. If an agreement has been reached, it is important to summarise what has been agreed, review the key points to ensure they have been understood by all parties, confirm any areas where agreement was not reached and, if necessary, document the agreement for signature (de Janasz et al., 2012).

Management and negotiation

While many negotiators may use tactics to try to win a negotiation, negotiators should display ethical behaviour. Spangle and Isenhart (2003, p. 172) identify the following unethical negotiating tactics:

- withholding information that has a substantial influence on the available options
- making false statements or lying to mislead the other party
- offering bribes or kickbacks
- insulting or demeaning the other party
- making promises that will not be met.

> **Negotiating in bad faith:** To continue to negotiate despite having no intention of making any compromises

Unethical negotiation includes **negotiating in bad faith**. De Janasz and colleagues (2012) advise that if the person with whom one is negotiating uses unethical means, it is 'better to end the negotiation without a resolution or contract than participate in a negotiation that compromises your values or reputation and causes you to be a victim' (p. 199).

Negotiation skills improvement

Researchers have spent time identifying how individuals can improve their performance in negotiating. As early as 1990, it was suggested that improving integrative abilities, through greater accuracy in judgements about the interests of the other party and high aspirations for the negotiation outcomes, is associated with better negotiation performance (Thompson, 1990). A more recent study reports a 24 per cent decrease in negotiation time when a professional negotiator is used. More recently, the use of automated negotiation agents has been identified as assisting humans to improve their negotiations (Aydogan, Keskin & Çakan, 2022), a trend likely to increase. Also, contrary to expectation, there is no connection between the nature and duration of the relationship sustained by the negotiating parties and the time taken to reach a successful conclusion of negotiations (Malatesta, 2012). Having a great relationship does not necessarily make reaching agreement any easier.

The most important message from expert negotiators is to look for positives in all possible circumstances (Bazerman & Neale, 1992). The research has explored why negotiators do not always make rational decisions, and negotiators are advised to focus on meeting their own interests as well as those of their negotiating partner (Stamato, 2004). Margaret Neale (cited in Buell, 2007) says, 'If I can trade off issues that I care about more and you care about less, then we've been able to create value in a transaction' (p. 1).

Finally, the literature suggests that women are less likely than men to engage in negotiation (Stamato, 2004); this includes negotiation regarding their salary and working conditions. In general, women do not perceive negotiating opportunities as often as men (Babcock & Laschever, 2009). It is particularly important for women leaders and managers to develop their skills in negotiation.

Summary

- Practise, practise and practise to improve negotiating skills.
- Plan a negotiation strategy that involves considering the information available to confirm and frame one's own interests and those of the other party.
- To achieve a win–win solution, consider how to increase the size of the pie.
- Never use unethical negotiating.
- Walk away from a negotiation that does not meet your BATNA.

Reflective questions

1. Why is it important to separate the interests from the positions of people involved in a negotiation?
2. How would you find out these interests in a negotiation using a virtual venue?
3. How would you find out how culture influences these interests?

4. How might you calculate and use a BATNA when trying to decide whether to accept a job? What information apart from the job offer would be useful to your BATNA?
5. Expert negotiators see negotiation as joint problem-solving. What could you do to reorient a negotiation from adversarial to collaborative?

Self-analysis questions

Think about times when you have attempted to negotiate an agreement with someone, either informally or formally. Identify two agreements that from your perspective were successful and two that were unsuccessful. Write a brief description of each negotiation and look for commonalities between them. What were the conditions when you were successful? What were the conditions when you were unsuccessful? Who was involved? What preparation did you do? What can you learn from this about your negotiating style? What might you do differently in the future?

References

Adair, W. L., Taylor, M., Chu, J., Ethier, N., Xiong, T., Okumura, T. & Brett, J. (2013). Effective influence in negotiation: The role of culture and framing. *International Studies of Management & Organization*, *43*(4), 6–25.

Akpinar, N. J., Alfano, S., Kersten, G. & Yu, B. (2017). The role of sentiment and cultural differences in the communication process of e-negotiations. *International Conference on Group Decision and Negotiation: A Socio-technical Perspective.* (pp. 132–144). Springer International Publishing.

Ardianto, R. N. & P. Hermawan (2022). Systematic literature review of strategic behavior in negotiation. *Management and Economics Review*, *7*(3), 310–329.

Aydogan, R., Keskin, M.O. & Çakan, U. (2022). Would you imagine yourself negotiating with a robot, Jennifer? Why not? *IEEE Transactions on Human-Machine Systems*, *52*(1), 41–51.

Babcock, L. & Laschever, S. (2009). *Women don't ask: Negotiation and the gender divide*. Princeton University.

Bazerman, M. & Neale, M. (1992). *Negotiating rationally*. Free.

Bjola, C. & Coplen, M. (2022). Virtual venues and international negotiations: Lessons from the COVID-19 pandemic. *International Negotiation*, *28*(1), 69–93.

Buell, B. (2007). Negotiation strategy: Seven common pitfalls to avoid. Retrieved from: http://www.gsb.stanford.edu/insights/negotiation-strategy-seven-common-pitfalls-avoid

de Janasz, S. C., Dowd, K. O. & Schneider, B. Z. (2012). *Interpersonal skills in organizations* (4th ed.). McGraw-Hill Irwin.

Fisher, R., Ury, W. & Patton, B. (2012). *Getting to yes: Negotiating an agreement without giving in*. Random House Business.

——(1991). *Getting to yes*. Penguin.

Gettinger, J. & Koeszegi, S. T. (2015). More than words: The effect of emoticons in eElectronic negotiations. In B. Kamiński, G. E. Kersten & T. Szapiro (eds), *Outlooks and insights on group decision and negotiation: 15th International Conference, GDN 2015, Warsaw, Poland, June 22–26, Proceedings* (pp. 289–305). Springer International Publishing.

Hart, E. & Schweitzer, M. E. (2022). When we should care more about relationships than favorable deal terms in negotiation: The economic relevance of relational outcomes (ERRO). *Organizational Behavior and Human Decision Processes*, *168*, 104–108.

Higazee, M. Z. A. & Gab Allah, A. R. (2022). The relationship between the political skills and negotiation behaviors of front-line nursing managers. *Nursing Forum*, *57*(6), 1240–1248.

Malatesta, D. (2012). The link between information and bargaining efficiency. *Journal of Public Administration and Theory*, *22*(3), 527–551. https://doi.org/10.1093/jopart/mur028

Marques, I., Norgueira, F., Gonçalves, S. P. & Rocha, R. (2023). Leadership and negotiation in public health management: A systematic review of the literature. *18th European Conference on Management, Leadership and Governance, Academic Conferences and publishing limited*, *259*(2).

Sebenius, J. K. (2017). BATNAs in negotiation: Common errors and three kinds of 'No'. *Negotiation Journal*, *33*(2), 89–99.

Spangle, M. L. & Isenhart, M. W. (2003). *Negotiation: Communication for diverse settings*. Sage.

Stamato, L. (2004). The new age of negotiation. *Ivey Business Journal*, (July–August), 1–3. http://iveybusinessjournal.com

Thompson, L. (1990). The influence of experience on negotiation performance. *Journal of Experimental and Social Psychology*, *26*(6), 528–544.

Tversky, A. & Kahneman, D. (1981). The framing of decisions and the psychology of choice. *Science*, *211*(4481), 453–458.

Part 5
Drives Innovation

23 Creativity and visioning

Godfrey Isouard

Learning objectives

How do I:

- work with others in my organisation to develop an effective vision for the future?
- increase my ability to identify and explore creative solutions to organisational issues?
- foster creativity among the people I work with?
- assist my organisation to become a learning organisation?

Introduction

The healthcare sector is continually confronted with the issue of how to manage with less. In response, health leaders and managers must explore and use new ways to face such challenges. These issues ultimately affect the quality and safety, and the productivity and efficiency, of the health services delivered. Within each organisation, the effectiveness of the leadership and culture directly affect the quality of patient care delivered. To effectively address such challenges, leaders have begun to adopt new strategies and roles that focus on visioning and creativity.

Definitions

Creativity, or creative capital, is by far an organisation's most important asset. Creative-thinking employees are regarded as the key determinants of a successful organisation. The development of such individuals requires organisations to take positive steps towards encouraging employee participation, which then enables greater intrinsic motivation and engagement in work (Roshavati, Rahid & Siti, 2020; Aldabbas, Pinnington & Lahrech, 2023).

Visioning is regarded as an important element that provides clear direction to an organisation. When used strategically, it provides the organisation with a sound platform for planning, establishing goals and expanding and functioning into the future (Millett, 2006). The effective leader takes the essential role in building the appropriate culture through establishing the mission and **vision**, and developing plans that move beyond the certainties of today. At the organisational level, visioning is important for strategic-planning processes and assists in motivating employees to work toward shared goals.

Organisations

Creativity and visioning are vital to the success of an organisation. However, it is challenging for many organisations to encourage and foster new ideas, and to establish creativity and **innovation** that can benefit all concerned. Of relevance is that the need to be creative is not confined to commercial and non-health-based organisations. Innovation and creativity have an important place in **not-for-profit organisations** and in the public and government domains, where the drive has shifted to greater efficiency, effectiveness and productivity. There is increasing pressure on these latter organisations to find new and improved means of working and innovative solutions to current and future problems.

Systems-based approach

Effective leadership across all levels of government in Australia strengthens the capacity of the environment to enable real improvements and reforms in the health system. Through a **systems-based approach**, leading organisations use creativity and innovation to address the challenges, thereby building cultures which foster capacity for innovation and change. This change in culture is generally undertaken through leadership in the organisation, which adopts a systems-based approach.

Visioning: The process of assessing how fit an organisation is to grow and function in the future

Vision: A clear purpose that expresses a distinct sense of an organisation's future

Creativity: The act of generating new ideas and thoughts and transforming them into reality

Innovation: Represents the stage of using new knowledge to materialise into valued new product prototypes, processes or services (Castaner, 2016)

Not-for-profit organisation: An organisation that is not operating for the profit or personal gain of its individual members or shareholders

Systems-based approach: A leadership method that assumes an organisation is a convoluted interaction of dynamic parts that work together for a common purpose

In such organisations, there are common elements that characterise the culture. Achieving the desired organisational culture is a key factor in healthcare reform (Tierney, 2019). Such creativity, innovation and organisational change can only be achieved with a culture that encourages adaptability to change. Once such a culture is established, the rate of innovation is dependent on how the norms, social status and hierarchy influence employee behaviours. The existence of ample resources is also another factor determining the rate of innovation.

These are critical in ensuring that creativity and change are successfully introduced and maintained within the healthcare organisation setting. They include effective transformational leadership, adoption of a systems-based approach and clear understanding of how to develop organisational cultures that enhance and nurture the workplace environment to embrace creativity and change. These elements are discussed and analysed in this chapter.

Learning organisations

An important aspect in any organisation involves its learning capacity, by means of which the vision exists to ensure that all activities are aligned. **Learning organisations** are founded on uniform engagement and collaboration by all employees, who are committed and accountable to change, each directed towards shared principles. As originally described by Peter Senge (1990) in his book *The fifth discipline*, in learning organisations employees strive to achieve their target goals, new ideas are enhanced, team aspiration is allowed to reign, and all are inspired to learn to view the whole together. According to Senge, an emphasis on knowledge management is characteristic of learning organisations, which can change continuously as they learn from experience to improve overall performance. This is achieved through continuous development, retention and leveraging of both individual and collective learning. Senge also describes learning organisations as encouraging and supporting their workers towards ongoing learning while stressing information-sharing, teamwork and participation as important.

Learning organisation: An organisation in which employees strive to achieve their target goals, new ideas are enhanced, team aspiration is allowed to reign, and all are inspired to continuously learn to view the whole together

Learning organisations are readily adaptable to changes in the external environment (Budiyono, Bdiyanto & Suwitho, 2018). The existence of such a learning environment is fundamental to the development of creativity, and this has been shown to be achieved through a transformational approach to leadership. Transformation to a learning organisation provides the necessary culture to foster innovation, creativity and change (Aliev & Sigov, 2017; Joel et al., 2023).

Employees within an effective learning organisation are valued for their own contributions and are encouraged to improve and develop their individual skills and competencies. They benefit from each other's experience.

Leaders in these organisations play a significant role in enhancing and maintaining a learning environment. The leader tends to respect and treat all equally within the workplace environment. In turn, employees are motivated to work towards achieving the goals set by their leaders. This ultimately provides the appropriate culture for innovative solutions, enhanced creativity and new ideas (Gurlek & Cemberci, 2020). Recent research has identified the means by which learning organisations improve organisational learning capability (Rupcic, 2023).

The effect on employees within such organisations has been found to be highly positive (Rupcic, 2023). Individuals tend to acquire skills and knowledge above their position's described requirements. This enables them to accept and appreciate other roles and activities in the organisation. The leadership strategy to use flexible arrangements in the workplace gives employees the liberty to move freely, while removing the obstacles associated with a rigidly structured organisation. It also ensures that employees can cope successfully with a changing environment, as is found in health care today.

From time to time, the turbulence of the learning organisation's environment does affect the functioning of creative, knowledge-based organisations (Blaskova, Sokol & Figurska, 2023). However, these changes in the environment are often unpredictable and so quite difficult to prepare strategies for. The authors report that within these organisations leadership must creatively use their knowledge in response to these changes.

Management and innovation

Creating the required culture

In this context, culture is regarded as the norms and beliefs of an organisation, and the ways in which it acts collectively. The culture provides the key catalyst to introducing innovation and change, and together with leadership is a main factor in providing the receptive environment for change (Tierney, 2019).

For a leader and manager to create a learning organisation, they must be competent in transforming and building the organisation's culture and understand how to create a culture that supports innovation and change. However, although it is widely recognised that creativity and visioning are key ingredients in a high-performing organisation, it is often difficult to introduce, manage and sustain the required cultural change. The key activities that provide beneficial outcomes in cultural change include motivating change, creating a vision, developing political support for change, managing the transition and sustaining momentum (Smith & Green, 2020; Emami, Rezaei, Valaei & Gardener, 2023).

The key elements needed to create the necessary culture include:

- a workplace environment enabling support mechanisms that encourage employees to develop and trial new ideas
- flat structures with flexible teams, incorporating rewards and incentives for creative and innovative actions
- teams of managers who feel comfortable guiding flexible teams that take acceptable risks
- open communication channels that build trust
- managers who play a significant role with regard to facilitating learning and more effectively use their knowledge and experience.

LEADING FOR CREATIVITY AT CARE LINE HOSPITAL

John is the new chief executive officer of Care Line Hospital, a tertiary referral publicly funded hospital located in metropolitan Sydney. On commencing employment, John uncovers several serious issues in performance and service delivery, with decreased efficiency, low productivity and ineffectiveness throughout the organisation. Specifically, there is poor financial management and performance, a high turnover of senior management staff, a high level of dissatisfaction among the employees and increased demands for services.

> ### LEADING FOR CREATIVITY AT CARE LINE HOSPITAL Continued
>
> After wide consultation and analysis, John determines that the situation requires a new and creative model of organisation, management and service delivery. In consultation with his senior executive team, John's response is to form the following set of strategies:
>
> - Introduce measures to change the culture so that creativity is fostered throughout the organisation by encouraging and supporting new ideas.
> - Make plans to transform the culture to that of a learning organisation.
> - Establish a new leadership group for the organisation, including the appointment of designated 'ideas champions', whose roles are to develop new and creative initiatives while actively targeting improvements and challenging the existing norms and processes of the organisation.
> - Base the new culture on uniform engagement and collaboration by all employees who are committed and accountable to change, each being directed towards shared principles.
> - Include in the implementation plan initiatives to introduce change, develop the vision, secure political agreement for change, manage the period of change and maintain the change achieved.
> - Establish a process through which all employees will be encouraged to learn from experience in an environment that encourages discussion and disagreement.
> - Develop ideas on how best to negotiate change processes.

Challenges

Not all leaders and managers who seek a creative culture are successful in attaining it. Numerous challenges exist along the way, which could jeopardise its development at the organisational level. These include difficulty in converting individual creativity to organisational creativity, lack of effective leadership to encourage employees to learn from experience, insufficient stimulus and motivation to generate new ideas, and barriers such as poor organisational structure, lack of clarity and unclear vision for the organisation that impede creativity (Smith & Green, 2020; Emami et al., 2023).

Structure

The organisational structure in use has a clear effect on employees' ability to contribute to ideas and creativity. Vertically structured organisations tend to be rigid and often result in employees feeling stifled in what they can and cannot undertake. Although horizontally structured organisations are less efficient, there are fewer rules, and they provide employees with a sense of identification with the organisation. Employees in such work environments normally strive to achieve their target goals; through this, new ideas are fostered, and team and group aspiration flow readily (Alipoor, Ahmadi, Pouya, Ahmadi & Mowlaie, 2017; Smith & Green, 2020; Emami et al., 2023).

Strategies need to be established by the leader to incorporate smaller units with a clear direction and enable structures that facilitate the development and trialling of new ideas. These are often referred to in the literature as 'innovation factories'. They provide the mechanism by which to enhance innovative thinking in organisations with more traditional norms.

Organisations with modern norms are generally technologically developed, rational, empathic and change-oriented, whereas those with traditional norms are the direct opposite. Those organisations embracing traditional leadership and structural domains have been found to stifle creativity and innovations. In comparison, organisations that have established a work environment perceived by its employees to have strong work processes and clear vision have enabled creativity related processes to thrive (Smith & Green, 2020).

Leadership

Learning organisations need a designated person to be assigned to a leadership role in developing individuals and teams to produce new and creative initiatives. These people are often called 'ideas champions'. They aim to achieve improvements and challenge current norms and processes.

While poor leadership can result in little or no uptake of innovation or creativity within the organisation, effective leadership has been shown to foster employee creativity and innovation, and to the success of work teams that are largely facilitated through their creative self-efficacy (Mittal & Dhar, 2015).

Effective leadership in healthcare is critical to developing a culture that enhances and supports innovation and change for sustainability. To secure continuous improvement, leaders of learning organisations in health care should build a workplace climate that promotes the generation and implementation of new ideas. Effective leaders facilitate the achievement of a supportive workplace climate which, in turn, enhances innovation and organisational performance (Wikhamn & Selart, 2019; Gil, Garcia-Alcaraz, Mataveli & Tobias, 2023).

Converting creativity

One significant challenge for a leader is converting individual creativity into organisational creativity. As organisations aim to become more creative and innovative, the strategies employed can often lead to conditions that encourage individual effort more than team creativity. This can result in pockets of creativity but not an overall commitment to the organisation's goals. To attain the appropriate culture, the process must be seen as long term in nature rather than as an instant solution (Blaskova et al., 2023).

While it is important to commence at the individual level to build capacity within an organisation, creativity must then spread across all work functions and teams for the organisation to become more creative and effective. Individual effort needs to be converted across the organisation and in line with the organisation's mission and vision

Converting individual creativity to sustainable organisational creativity requires leadership in the workplace to remove barriers that obstruct the optimal climate needed for creativity to prosper (Blaskova et al., 2023). The following strategies are recommended by the authors for senior management to achieve such organisational creativity:

- empowerment of individuals' motivation at work
- increasing leaders' motivation at work
- introducing appropriate change management
- removing barriers and restrictive practices in the workplace
- enhancing organisational memory and learning

- maintaining employee commitment to the overall mission and vision
- enhancing information-gathering and dissemination throughout the organisation
- encouraging and valuing employee views and ideas.

Leadership and innovation

Effective leadership

Healthcare leaders appreciate their responsibility in providing clear direction into the future. They need to ensure that their organisation adapts in an environment of limited resources and increased demands for services. To operate effectively in the long term, a visioning process should be undertaken (Zhou, Zhao, Tian, Zhang & Chen, 2018).

The quality of leadership within an organisation has been shown to affect its culture, which in turn affects creativity, innovation and performance (Nasir et al., 2022). It ultimately affects employees and their commitment and trust, the overall effectiveness of the team, and therefore personal and collective performance. In essence, effective leadership requires a vision of the future that inspires employees of the organisation. The vision must be both effective and realistic. Successful leaders are those who work towards a shared and common vision to achieve the organisation's goals. In this context, the vision forms the unifying thread and acts as a shared goal for all employees. The leader must consider how to meet employees' needs for expression in order to encourage innovation and creativity within the workplace (Mittal & Dhar, 2015).

Many leaders today foster lateral thinking among employees in an attempt to enhance creativity within the organisation. The optimal strategies target employees who work across various levels, including staff and line managers, and the planning and strategy units. Such leaders are considered to be demonstrating a vision, trustworthiness and the capability to motivate (Bleich, 2019).

There are several ways for leaders to enhance lateral thinking among employees. Within healthcare, leaders may establish interested teams of colleagues who collaborate to use lateral thinking to address complex issues, identify new innovative solutions and explore new opportunities outside traditional problem-solving domains (Bleich, 2019). In these instances, lateral-thinking leaders select teams of healthcare staff from various professional backgrounds who are committed to exploring creativity. The authors report that the leaders empower each staff member to maximise use of their abilities.

Transformational leadership

Transformational leadership: A leadership style that can inspire positive changes in followers

The changing role of today's leaders follows contemporary leadership theories, which account not only for the leader but also for the people they lead. In particular, **transformational leadership** theories focus on the role that leaders play in transforming employees in terms of their personal values and goals, so that these are more consistent with those of the organisation. Transformational leadership has been found to comprise several key elements: individualised consideration, intellectual stimulation, inspirational motivation and idealised influence.

Transformational leadership has been shown to drive organisational innovation (Chen, Zheng, Yang & Bai, 2016). The researchers identified potential mediators in driving such innovation. These included empowerment of employees, support from senior leadership for innovation, the existence of a learning organisation and availability of adequate resources.

There is strong empirical evidence that transformational leadership develops optimal organisational culture and positive change (Minai, Jauhari, Kumar & Singh, 2020). It has also been found to increase employee commitment and job satisfaction, and to decrease employee turnover and burnout. Transformational leaders are reported as inspiring their employees to higher levels of performance through transformation of their attitudes, beliefs and values (Nasir et al., 2022). Such leaders achieve change by creating shared understanding and acting as strong role models.

Vision is a key component of transformational leadership. It supports the notion that employees and others should strive to achieve goals at work. Transformational leaders leave a lasting effect on their employees, who are able to commit to the organisation's vision.

Certain aspects of transformational leadership, such as intellectual stimulation and common values, have been found to result in a culture of enhanced ideas, innovation and creativity, as well as greater trust and team togetherness. This contributes to continuous change due to an increased willingness by employees to accept and participate more readily in change. Such leadership transforms the organisational culture in a way that means creativity and change become the norm.

Summary

- Creativity and visioning are vital elements to the success of an organisation.
- Organisational visioning is used to provide clear direction to the organisation.
- Transformational leadership and a systems-based approach can help ensure that creativity and change are successfully introduced.
- Transformational leadership develops optimal organisational culture and positive change to drive innovation.
- Learning organisations provide the necessary culture to foster innovation, creativity and change.

Reflective questions

1. What do you understand creativity to be in an organisation? As a health leader, what measures would you take to enhance creativity in the workplace?
2. What is your understanding of organisational culture? As a health leader, what strategies would you consider to be nurturing of a workplace environment that embraces creativity and change?
3. Do you consider it important to identify factors that influence creativity and the generation of new ideas in the workplace? Why?
4. How do you encourage employees to share a common vision for the organisation? Describe the approach you would take and some of the challenges you are likely to encounter.
5. In what ways can becoming a learning organisation improve the performance and effectiveness of a healthcare organisation? What effect would it have on its employees?

Self-analysis questions

List the key leadership and management characteristics identified in this chapter. Self-assess your current status and development with regard to these. Discuss with colleagues and mentors your development in these areas and the areas that need to be focused on for future development.

References

Aldabbas, H. Pinnington, A. H. & Lahrech, A. (2023). Encouraging more creativity in organisations: The importance of employees' intrinsic motivation and work engagement. *International Journal of Organisational Analysis*, *31*(6), 2337–2358. https://doi.org/10.1108/IJOA-11-2021-3038

Aliev, I. M. & Sigov, V. I. (2017). Creating a learning organisation as an increase in the adaptability of a company's human capital to the volatility of the external environment. *European Research Studies Journal*, XX (4B), 57–69.

Alipoor, H. Ahmadi, K. Pouya, S. Ahmadi, K. & Mowlaie, S. (2017). The effect of organisational structure on employees' job performance in private hospitals of Ahvaz. *Journal of ecophysiology & occupational health*, *17*(3/4), 119–123. https://doi.org/10.18311/jeoh/2017/19831

Blaskova, M. Sokol, A. & Figurska, I. (2023). Organisational barriers of a knowledge-based organisation in the aspect of sustainable creativity development. *Journal of Vasyl Stefanyk Precarpathian National University*, *10*(4), 46–62.

Bleich, M.R. (2019). Advancing lateral leadership in health care. *The Journal of Continuing Education in Nursing; Thorofare*, *50*(9), 389–391. https://doi.org/10.3928/00220124-20190814-03

Budiyono, B., Bdiyanto, B. & Suwitho, S. (2018). The influence of leadership and external environment on performance through learning organisation, and the influence towards competitiveness through performance of institute of economic science in Java. *International Review of Management and Marketing*, *8*(4), 36–44.

Castaner, X. (2016). Redefining creativity and innovation in organisations: Suggestions for redirecting research. *International Journal of Innovation Management*, *29*(4), 1640001.

Chen, L., Zheng, W., Yang, B. & Bai, S. (2016). Transformational leadership, social capital and organizational innovation. *Leadership and Organization Development Journal*, *37*(7), 843–859.

Emami, M., Rezaei, S., Valaei, N. & Gardener, J. (2023). Creativity mindset as the organisational capability: The role of creativity-relevant processes, domain-relevant skills and intrinsic task motivation. *Asia-Pacific Journal of Business Administration*, *15*(1), 139–160.

Gil, A. J. Garcia-Alcaraz, J. L., Mataveli, M. & Tobias, C. (2023). The interrelationships between organisational climate and job satisfaction and their impact on training outcomes. *Journal of Workplace Learning*, *35*(7), 613–631. https://doi.org/10.1108/JWL-03-2023-0050

Gurlek, M. & Cemberci, M. (2020). Understanding the relationships among knowledge-oriented leadership, knowledge management capacity, innovation performance and organisational performance: A serial mediation analysis. *Kybernetes*, *49*(11), 2819–2846. https://doi.org/10.1108/K-09-2019-0632

Joel, O. O., Moses, C. L. Igbinoba, E. E. Olokundun, M. A. Salau, O. P., Ojebola, O. & Adebayo, O. P. (2023). Bolstering the moderating effect of supervisory innovative support on organisational learning and employees' engagement. *Administrative Sciences*, *13*(3), 81. https://doi.org/10.3390/admsci13030081

Millett, S. M. (2006). Futuring and visioning: Complementary approaches to strategic decision making. *Strategy and Leadership*, *34*(3), 43–50. https://doi.org/10.1108/10878570610660591

Minai, M. H., Jauhari, H., Kumar, M. & Singh, S. (2020). Unpacking transformational leadership: Dimensional analysis with psychological empowerment. *Personnel review*, *49*(7), 1419–1434.

Mittal, S. & Dhar, R. L. (2015). Transformational leadership and employee creativity. *Management Decision*, *53*(5), 894–910.

Nasir, J., Ibrahim, R. M., Sarwar, M. A., Sarwar, B., Al-Rahmi, W. M., Alturise, F., Samed Al-Adwan, A. & Uddin, M. (2022). The effects of transformational leadership, organisational innovation, work stressors, and creativity on employee performance in SMEs. *Frontiers in Psychology, 13*, 772104.

Roshavati, A. H., Rahid, M. R. & Siti, N. A. H. (2020). The effects of employee participation in creative-relevant process and creative self-efficacy on employee creativity. *Geografia: Malaysian Journal of Society and Space, 16*(2).

Rupcic, N. (2023). Means to improve organisational learning capability. *The Learning Organisation. 30*(1), 101–109.

Senge, P. (1990). *The fifth discipline: The art and practice of the learning organisation.* Century Business.

Smith, N. L. & Green, B. C. (2020). Examining the factors influencing organisational creativity in professional sport organisations. *Sport Management Review, 23*(5), 992–1004.

Tierney, M. (2019). Creating a culture of improvement for better care. *International Journal of Integrated Care, 19*(4), 279. https://doi.org/10.5334/ijic.s3279

Wikhamn, W. & Selart, M. (2019). Empowerment and initiative: The mediating role of obligation. *Employee relations, 41*(4), 662–677.

Zhou, L. Zhao, S., Tian, F., Zhang, X. & Chen, S. (2018). Visionary leadership and employee creativity in China. *International Journal of Manpower, 39*(1), 93–105. https://doi.org/10.1108/IJM-04-2016-0092

24 Evidence-based practice

Sandra G. Leggat
With acknowledgement to Denise M. Jepson

Learning objectives

How do I:

- source evidence for my decision-making?
- critically appraise evidence?
- apply relevant evidence?

Introduction

Building on the concepts of evidence-based medicine, evidence-based management (EBMgmt) suggests that leaders and managers find, evaluate and use the best available scientific evidence to inform their practice. This chapter discusses when and how to look for evidence and outlines how to apply it.

Use of evidence

While there are studies linking doctors who practise evidence-based medicine with better clinical outcomes than those who do not (Pfeffer & Sutton, 2006), and despite the logic of basing decisions on evidence, we could find no experimental studies linking **evidence-based management** with better organisational outcomes. The large body of research that suggests that managers have difficulty finding and applying evidence to their management practice, in general (Hemsley-Brown & Sharp, 2003), and to healthcare leadership and management specifically (Finkler & Ward, 2003) remains. Much of the current research focuses on facilitators and barriers to EBMgmt (Shafaghat et al., 2021).

> **Evidence-based management:** 'Translating principles based on best evidence into organisational practices' (Rousseau, 2006, p. 256)

Health-service managers believe that using evidence will improve their effectiveness as managers (Liang, Howard, Leggat & Murphy, 2012), and most report a desire to use and apply evidence (Mitton & Patten, 2004). 'However, they make little regular use of evidence in their decision-making, especially neglecting scientific or research evidence' (Liang et al., 2012, p. 285). A systematic review confirms that most empirical studies focus on opinion as evidence, with limited use of administrative data and other sources, such as social media (Roshanghalb et al., 2018).

Management research has had a shorter timeframe than other areas of research (Axelsson, 1998), which has led to the dearth of robust evidence. In addition, many articles outline the divide between those who use the evidence and those who produce the evidence, with suggestions that researchers need to better understand context and decision-making processes (Shafaghat et al., 2021), providing systematic research reviews and meta-analyses (Axelsson, 1998) that clearly describe what is known and what is still to be learned. A framework for improving the use of evidence in managerial decision-making is proposed by Liang and colleagues (2012). As outlined in Figure 24.1, the writers suggest roles for a range of players in the healthcare system.

Recent research has found that an organisational culture, and policies and procedures, that support EBMgmt is essential (Daouk-Öyry, Sahakian & van der Vijver, 2021; Shafaghat et al. 2021). To bridge the research–practice gap (Walshe & Rundall, 2001), managers should actively seek to participate in scholarly or scientific management research. Further, managers can work with educational institutions to learn the skills and techniques to find, evaluate and apply evidence.

Organisations must have a coherent approach to foster EBMgmt. This will encourage a power shift in organisations, replacing formal power and opinion with facts and data (Pfeffer & Sutton, 2006). Organisational factors critical to the success of evidence-informed decision-making in health service management are supportive systems for access to evidence and information-sharing (Lavis et al., 2005) and provision of incentives to promote the

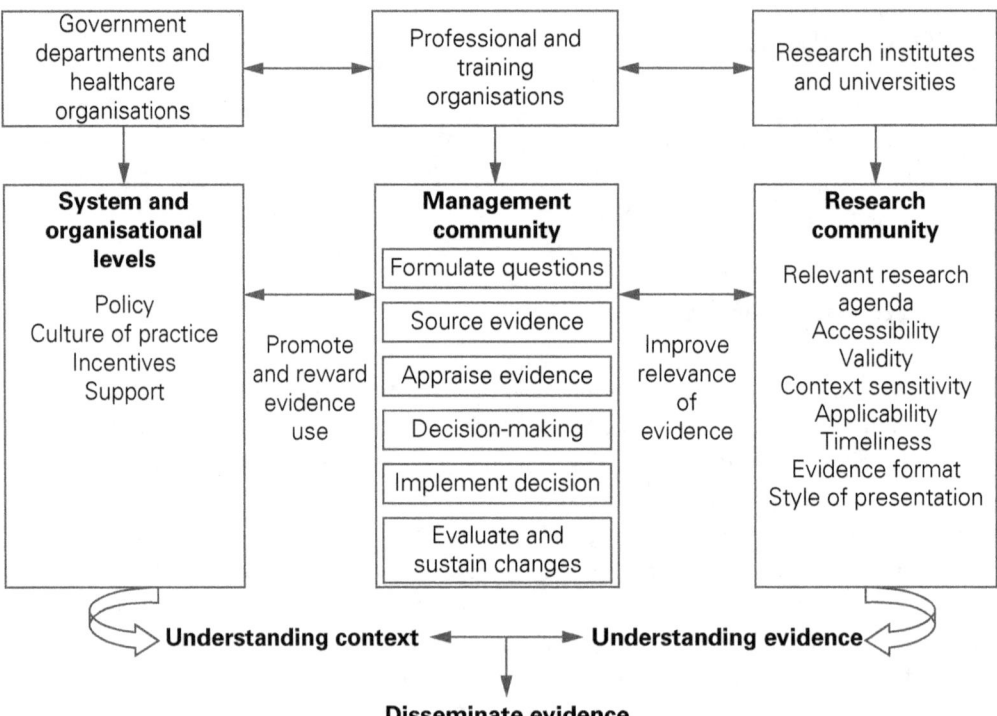

Figure 24.1 Framework for improving the use of evidence in managerial decision-making
Source: Liang et al. (2012).

use of evidence (Nutley & Davies, 2000). Shortell (2006) highlights the important role of health service boards in driving the necessary cultural change to implement supportive organisational systems.

Frameworks for evidence-based management

Barends, Rousseau and Briner (2014, p. 2) suggest six steps to evidence-based management:

1. Asking: translating a practical issue or problem into an answerable question
2. Acquiring: systematically searching for and retrieving the evidence
3. Appraising: critically judging the trustworthiness and relevance of the evidence
4. Aggregating: weighing and pulling together the evidence
5. Applying: incorporating the evidence into the decision-making process
6. Assessing: evaluating the outcome of the decision taken.

Pfeffer and Sutton (2006) suggest that everyone in an organisation needs to take responsibility for evidence-based management. They propose that managers ask for evidence of efficacy every time someone proposes a change. In fact, Rousseau and ten Have (2022) identify the need for a subset of EBMgmt in evidence-based change management, suggesting that planned change is more likely to succeed when informed by science. Managers should also ensure that decision-makers have all the available supporting (and non-supporting) data.

Source the evidence

Managers should consider all sources of evidence, ranging from scientific to opinion or stakeholder evidence (Barends et al., 2014). It is important to acquire the *best* available evidence to address the issue at hand, while recognising that in most instances issues such as time and access mean that not *all* available evidence will be included in a review. Four specific sources of evidence, and questions to ask when considering them, are provided here.

Scientific, scholarly or academic research findings

What has been studied, researched and established in peer-reviewed studies on this topic? Which databases should we search? How might a librarian help us find out about this topic?

Stakeholders' values and concerns

Who may be affected by this decision? Whose views are important when coming to this decision? Whom should we involve in interviews or discussions about this topic?

Organisational data, facts and figures

What do we know about this issue within our organisation? What information and metrics are available to inform and support our decision-making? Which reports could we use that would help our deliberations?

Professional experience and judgement

Who has experience or expertise in this area, either within or outside this organisation? Who has experience or expertise in a similar area and therefore could usefully inform this decision? With whom else might we discuss this topic?

POLICY IMPLEMENTATION ENHANCED BY EVIDENCE

In many jurisdictions, healthcare boards are advised to measure the safety culture of their organisations. Often, the policy directive includes a reading list to justify the policy, but no resources have been supplied on how to measure safety culture.

The quality management team has many questions as they explore how best to measure safety culture in their organisation. They want to know, for example: What is the agreed definition of safety culture? What is the evidence that a high rating on safety culture results in better patient care and outcomes? What tools are available to measure safety culture? Which of these tools have been found to have an association with an improvement in patient safety? Are there particular variables within the safety culture measurement tools that are linked with better safety culture? Can safety culture be measured using existing data?

The managers planning the safety culture implementation are all former clinicians now working in management roles, well used to routinely checking evidence-based sources for clinical treatments and treatment options. However, these managers have not been trained in how to design, implement or measure safety culture. Their typical way of implementing a management intervention is to discuss similar interventions with other healthcare services,

> **POLICY IMPLEMENTATION ENHANCED BY EVIDENCE** Continued
>
> ask about their successes and learnings, and adapt those experiences to their own situation. Sometimes, they may ask to see what books on the topic are available in their institutional library.
>
> After reflecting on the lack of advice from the government department and their peer health services, the team wants to find robust evidence before they spend the time and effort to implement a measurement system that will not meet their needs. They specifically look for recent systematic literature reviews to ensure summaries of peer-reviewed literature are included in the evidence upon which they are planning the program. The team will likely have to provide advice to the board with regard to the evidence for measurement of safety culture.

Appraise the evidence

While all types of evidence can be useful for decision-making, managers must be aware of how the evidence applies to their situation and the inherent strengths and weaknesses. That is, where the evidence was gathered, and under what conditions. Who conducted the research or spoke of the experience, and what biases or other limits might have applied in that instance? What else might provide an alternative explanation for the results?

Evidence can be of variable quality, even within the scientific literature, and difficulties arise when comparing studies using different methodologies. There is debate between researchers who see the randomised controlled trial, systematic review or meta-analysis as the gold standard for research evidence, and those who privilege other forms of evidence (see e.g. O'Halloran, Porter & Blackwood, 2010). On the other hand, research organisations acknowledge that many questions are best answered by qualitative and cross-sectional studies (National Institute for Health and Clinical Excellence, 2009). A hierarchy of evidence is commonly used by researchers (Murad, Asi, Alsawas & Alhadab, 2016). This hierarchy lists the higher-volume stakeholder evidence, such as background and organisational information and expert opinion, at the bottom of the pyramid and the empirically based, lower-volume information at the top.

Apply the evidence to decision-making

Some decisions are novel and apply at one time to unknown or uncertain circumstances. Consider, for example, the implementation of a safety culture measure discussed earlier, which needs a series of decisions at the implementation stage. Other decisions are applied routinely as a matter of normal business practice, such as recruiting or other selection decision-making. In both these circumstances, it is preferable to consider the best available evidence, critically appraised, that can be applied.

Biases may influence decision-making processes. While it is beyond the scope of this chapter to provide detailed discussion of decision-making biases, there are two to which managers should pay attention. The first is **group think**, which occurs when an individual feels pressure (real or imagined) to agree with the group. Group think is dangerous because

Group think: A bias that occurs when an individual feels pressure (real or imagined) to agree with the group

the group can be lulled into believing that because many think this way, it is the best way. The second is **sunk-cost bias**, which means that a wrong decision was made on the basis of what had previously been invested, be it financial resources or time. It is sunk cost because resources have already been expended and which are unlikely to be recovered, so it becomes irrelevant for the next decision.

Sunk-cost bias: A bias that occurs when an individual wrongly makes a decision based on what they have previously invested

The role of knowledge management

Although knowledge was considered a business asset as early as the 1900s, application to health care has been slower (Kothari, Hovanec, Hastie & Sibbald, 2011). The context of healthcare has limited **knowledge management** (KM) implementation, with databases that are designed for specific purposes limiting opportunities for sharing and synthesis and, unlike for-profit businesses, public health care rarely has the resources to invest in sophisticated KM. This has led to single initiatives, such as communities of practice, a popular KM strategy, which are largely created to respond to specific issues, with limited long-term sustainability. KM has the potential to assist in implementation of EBMgmt but requires managers to invest in a comprehensive plan and implementation.

Knowledge management: Encompasses mechanisms to provide 'the right information, to the right person, at the right time, with the potential of attaining greater competitive advantage' (Kothari et al. 2011, p.1)

Summary

- Managers need to look for evidence when they or others plan a significant change in the workplace.
- Evidence is acquired from four areas: scientific research findings; stakeholders' values and concerns; organisational data, facts and figures; and professional experience and judgement.
- The quality of the different forms of evidence must be considered by examining aspects such as the source, method, context and analyses used.
- Relevant evidence should be used appropriately in decision-making strategies.

Reflective questions

1. Even scientifically rigorous studies can often be contradictory, leading to apparently opposite results. How might you deal with conflicting evidence?
2. How might you justify your selection of experts when you call on people in your personal network to give you advice?
3. To what extent does your own experience with an issue or topic form part of the evidence base?
4. Many scholarly studies include sophisticated statistical analyses to reach their conclusions. How might you deal with this evidence when you do not understand the statistics used?
5. How do you access data within your organisation? Are there strategies in place for knowledge management?

Self-analysis question

Lynn McVey (2013, para. 10), chief executive officer and president of Meadowlands Hospital Medical Center in New Jersey in the United States, claims that

> [w]hen a [doctor] tells me, 'The nurses on the 3rd floor suck.' Immediately I know he hasn't yet been baptized by evidence-based management. After I drill down his statement several layers, I ultimately discover he could not find nurse Janie Friday morning when he needed her. I then explain I can actually help him when he uses evidence-based statements, but nobody can do anything with, 'The nurses on the 3rd floor suck'.

How does this relate to your understanding of evidence-based management in healthcare?

References

Axelsson, R. (1998). Towards an evidence based health care management. *International Journal of Health Planning and Management*, *13*(4), 307–317. https://doi.org/10.1002/(SICI)1099-1751(199810/12)13:4<307::AID-HPM525>3.0.CO;2-V

Barends, E., Rousseau, D. M. & Briner, R. B. (2014). *Evidence-based management: The basic principles*. Center for Evidence-Based Management.

Daouk-Öyry, L., Sahakian, T. & van der Vijver, F. (2021). Evidence-based management competency model for managers in hospital settings. *British Journal of Management*, *32*(4), 1384–1403.

Finkler, S. A. & Ward, D. M. (2003). The case for the use of evidence-based management research for the control of hospital costs. *Health Care Management Review*, *28*(4), 348–365. https://doi.org/10.1097/00004010-200310000-00007

Hemsley-Brown, J. V. & Sharp, C. (2003). The use of research to improve professional practice: A systematic review of the literature. *Oxford Review of Education*, *29*(4), 449–470. https://doi.org/10.1080/0305498032000153025

Kothari, A., Hovanec, N., Hastie, R. & Sibbald, S. (2011). Lessons from the business sector for successful knowledge management in health care: A systematic review. *BMC Health Services Research*, *11*(1), 1–11.

Lavis, J. N., Davies, H., Oxman, A., Denis, J., Golden-Biddle, K. & Ferlie, E. (2005). Towards systematic reviews that inform health care management and policy-making. *Journal of Health Services Research & Policy*, *10*(1), 35–48. https://doi.org/10.1258/1355819054308549

Liang, Z., Howard, P. F., Leggat, S. G. & Murphy, G. (2012). A framework to improve evidence-informed decision-making in health service management. *Australian Health Review*, *36*(3), 284–289. https://doi.org/10.1071/AH11051

McVey, L. (2013). Lessons from Beyonce: Hospitals Need Evidence-based Management. Retrieved from: https://www.fiercehealthcare.com/healthcare/lessons-from-beyonce-hospitals-need-evidence-based-management

Mitton, C. & Patten, S. (2004). Evidence-based priority-setting: What do the decisionmakers think? *Journal of Health Services Research & Policy*, *9*(3), 146–152. https://doi.org/10.1258/1355819041403240

Murad, M. H., Asi, N., Alsawas, M. & Alahdab, F. (2016). New evidence pyramid. *BMJ Evidence-Based Medicine*, *21*(4), 125–127.

National Institute for Health and Clinical Excellence (NIHHCE). (2009). *The guidelines manual*. NIHHCE.

Nutley, S. & Davies, H. T. O. (2000). Making a reality of evidence-based practice: Some lessons from the diffusion of innovation. *Public Money and Management,* (October–December), 35–42. https://doi.org/10.1111/1467-9302.00234

O'Halloran, P., Porter, S. & Blackwood, B. (2010). Evidence based practice and its critics: What is a nurse manager to do? *Journal of Nursing Management*, *18*(1), 90–95. https://doi.org/10.1111/j.1365-2834.2009.01068.x

Pfeffer, J. & Sutton, R. I. (2006). Evidence-based management. *Harvard Business Review*, *84*(1), 62–74.

Roshanghalb, A., Lettieri, E., Aloini, D., Cannavacciuolo, L., Gitto, S. & Visintin, F. (2018). What evidence on evidence-based management in healthcare? *Management Decision*, *56*(10), 2069–2084.

Rousseau, D. M. (2006). Is there such a thing as 'evidence-based management'? *Academy of Management Review*, *31*(2), 256–269. https://doi.org/10.5465/AMR.2006.20208679

Rousseau, D. M. & ten Have, S. (2022). Evidence-based change management. *Organizational Dynamics*, *51*(3), 100899.

Shafaghat, T., Imani Nasab, M. H., Bahrami, M. A., Kavosi, Z., Roozrokh Arshadi Montazer, M., Rahimi Zarchi, M. K. & Bastani, P. (2021). A mapping of facilitators and barriers to evidence-based management in health systems: a scoping review study. *Systematic Reviews*, *10*(1), 1–14.

Shortell, S. M. (2006). Promoting evidence-based management. *Frontiers of Health Services Management*, *22*(3), 23–29.

Walshe, K. & Rundall, T. G. (2001). Evidence-based management: From theory to practice in health care. *Milbank Quarterly*, *79*(3), 429–457. https://doi.org/10.1111/1468-0009.00214

25 Successfully managing conflict

Gary E. Day

Learning objectives

How do I:

- recognise the types and origins of conflict in my workplace?
- determine which is the best approach to managing conflict?
- develop my skills to be more successful in managing conflict within my workplace?
- analyse conflict situations and design an appropriate conflict-management strategy?

Introduction

A 2021 report on a study of workplace conflict in the United Kingdom concludes that, in 2018–19, more than 35 per cent of respondents reported workplace conflict, with an estimated 485 000 employees resigning as a result (Advisory, Conciliation and Arbitration Service, 2021). Managers need to understand that conflict does not resolve itself; rather, it tends to gather intensity and energy. Gupta, Boyd and Kuzmits (2011) have found that 'employees spend as much as 42 per cent of their time engaging in or attempting to resolve conflict and 20 per cent of managers' time is taken up by conflict-related issues' (p. 395). Managing conflict is one of the primary responsibilities of managing staff and teams, particularly in multicultural work environments. Understanding what is 'culturally normative in terms of self-worth, confrontation, emotional expression, and managerial intervention can help [staff] involved in workplace conflict understand what they are experiencing' (Brett, 2018, p. 32). Additionally, it can help managers intervene appropriately (Brett, 2018). In this chapter, different types and origins of conflict are discussed, as well as approaches to managing and resolving conflict.

Types and origins of conflict

Conflict is best defined as unresolved, protracted disagreements between individuals or groups that negatively affect staff, organisations and working relationships. Conflict between team members and work groups can be highly disruptive and can lead to poor team outcomes and lack of team cohesion and trust. At its worst, conflict can lead to staff turnover (McKibben, 2017); absenteeism (Vivar, 2006); negative patient outcomes, organisational loyalty and work commitment (McKibben, 2017; Jehn, 1995; Jehn & Chatman, 1999); low staff morale (Iglesias & Vallejo, 2012); and a negative workplace culture.

There are numerous ways of defining the types, levels and origins of **conflict**. Gupta and colleagues (2011) divide conflict into four areas, which 'recognises that entities (people, parties, groups) might become involved at different points in time in conflict, and that conflict can be between organizations (inter-organizational), groups (inter-group), individuals (inter-personal) and also with oneself (intra-personal)' (p. 396). Malloch and Porter-O'Grady (2005) offer a different perspective on the origins of conflict by highlighting five primary causes, which are discussed in the following section. Irrespective of the causes, conflict usually goes through four distinct phases: frustration of one or more parties involved in conflict, conceptualisation or rationalisation of cause, expression of behaviours, and behaviours resulting in negative outcome (Piryani & Piryani, 2018). Healthcare managers should be cognisant that any given conflict may originate from a combination of two or more of these causes.

Conflict: Unresolved, protracted disagreements between individuals or groups that negatively affect staff, organisations and working relationships

Relationship-based conflict

Relationship-based conflict involves a fundamental and intractable difference between two individuals and is probably most commonly seen between staff members within a department. The conflict might be quite heated or quietly insidious, and outwardly manifested through harassing, bullying, gossiping or denigrating behaviours.

Values-based conflict

This is seen in a clash of values between the organisation and the staff. Commonly, the organisation's 'lived' values will be at odds with its 'espoused' values, which causes friction with staff. Conflict concerning values can occur when staff members feel the organisation is not true to its stated values or deviates from the reason they decided to join the organisation.

Interest-based conflict

Interest-based conflict can be seen when different professional groups in an organisation have conflict over a common issue. While there may be mutual commitment to the overall aims of the organisation, there remains conflict based on a shared interest. This might be seen, for example, if nursing and medical staff identify a different solution or approach to the same problem. The conflict arises when each professional group is unwilling to move from their stated or professional position.

Structure-driven conflict

Structure-driven conflict happens when inequities in the system cause discordance between groups. It may be a result of inadequate or unfair polices, rules, practices or protocols, or of contextual or organisational factors that inhibit cooperative professional relationships (Malloch & Porter-O'Grady, 2005). This may occur in the unequal treatment of different groups within a health system or hospital, when one group receives favourable treatment in terms of services, pay increases or privileges over other clinical groups that are working under the same conditions in the same organisation.

Data-based conflict

Differences of opinion can be based on the use of data to support a given argument or point of view. Data may be used or manipulated to support a position, and this may be the source of conflict between groups. Alternatively, one group may be given more access to data than another group, or one group may not be given the same information to assist in a decision-making process.

Is all conflict bad?

While it is often thought that all conflict is inherently bad and that organisations should always be peaceful and harmonious, conflict can in fact be functional as well as dysfunctional. Parkin (2009) claims that functional conflict focuses on disagreements about content and issues of tasks, with their surrounding decisions, opinions, ideas and points of view. In the right surroundings and with the correct management, functional conflict can energise groups, bring new perspectives to the surface and improve team performance. According to Parkin, functional conflict can increase understandings of alternative and multiple views, stimulate questioning and effective use of information, improve the evaluation of alternatives and enhance critical thinking.

Functional conflict can be achieved only when there is mutual respect for all parties involved, maturity among the team members and open and honest communication throughout; however, not when teams are in turmoil or are harbouring dysfunctional, unresolved conflict. Heifetz, Grashow and Linsky (2009) go further, suggesting that managers can orchestrate functional conflict to achieve deep, not superficial, harmony within teams.

Management of conflict

Most people dislike dealing with conflict or actively avoid it, because it is often heated, takes considerable emotional capital and is confronting. Human nature, through the 'fight or flight' mechanism, either encourages people to run away from conflict or, when cornered, compels them to fight.

Managers often avoid dealing with conflict, hoping that it will self-rectify, disappear or calm down. Unfortunately, failure to adequately address and actively manage conflict can lead to its escalation. Health managers need the correct tools and approaches to adequately address and manage conflict. Just as one type of fire extinguisher will not extinguish every type of fire, so a single approach to conflict resolution will not manage every type of conflict, and health managers need to develop a suite of methods to deal with the range of conflicts they will face. Lencioni (2005) claims that avoiding conflict is one of the main types of team dysfunctions and that a fundamental requirement of managers is to address and deal with conflict.

Katz and Flynn (2013) suggest that leaders and employees give different definitions of conflict and have varying opinions on the effectiveness of the systems in place. There is also little awareness of the tools and strategies available to mitigate conflict in the workplace. It is therefore critical that health managers have open conversations with staff to discuss conflicts that detract from the team's performance and how to adequately address them.

Health managers need to be in a position to actively deal with or 'call' conflict when they see it. By making it explicit within the team that the manager will address conflict, the team effectively gives permission for conflict management and resolution to occur. Openly discussing conflict also demonstrates to the team that dealing with conflict is another management function, just like staffing and budgeting. This active approach can take the mystique and stress out of managing conflict at the local level.

While it is important to consider the health manager's role in managing and dealing with conflict, there is also an important leadership function in conflict resolution, to prevent and deal with conflict situations as they arise. Demonstrating strong leadership is as important as developing sound management strategies to deal with conflict. Healthcare workers at any level can demonstrate leadership and effect positive strategies to prevent conflict from occurring or escalating.

LEADING THROUGH CRISIS: A CASE STUDY IN CONFLICT PREVENTION DURING THE COVID-19 PANDEMIC IN A HOSPITAL SETTING

Introduction

The COVID-19 pandemic brought unprecedented challenges to healthcare systems worldwide. This case study delves into a hospital's leadership response to mitigate conflicts among its staff during this crisis, emphasising the critical role of leadership in fostering resilience and unity.

Proactive communication

Recognising the heightened stress and uncertainty, the hospital leadership prioritised transparent and frequent communication. Regular virtual town-hall meetings, email updates and a dedicated information hub were established to keep staff well-informed about the evolving situation, safety protocols and organisational decisions.

Support systems

Leadership implemented support mechanisms to address the emotional toll on healthcare workers. Mental health resources, counselling services and peer-support groups were introduced to provide outlets for staff to share experiences and cope with the unique stressors associated with the pandemic.

Resource allocation

Effective leadership ensured that resources, such as personal protective equipment and medical supplies, were equitably distributed. Transparent decision-making processes and regular updates on resource availability sought to alleviate concerns among staff, minimising potential conflicts related to resource shortages.

Recognition and appreciation

Leadership actively acknowledged and celebrated the dedication of frontline workers. Recognition programs were established to highlight individual and team efforts. This not only boosted morale but also fostered a sense of unity and shared purpose among the hospital staff.

Results

The hospital experienced a notable decrease in internal conflicts, with staff expressing greater cohesion and solidarity. Through visible leadership and by prioritising transparent communication, offering support systems, ensuring fair resource allocation and recognising the efforts of healthcare workers, leadership successfully prevented and mitigated conflicts during the challenging COVID-19 pandemic.

> ## Conclusion
> This case study underscores the pivotal role of leadership in navigating crisis situations. By adopting proactive measures and prioritising the wellbeing of staff, hospital leadership created a resilient and united workforce, ultimately enhancing the hospital's capacity to provide effective patient care during the COVID-19 pandemic.

Approaches to conflict resolution

The seminal works of Kenneth Thomas and Ralph Kilmann (1974) and of M. Afzalur Rahim (1983) categorise approaches to conflict resolution based on a dynamic interaction between cooperation and assertiveness. Before being discussed in detail, Thomas and Kilmann's (1974) categorisations are listed here, followed in parentheses by the corresponding categorisations of Rahim (1983):

- avoiding (avoiding)
- compromising (compromising)
- collaborating (integrating)
- accommodating (obliging)
- competing (dominating).

When all parties in a conflict feel they have achieved a win–win result and that each party was treated with respect, and when none of the parties feels they have had to compromise their own position, the conflict has been adequately addressed. But when one group feels they have lost out in the negotiations, there is a high probability that the conflict will recur. Conflict resolution can be seen as a balance between assertiveness and cooperativeness. (see Figure 25.1).

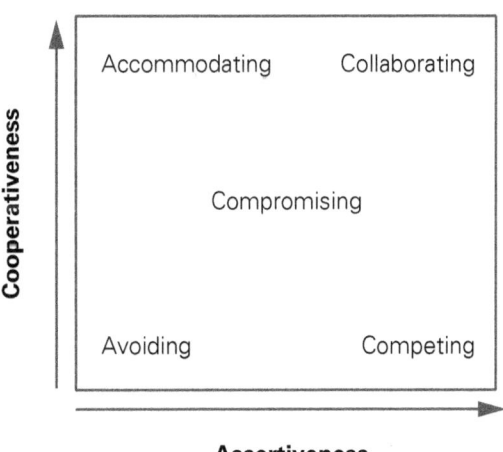

Figure 25.1 Conflict-resolution matrix

Source: Adapted from Smiley (2018).

Unfortunately, managers can often choose the wrong approach when attempting to manage conflict. In a recent systematic review, nurses most frequently used a collaborative (or integrating) style of conflict resolution, followed by accommodating (Labrague, Al Hamdan & McEnroe-Petitte, 2018).

Avoiding

Unfortunately, avoidance is a common approach to conflict resolution. It should be noted that avoidance may be used as a deliberate stalling or delaying tactic; however, it usually ends in a lose–lose situation for the conflicted parties. This approach is low assertiveness and low cooperation. The leader withdraws from the conflict, and therefore no one wins. The leader may deal with the conflict in a passive attitude in the hope that the situation will just 'resolve itself' (Smiley, 2018, p. 127). Avoidant behaviours can be seen as reducing the importance of the issues causing the conflict, and the approach exhibits a low concern for others. Avoidance is failure to address the issues and to look for suitable solutions.

Compromising

Conflict-resolution strategies that rely on compromise result in an outcome in which there is moderate concern for each party (Rahim, 2011). This approach is:

> moderate assertiveness and moderate cooperative. It is often described as "giving up more than one would want" to allow for each party to have their concerns partially fulfilled. This can be viewed as a situation where neither person wins or losses, but rather as an acceptable solution that is reached by either splitting the difference between the two positions, trading concerns, or seeking a middle ground. (Smiley, 2018, p. 128)

While relationships are left largely intact, parties may feel emotionally or professionally deflated. It could be argued that a compromised solution produces a lose–lose outcome for the parties.

Collaborating (integrating)

Collaborating strategies are used when parties have a high level of concern for each other. This mode is high assertiveness and high cooperation. This approach will 'require a lot of time, energy and resources to identify the underlying needs of each party' (Smiley, 2018, p. 128). An outcome is reached that satisfies the needs of all parties, meaning a win–win result. Gupta and colleagues (2011) say that the collaborative approach to conflict resolution is superior, as it 'promotes creative problem solving and fosters mutual respect and rapport' (p. 397).

Accommodating (obliging)

This mode is 'low assertiveness and high cooperation. The leader ignores their own concerns in order to fulfill the concerns of others. They are willing to sacrifice their own needs to "keep the peace" within the team' (Smiley, 2018, p. 127). Therefore, the leader loses and the other party wins. Obliging is often associated with self-effacing or timid behaviour by one party and results in unilateral possessions and unconditional promises. Accommodating produces lose–win outcomes in which one party must give up ground or their position at the expense of the other. In some cases, accommodating resolution strategies are used to maintain harmony. Managers may adopt an accommodating (or avoiding) approach to reduce the immediate heat in the issue until a more appropriate, long-term strategy is developed.

Competing (dominating)

This mode is 'high assertiveness and low cooperation'. The leader 'fulfills their own concerns at the expense of others. The leader uses any appropriate power they have to win the conflict' (Smiley, 2018, p. 127). It is worth noting that both competing and accommodating strategies may be heavily influenced by power dynamics in the workplace and used to either keep the peace or demonstrate superiority. Neither strategy achieves lasting resolution, as they divide rather than unite the parties.

Conflict-resolution strategies

When considering an approach to conflict resolution, it is important to understand the influence of culture on the different parties. Brett (2018) argues that 'when people from dignity, face, and honor cultures are working together the fundamental differences in the logic of self-worth in these three types of culture may cause conflict. People from dignity and honor cultures are likely to confront conflict directly, while those from face cultures are more likely to confront conflict indirectly' (p. 32).

A contemporary conflict-resolution tool is called the evaporating cloud approach (Gupta et al., 2011; see Figure 25.2). It involves three key steps: identifying and displaying all elements of a conflict situation, identifying all underlying assumptions that cause the conflict to exist and developing solutions that invalidate one or more of the assumptions.

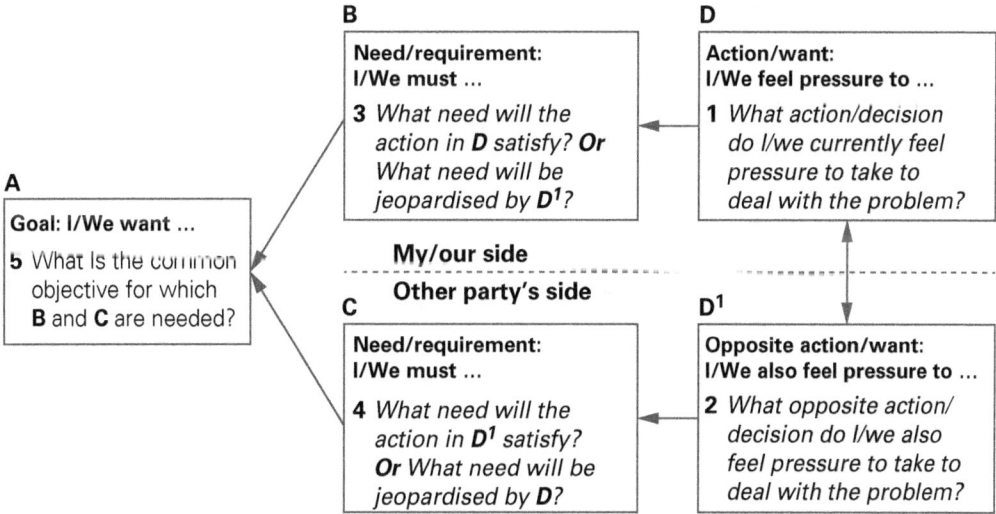

Figure 25.2 Evaporating cloud framework

Source: Adapted from Gupta et al. (2011).

The evaporating cloud framework, as described by Gupta and colleagues (2011), provides structure to a formal discussion to work through conflict situations. One of the issues with unresolved conflict is that the parties often do not want to or know how to go about resolving the matter. By using the framework to guide the discussion, a structured solution can be reached. The framework leads the parties through the following process: 'D and D^1 represent two opposing wants or actions … B and C represent the basic needs to be satisfied, and … A represents the common objective for which B and C are needed' (p. 399).

In using the evaporating cloud approach, the manager must take an active role in bringing the conflicted parties together. The process requires each party to verbalise what they need or require, and at the end of the process to identify common objectives. The process enables the manager to depersonalise the conflict by separating the issue from the personalities involved and by concentrating on the shared interests rather than the individual positions of each party. It also focuses the parties on possibilities, options and solutions. This approach is useful for interest-driven, structure-driven and data-based conflicts, and stops the issue from becoming relationship-based.

Considerations when managing conflict

Managers must be able to step outside the conflict they are managing. If the manager is central to the conflict and a party to it, they should consider asking someone else to mediate and negotiate an outcome.

It is essential to collect all the data and clarify all the concerns and questions before developing a strategy to resolve the conflict. In relationship-based conflicts, it may be necessary to remove one or more of the parties for a time to bring the team back into equilibrium. The manager should also set out the ground rules and process by which the negotiation will take place. Each group must be heard by the other, and there should be mutual respect and honesty between the parties.

During negotiations it is important to concentrate on the similarities shared by the parties rather than on the differences between them; in many situations there will be more of the former than of the latter. Establishing the similarities between the parties changes the management of conflict into a more positive exercise, from which it is easier to work through the points of misalignment. This approach is particularly successful with interest-based and structure-driven conflict situations.

Managers need to look for small wins and then build on them. Having 'wins' in conflict negotiations enables all parties to see that progress is being made. Wins also develop trust between the parties and the manager.

Finally, after the conflict has been resolved, the manager can play an important role in refocusing the team and rebuilding trust within it. This is essential to re-establish trusting, robust, professional working relationships and team norms, and to ensure the team is focused on its core business. The manager also needs to continually monitor the team's progress, so it does not slip back into the conflict situation.

Summary

- Conflict can be intrapersonal, interpersonal, intergroup and interorganisational.
- Conflict is a major cause of team dysfunction and the basis of negative team, organisational and patient outcomes. Managers need to take a leadership role in identifying conflict and constructively dealing with it.
- Preventing and de-escalating conflict is both a management and leadership function.
- Managers need to be able to draw from a range of approaches when dealing with conflict, including avoiding, compromising, collaborating, accommodating and competing, and must choose the correct approach for each conflict situation.
- Conflicts can be relationship-based, values-based, interest-based, structure-driven, data-based or a combination of these. Management of a conflict may therefore mean addressing more than one root cause.

Reflective questions

1. In what way is preventing or de-escalating conflict a leadership and a management function?
2. Why is it important to understand the different types of conflicts that occur in the workplace?
3. Based on your experience (both professionally and personally), what is your predominant style in dealing with conflict, and why?
4. Which among the types of conflicts discussed in this chapter would you find most difficult to manage, and why?
5. Can all conflict in the workplace be categorised as bad? Justify your answer.

Self-analysis questions

Consider the last time you were involved in a conflict situation (at home or at work). What sort of conflict was it, and how would you categorise it? What role did you play? What did the situation tell you about your leadership and management style? What did you learn from the situation?

References

Advisory, Conciliation and Arbitration Service. (2021). Estimating the Cost of Workplace Conflict. Retrieved from: https://www.acas.org.uk/research-and-commentary/workplace-conflict

Brett, J. (2018). Intercultural challenges in managing workplace conflict – A call for research, *Cross Cultural & Strategic Management*, 25(1), 32–52. https://doi.org/10.1108/CCSM-11-2016-0190

Gupta, M., Boyd, L. & Kuzmits, F. (2011). The evaporating cloud: A tool for resolving workplace conflict. *International Journal of Conflict Management*, 22(4), 394–412. https://doi.org/10.1108/10444061111171387

Heifetz, R., Grashow, A. & Linsky, M. (2009). *The practice of adaptive leadership: Tools and tactics for changing your organization and the world*. Harvard Business.

Iglesias, M. E. L. & Vallejo, R. B. (2012). Conflict resolution styles in the nursing profession. *Contemporary Nurse*, 43(1), 73–80. https://doi.org/10.5172/conu.2012.43.1.73

Jehn, K. (1995). A multimethod examination of the benefits and detriments of intragroup conflict. *Administrative Science Quarterly, 40*(2), 256–282.

Jehn, K. & Chatman, J. (1999). The influence of proportional and perceptual conflict composition on team performance. *International Journal of Conflict Management, 11*, 56–73. https://doi.org/10.1108/eb022835

Katz, N. H. & Flynn, L. T. (2013). Understanding conflict management systems and strategies in the workplace: A pilot study. *Conflict Resolution Quarterly, 30*(4), 393–410. https://doi.org/10.1002/crq.21070

Labrague, L. J., Al Hamdan, Z. & McEnroe-Petitte, D. M. (2018). An integrative review on conflict management styles among nursing professionals: Implications for nursing management. *Journal of Nursing Management, 26*, 902–917. https://doi.org/10.1111/jonm.12626

Lencioni, P. (2005). *Overcoming the five dysfunctions of a team: A field guide for leaders, managers and facilitators*. Jossey-Bass.

Malloch, K. & Porter-O'Grady, T. (2005). *The quantum leader: Applications for the new world of work*. Jones & Bartlett.

McKibben, L. (2017). Conflict management: Importance and implications. *British Journal of Nursing, 26*(2). https://doi.org/10.12968/bjon.2017.26.2.100

Parkin, P. (2009). *Managing change in healthcare: Using action research*. Sage.

Piryani, R. M. & Piryani, S. (2018). Conflict management in healthcare. *Journal of Nepal Health Research Council, 16*(41), 481–482. http://dx.doi.org/10.33314/jnhrc.v16i41.1703

Rahim, M. A. (2011). *Managing conflict in organizations* (4th ed.). Transaction.

——— (1983). A measure of styles of handling interpersonal conflict. *Academy of Management Journal, 26*, 368–376.

Smiley, F. (2018). Leadership guide to conflict and conflict management. In J. Applegate et al. (eds). *Leadership in healthcare and public health*. Retrieved from: https://ohiostate.pressbooks.pub/pubhhmp6615/chapter/leadership-guide-to-conflict-and-conflict-management/2024

Thomas, K. W. & Kilmann, R. H. (1974). *Thomas-Kilmann conflict mode instrument*. Xicom.

Vivar, C. G. (2006). Putting conflict management into practice: A nursing case study. *Journal of Nursing Management, 14*, 201–206. https://doi.org/10.1111/j.1365-2934.2006.00554.x

Building positive workplace cultures

26

Gary E. Day and Kirsty Marles

Learning objectives

How do I:

- identify barriers associated with workplace culture to be able to create the conditions for the desired culture in my workplace?
- identify the effects of positive and negative workplace cultures on the functioning of an organisation, particularly in the area of patient safety and quality?
- identify different types of workplace cultures?
- understand the impact a health manager or leader can have on the culture of an organisation or department?
- build positive workplace cultures?
- identify and address burnout and stress in my workplace and team?

Introduction

Understanding, managing and building positive culture within a workplace are key responsibilities of leadership and management. This chapter outlines what workplace culture is, the effects of poor culture on an organisation and what managers can do to improve workplace culture.

The Austrian American management theorist Peter Drucker (as cited in Fernández-Aráoz, 2014) once famously said, 'Culture eats strategy over breakfast' (para. 2). This might seem implausible, because there is an expectation that healthcare managers plan, set out, implement and then evaluate strategy. Drucker's point is that unless there is a positive workplace culture, seeing a strategy move to successful implementation and adoption is very difficult, sometimes impossible.

Definitions

Workplace culture (also called organisational or corporate culture) has been well defined in the literature. Culture has often been described as the particular beliefs or values of an organisation that distinguish it from other similar organisations. Local definitions include 'the way we do things around here' and 'our corporate DNA'. These descriptions of workplace culture hold true and describe the unique and often hard-to-define 'feel' of an organisation. Groysberg, Lee, Price and Cheng (2018) describe workplace culture as 'the tacit social order of an organization: It shapes attitudes and behaviours in wide-ranging and durable ways. Cultural norms define what is encouraged, discouraged, accepted, or rejected within a group' (p. 4).

While we may talk about a single defining culture, the truth is that in larger organisations there may be several cultures or subcultures. Manley, Sanders, Cardiff and Webster (2011) state that 'organisational culture in the past has been assumed to be singular and pervasive, monolithic and integrative, but all organisations have multiple cultures usually associated with different functional groupings or geographical locations' (p. 4). Subcultures can be routinely seen in large hospitals, where individual departments may have cultures that are slightly different from, but aligned with, that of the organisation overall. Subcultures are commonplace and contribute to the overall feel, function and direction of an organisation.

On the other hand, countercultures – a form of organisational incivility – work at odds with the organisation and can be quite disruptive or destructive to its overall functioning. Andersson and Pearson, as cited in Namin, Øgaard and Røislien (2022), describe organisational incivility as 'low-intensity deviant behavior with ambiguous intent to harm the target, in violation of workplace norms for mutual respect. Uncivil behaviors are characteristically rude and discourteous, displaying a lack of regard for others. There is some overlap between workplace incivility and other negative treatments in the organization, including aggression, social undermining at work, deviance, antisocial behavior and violence'. One of the key responsibilities of a healthcare manager and leader is the cultivation of positive, productive workplace cultures. Spence (2024) argues that 'leaders profoundly influence culture by setting a vision that unites employees and creating a purpose-driven

---

Workplace culture: The beliefs, norms or values of an organisation that distinguish it from other similar organisations

work environment that supports them as they work to achieve that vision. Their actions shape organizational behaviors, making their role in culture strategically imperative for sustained excellence' (n.p.).

Typology of workplace cultures

While setting the culture of an organisation is the primary responsibility of the chief executive officer and the executive team, managers are expected to support and promote the desired culture. To understand what sort of culture prevails in an organisation, it is necessary to be able to categorise culture types. Categorisation enables the health manager to determine whether there is a need to redefine and change the culture in which they work. Self-aware health managers also need to ask themselves the following questions: How am I contributing to the culture in this organisation? If I assess the current culture in the organisation to be negative or counterproductive, what am I going to do to change it?

The literature categorises culture in many ways, ranging from three-culture models (Westrum, 2004) to quadrant models (Quinn and Rohrbaugh, 1983; Wolniak, 2013) to cultures depicted as animal types (Line, 1999). A cultural framework that has been used widely in a number of industries, including health, is the **Competing Values Framework** (Cameron & Quinn, 2011; see Figure 26.1). It categorises four main cultural types and describes how each of these predominantly functions.

Competing Values Framework: A research-informed framework describing four key culture types: clan, hierarchy, adhocracy and market (Cameron & Quinn, 2011)

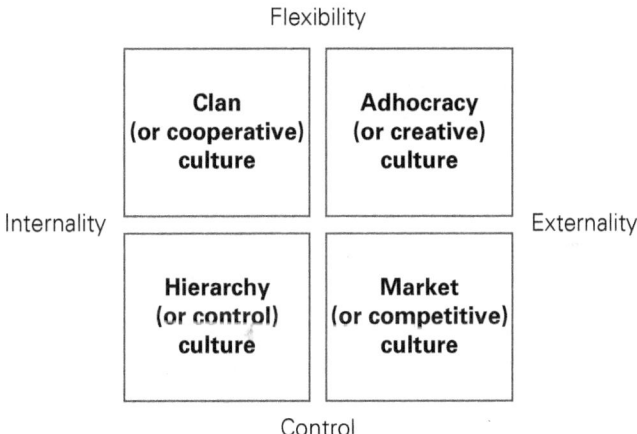

Figure 26.1 Competing Values Framework
Source: Adapted from Cameron & Quinn (2011).

The Competing Values Framework runs along two axes forming a cross. The vertical axis focuses on organisations that have flexibility and discretion through to those with high levels of stability and control. The horizontal axis highlights organisations with a strong internal focus and integration through to those that are externally focused and differentiated. Using these axes, Cameron and Quinn (2011) have categorised four predominant cultures, which are discussed in this section. Staff within healthcare organisations may identify any one of these types. Each has its benefits and limitations depending on the type of organisation and the direction in which a healthcare facility is heading. Healthcare managers need to be aware of how they influence the culture and how they should support staff in their specific cultural type.

Clan (or cooperative) culture

This culture is characterised by a strong internal focus and flexibility. Organisations with a clan culture exhibit strong family-like, nurturing, cohesive and collaborative traits. Teams within such organisations work with a level of autonomy and self-direction.

Hierarchy (or control) culture

The hierarchy culture is characterised by an internal focus with strong control processes. Organisations with a hierarchy culture have defined hierarchies or bureaucracies, and command-and-control structures that focus on policies, procedures, processes and protocols. They aim to be stable, consistent and dependable.

Adhocracy (or creative) culture

This culture is characterised by flexibility and an external focus. Organisations with an adhocracy culture promote rapid change, creativity and innovation, and they can be high-pressured, as they search for the next new product and aim to be 'ahead of the game'.

Market (or competitive) culture

The market culture has strong internal control and is externally focused. Organisations with a market culture focus on the external customer rather than staff and can be highly competitive, as they seek new customers and have an emphasis on customer service.

Measuring workplace culture

There are several ways in which to measure culture within organisations, from the subjective (having a general sense of what the organisation is like) to the objective (validated survey instruments and other qualitative approaches). Researchers have tried to understand the scope and range of quantitative instruments to measure workplace culture in healthcare organisations, and Scott and colleagues (2003) have identified 13 such instruments. However, while all examined employee views, perceptions and opinions of their working environments, only two considered the values and beliefs that might inform those views. The authors conclude that 'it is unlikely that any single instrument will ever provide a valid, reliable, and trustworthy assessment of an organisation's culture, and so a multi-method approach will always be desirable' (p. 942). Organisations tend to use a range of approaches to measure their culture, including measurements focusing on staff and patients. Sutherland and Watters (2024) point to simple 'proxy' measurements of workplace culture including the number of staff engaged in safety and quality or quality improvement projects, or the levels of sick leave or employee turnover.

Organisational implications of different workplace cultures

The healthcare manager's role in proactively managing culture is critical to the overall functioning and success of the organisation. The culture of an organisation can have a positive effect on its operation, profitability and ability to work through challenging circumstances. While the culture of an organisation may seem a soft, non-core issue to some, the positive and negative influences of culture can have substantial financial and operational implications.

Workplace culture can lead to positive outcomes in many areas of a health organisation. 'Positive organisational and workplace cultures were consistently associated with a wide range of patient outcomes such as reduced mortality rates, falls, hospital acquired infections and increased patient satisfaction' (Braithwaite, Herkes, Ludlow, Testa and Lamprell, 2017, p. 1) and lower risk-standardised mortality rates (Curry et al., 2017). Research also shows that workplace cultures are positively and directly related to organisational attractiveness and employees' individual innovative behaviour (Mutonyi, Slåtten, Lien & González-Pieñero, 2022). This also includes lowering patient mortality and improving nurses' health, job satisfaction, organisational commitment, emotional exhaustion and intention to stay (Laschinger, Cummings, Wong & Grau, 2014).

Positive culture also leads to increased optimism among staff about the organisation's ability to meet future challenges, improved working relationships, greater accountability and efficiency, better cost-management, increased devolvement of management to clinicians, and facilities that are more strategically placed and patient-focused (Braithwaite et al., 2005).

However, negative workplace culture, the consequences of which are regularly discussed in healthcare reports and reviews, can manifest through unethical and possibly illegal activity (Casali & Day, 2010), higher staff turnover and lower staff morale and productivity (Siourouni, Kastanioti, Tziallas & Niakas, 2012). It can also result in a lower quality of care (Mid Staffordshire NHS Foundation Trust Public Inquiry, 2010) and higher levels of workplace bullying (O'Farrell & Nordstrom, 2013).

There has also been recent debate about how the COVID-19 pandemic has disrupted organisational culture, especially with the move to working from home. Spicer (2020) suggests that because of the COVID-19 lockdown and the changes in work practices, managers may need to reimagine and redefine organisational culture. Spicer (2020) posits that due to the fundamental change to work practices, working from home and social distancing, our traditional, cultural and social norms at work may have changed. For example, is there a change in work culture due to working together in a physical space as opposed to working remotely from home? Does working online change work norms or symbols, and does the work culture that has been built up over some time become degraded by physical separation of the team?

> ### THE EFFECT OF CULTURE ON THE PROVISION OF CARE
>
> Several commissions of inquiry in Australia have shed light on the link between organisational culture and patient care. Australia's Royal Commission into Aged Care Quality and Safety (2021) noted that 'poor workplace culture has … contributed to poor care' (p. 75). The Royal Commission found that 'values and behaviour of people in senior positions have a significant impact on workplace culture and the quality of care that is delivered. When these values and behaviours are poor, so may be the care that people receive' (p. 75).
>
> These issues are not unique to Australian healthcare facilities, and similar cultural and patient-care issues have been raised in the United Kingdom. The Francis Inquiry, which began in 2010, highlighted poor clinical outcomes attributed to inappropriate culture within the Mid Staffordshire NHS Trust. Examples of poor culture leading to substandard and dangerous care can be seen in these excerpts from one of the inquiry's reports (Mid Staffordshire NHS Foundation Trust Public Inquiry, 2010):
>
> > [The chief executive of the trust] described the Trust's culture as being inwardly focused and complacent, resistant to change and accepting of poor standards (p. 22):
> >
> > When [a patient's daughter] was asked to describe the nursing culture on Ward 11, she said, 'They were bullies. They bullied … the other staff and they bullied the patients. There was no word for it. … particularly during the two weeks that Mum was dying, effectively, they were calling out for the toilet and they would just walk by them.' (p. 45)

Management imperatives in building positive workplace cultures

The contemporary literature highlights several critical success factors for creating and maintaining positive workplace cultures, of which four are mentioned regularly: positive and supportive leadership, workplace learning, collaboration and a focus on the patient or client.

Lamb, Burford and Alberti (2022) claim that 'role modelling has a crucial impact on the future [health] workforce, with the potential to shape perceptions, to attract and deter individuals from the career, and to support their development as professionals' (p. 265). Laschinger and colleagues (2014) report that positive and supportive leadership empowers staff, lowers patient mortality, improves nurses' health and job satisfaction, and reduces absenteeism, staff turnover and incivility. Also, managers who build emotional resilience in their workforce and team members create a healthier workplace culture, thereby reducing absenteeism, improving teamwork and raising morale (Sergeant & Laws-Chapman, 2012). To ensure that staff feel engaged, managers need to be highly visible, provide feedback and coaching to employees and make sure that doctors are included as part of developing the culture (Hegland, Tarcon & Krueger, 2010).

The literature also emphasises the development of staff as a key component in developing positive workplace cultures. Tomlinson (2010), when reviewing an organisation with a culture of high employee engagement, identifies emphases on leadership, employee and organisational development, employee recognition and internal communication. Similarly,

Goh, Chan and Kuziemsky (2013) suggest that to develop positive workplace cultures, managers need to foster collaborative learning among staff to rid their organisation of a blame culture and to prioritise patient safety. Organisational leaders need to 'implement fair processes and reward staff for providing safety information, and staff are responsible for reporting adverse events, speaking up for safety, and coming to work with good intentions' (Safer Care Victoria, n.d., p. 1).

Changing an organisation's culture

Changing organisational culture is not easy; it takes time and effort. There are often long-held, deeply taken-for-granted behaviours, attitudes and values that form the cultural reality of the organisation (Schedlitzki & Edwards, 2014). Any attempt to effect a change in culture requires relationships and leadership that use systems to embed shared values, beliefs and purpose in everyday practice.

Changing to a more desired culture takes concerted and persistent effort by all levels of management over an extended period. It probably took years for the culture to reach its current state, so any attempt to change it is likely to take as long again. Building trust with the organisation's staff, creating new norms, rewarding new behaviours, establishing new customs and rituals: these all take time, effort and consistent messages from the executive.

When embarking on major cultural change, continuing and continual communication from the executive to the staff should be implemented. The executive team needs to be adept at 'selling the vision', creating a level of excitement and anticipation about where the organisation is heading and making sure staff buy into this. Both formal and informal approaches may be used to ensure staff are aware of what is being proposed. Also, the espoused vision of the organisation must match the lived vision: the leadership and management should make sure that what they are doing is in line with what they say they are doing. For example, new staff should be selected and recruited in line with the organisation's values and beliefs. Failure in this area leads to staff confusion and lack of trust.

Managers should maintain or create rituals and customs that are unique to the organisation. This might be as simple as celebrating birthdays or anniversaries and celebrating 'wins' in the organisation. The leadership needs to be specific about the kinds of behaviours that are in line with the new culture and be proactive about addressing behaviours that are not in line with the organisation's vision and values.

Leadership imperatives in building positive workplace cultures

Leadership and culture are often discussed within the organisational development literature as being mutually dependent. Many researchers believe that the most important role of a formal leader is to create and manage culture (Schedlitzki & Edwards, 2014). To understand workplace culture, to know what is a positive culture and to know how to develop a positive culture are essential knowledge required of formal leaders in healthcare settings.

Leaders must be clear about the type of culture they want for their organisations. They must strategise and plan to create the conditions required to support a positive workplace culture. It is essential to deliver consistent messages through all the workplace mechanisms so as to contribute to building positive organisational culture.

Edgar Schein is recognised for his notable research into organisational development. In his text *Organizational culture and leadership*, Schein (2010) describes primary and secondary embedding mechanisms. These are drawn upon in the following discussion to describe the role of the formal leader in building and embedding positive workplace cultures.

'What leaders pay attention to, measure, and control on a regular basis has a critical impact on organisational culture' (Schein, 2010, p. 237). Schein's observation about what leaders pay attention to is mirrored by the former Australian Chief of Army, David Morrison (2013), in a nationally broadcast speech, 'The standard you walk past is the standard you accept. That goes for all of us, but especially those who, by their rank, have a leadership role.' This is a particularly powerful mechanism in highly regulated industries such as health and aged care, which have tight measures and controls set by independent regulators. In creating a positive workplace culture within these industries, the leader must be conscious of how compliance measures, such as legal, ethical, clinical and quality measures as well as their own behaviours, affect the culture within the organisation.

'Deliberate role modelling, teaching, and coaching' contribute to dispersing a positive workplace culture (Schein, 2010, p. 246). Leaders must themselves be conscious of the behaviour they are modelling. Similarly, those who are promoted to supervisory positions or who are responsible for training or coaching others must be champions of the positive workplace culture. This is particularly important when inducting or orientating new staff.

'How leaders allocate rewards and status' can also influence workplace culture (Schein, 2010, p. 247). However, this needs to be considered within the context of the quantity of resources that are available and the financial risks involved. Carney (2011) states that health leaders need to be able to 'place excellence at the forefront of care delivery, whilst at the same time being capable of managing the tensions that exist between cost effectiveness and the quality of care' (p. 523). Decisions about how to allocate scarce resources are not value-free or risk-free. It is the act of deciding how they are allocated that will reveal important aspects of an organisation's culture and attitude to risk. Organisations that cut costs often affect both patient safety and the engagement of staff. 'These challenges caused individual resource loss, and as stress arises from resource depletion, each turn of the stress spiral left the individuals and organization with fewer resources to counteract the loss, causing loss spirals to intensify in momentum and scale' (Rauf, Rook, Rajapakse, Lartey & Almeida, 2024, n.p.).

The use of the performance-appraisal process by managers and leaders acts as an important means for linking rewards and behavioural change to the type of culture and organisational values that they wish to promote. Performance appraisal is an activity that, if used proactively, can to 'enhance and boost the performance of employees and pave a way for career opportunity, promotion and further rewards' (Rana, Mukhtar & Mukhtar, 2022, p. 2351).

'How leaders recruit, select, promote and excommunicate' has a significant effect on changing, reinforcing and promoting an organisation's culture (Schein, 2010, p. 249). In the first instance, managers and organisations need to look at recruiting practices. 'Creating cultures starts with hiring the right people and then helping them develop critical relationships' (Hegland et al., 2010, p. 57). Ideally, leaders should use their selection and recruitment process to recruit and advance those they perceive as having the values they wish to cultivate and to remove those they consider as not sharing these values.

Managing stress and burnout: Strategies for health managers

The prevalence of work stress and **burnout** in the healthcare industry is a well-known and accepted problem. De Hert (2020) points out that 'healthcare workers … seem to be at particular risk for burnout' (p. 171). He notes that this can give rise to significant negative personal (substance abuse, broken relationships and even suicide) and professional consequences such as lower patient satisfaction, impaired quality of care, and medical errors. Further research on nurse burnout has reported negative impacts on patient satisfaction, increased risk in relation to safety and quality, and reduced nurses' organisational commitment and productivity. Traditionally, burnout is viewed as an individual issue (Jun, Ojemeni, Kalamani, Tong & Crecelius, 2021). It is clear that, left unaddressed, staff burnout and stress not only compromise patient safety and quality, but also result in organisational costs of reduced productivity and staff recruitment.

> **Burnout:** A 'work-related stress syndrome resulting from chronic exposure to job stress' (De Hert, 2020, p. 171). Burnout consists of dimensions including 'exhaustion, cynicism, and inefficiency' (Maslach, Shaufeli & Leiter, 2001, p. 397), and a sense of low personal accomplishment that leads to decreased effectiveness at work

Stress, burnout and psychological distress of healthcare workers during the COVID-19 pandemic has been well documented in Australian and international studies (Restauri & Sheridan, 2020; Murat, Köse & Savaser, 2020; Vizheh et al., 2020; Ehrlich, McKenney & Elkbuli, 2020; Smallwood et al., 2021). While burnout and stress of healthcare workers was well understood and documented before 2020 (Bridgeman, Bridgeman & Barone, 2018), the pandemic worsened its prevalence and harmful effects (Razai, Kooner & Majeed, 2023). A large Australian study of more than 9500 frontline healthcare workers shows that during the pandemic, 59.8 per cent of respondents self-reported mild to severe anxiety, 70.9 per cent reported moderate to severe burnout and 57.3 per cent reported mild to severe depression (Smallwood et al., 2021).

There are several factors (both personal and organisational) that contribute to the burnout and stress of healthcare staff (Leo et al., 2021), from personal resilience and coping mechanisms to organisational and structural barriers. It has been the long-term norm for individual healthcare workers to recognise and develop strategies to address their own stress, burnout and depression (Søvold et al., 2021). What health managers need to acknowledge is that being a frontline healthcare worker is a stressful job. They need to understand the strategies they can implement or influence to reduce the stress, burnout and depression. With Australia calculating a nursing shortage of more than 130 000 by 2030 (Duckett & Meehan, 2022), every effort should be made to provide safe, positive workplaces to minimise psychological or moral injury and reduce turnover rates. While the research suggests that there are several stress- and burnout-reducing strategies that can be controlled or initiated by the individual, managers still can promote these with staff. Specific individual or personal strategies include:

- increased physical activity, balanced diet, good sleep hygiene, family support, meaningful relationships, reflective practices and small group discussions (Leo et al., 2021)
- exercise and yoga (Cocchiara et al., 2019)
- increased individual levels of resilience and the ability to tolerate uncertainty (Di Trani, Mariani, Ferri, De Berardinis & Frigo, 2021)
- exploring the value of practising self-care strategies (Søvold et al., 2021)

- prioritising self-care and creating and maintaining healthy workplace boundaries (Wolters Klewer, 2023)
- yoga, mindfulness-based intervention, visual thinking strategies and forest bathing to improve mental health (Di Mario et al., 2023).

In addition to supporting and promoting self-help strategies to staff, there are several organisational strategies that managers can play an active part in introducing. These strategies include:

- Creating and promoting 'blame-free environments for sharing experiences and [advice], broad involvement in management decisions, multi-disciplinary psychosocial support teams, safe areas to withdraw quickly from stressful situations, adequate time planning, social support, and cultural level involvement of healthcare workers in the development, implementation, testing, and evaluation of measures against burnout' (Leo et al., 2021, p 1).
- 'Creating a work environment and culture where mental illness is not stigmatized' (Restauri & Sheridan, 2020, p. 925).
- 'Counselling and mindfulness, should be made accessible by healthcare employers. However, they are an addition and not a substitute for occupational interventions such as ensuring adequate staffing and manageable workloads' (Razai, Kooner & Majeed, 2023, p. 1).
- 'Increased availability of supervisors, protected time to ensure that time off is really time off, and shared scheduling to avoid long stretches of uninterrupted shifts' (Duckett & Meehan, 2022).
- 'Managing workload is a crucial factor in reducing burnout among healthcare workers. Adequate staffing levels and flexible work schedules is essential in reducing workload. Realistic workload and expectations with appropriate resources and training are crucial in reducing burnout and increasing engagement in the workplace' (Razai, Kooner & Majeed, 2023, p. 1).
- 'Organizational strategies to create a capable environment to reduce burnout could include the following interventions: improving workflow management, organizing services with an emphasis on reducing workload, improving communication skills, arranging discussion meetings, increasing interoperability, providing the opportunity for having adequate rest and exercise, holding workshops on coping skills, decreasing the clinical demand via schedule changes, and increasing teamwork' (Sharifi, Asadi-Pooya & Mousavi-Roknabadi, 2020, p. 4).
- 'Implementing evidence based interventions and organizational measures to help protect and support the mental health and well-being of the healthcare workforce. Lastly, we highlight systemic changes to empower healthcare workers and protect their mental health and well-being in the long run, and propose policy recommendations to guide healthcare leaders and health systems in this endeavour' (Søvold et al., 2021, p. 1).

Importantly, 'reframing burnout as an organizational and collective phenomenon affords the broader perspective necessary to address nurse burnout' (Jun et al., 2021, p. 1). No single strategy will likely significantly redress burnout and stress in the workplace; rather, a combination of several strategies is more likely to provide a workplace that promotes mental and psychological health.

Summary

- Workplace culture is formed by an organisation's unique behaviours, beliefs, values, ceremonies, experiences and history.
- A widely used approach to categorising workplace cultures is the Competing Values Framework, which identifies four main cultures: clan, hierarchy, adhocracy and market.
- A health manager's actions (or inactions) – their approach to organisational systems, policies and procedures, and customs and rituals – have a direct effect on the culture of a department or organisation.
- A health-service manager can build a positive workplace culture through role-modelling, teaching and coaching, by ensuring new staff are recruited, selected and promoted according to the organisation's stated values, and through clear, transparent, regular and purposeful communication with staff.
- Reframing stress and burnout of healthcare workers as an organisational and collective phenomenon affords the broader perspective necessary to address this issue. Also, no single strategy will likely significantly redress stress and burnout in the workplace; rather, a combination of several strategies is more likely to provide a workplace that promotes mental and psychological health and wellbeing.

Reflective questions

1. What are some of the rituals, beliefs, values and assumptions in your organisation that differentiate it from others?
2. Look at the mission, vision and values statements of your organisation. How is the culture reflected in them?
3. Are the actions of your organisation in line with its stated vision, values and mission? What is the impact of the lived and the espoused values on the culture of your organisation?
4. Using the Competing Values Framework as a guide, identify the type of culture in your department or organisation.
5. What change strategies could be adopted to create the conditions to enable the culture your workplace aspires to?

Self-analysis questions

Consider the culture in your organisation or in an organisation you have worked in. What role do you or the healthcare manager play in contributing to that culture? What would you do personally to change or improve the culture you are in? What leadership and management traits would you have to call on to make this change or improvement?

During the COVID-19 pandemic, what was the culture like in your organisation? Did it get worse? Stay the same? Get better? What factors influenced organisational culture at that time? Following the pandemic and lockdown, did the culture return to what it was before the pandemic? If not, why not? What did you see the hospital leadership team do to improve culture during the pandemic?

References

Braithwaite, J., Herkes, J., Ludlow, K., Testa, L. & Lamprell, G. (2017). Association between organisational and workplace cultures, and patient outcomes: Systematic review. *BMJ Open, 7*, e017708. https://doi.org/10.1136/bmjopen-2017-017708

Braithwaite, J., Westbrook, M. T., Iedema, R., Mallock, N. A., Forsyth, R. & Zhang, K. (2005). A tale of two hospitals: Assessing cultural landscapes and compositions. *Social Science and Medicine, 60*, 1149–1162. https://doi.org/10.1016/j.socscimed.2004.06.046

Bridgeman, P. J., Bridgeman, M. B. & Barone, J. (2018). Burnout syndrome among healthcare professionals. *American Journal of Health-System Pharmacy, 75*(3), 147–152. doi.org/10.2146/ajhp170460

Cameron, K. S. & Quinn, R. E. (2011). *Diagnosing and changing organizational culture: Based on the competing values framework* (3rd ed.). Jossey-Bass.

Carney, M. (2011). Influence of organizational culture on quality healthcare delivery. *International Journal of Health Care Quality Assurance, 24*(7), 523–539. https://doi.org/10.1108/09526861111160562

Casali, G. L. & Day, G. E. (2010). Treating an unhealthy organisational culture: The implications of the Bundaberg Hospital Inquiry for managerial ethical decision making. *Australian Health Review, 34*(1), 73–79. https://doi.org/10.1071/AH09543

Cocchiara, R. A., Peruzzo, M., Mannocci, A., Ottolenghi, L., Villari, P., Polimeni, A., Guerra F. & La Torre, G. (2019). The use of yoga to manage stress and burnout in healthcare workers: A systematic review. *Journal of Clinical Medicine, 8*(3), 284. https://doi.org/10.3390/jcm8030284

Curry, L.A, Brault, M.A., Linnander, E.L. et al. (2017). Influencing organisational culture to improve hospital performance in care of patients with acute myocardial infarction: A mixed-methods intervention study. *BMJ Quality & Safety, 27*, 207–217. https://doi.org/10.1136/bmjqs-2017-006989

De Hert, S. (2020). Burnout in healthcare workers: Prevalence, impact and preventative strategies. *Local and Regional Anesthesia, 13*, 171–183. https://doi.org/10.2147/LRA.S240564

Di Mario, S., Filomeno, L., Manai, M. V. et al. (2023). Strategies to reduce stress and burnout in healthcare workers: An RCT research protocol. *Journal of Public Health, 33*, 895–900. https://doi.org/10.1007/s10389-023-02080-3

Di Trani, M., Mariani, R., Ferri, R., De Berardinis, D. & Frigo, M. G. (2021). From resilience to burnout in healthcare workers during the COVID-19 emergency: The role of the ability to tolerate uncertainty. *Frontiers of Psychology, 16*(12), 646435. https://doi.org/10.3389/fpsyg.2021.646435

Duckett, S. & Meehan, E. (2022). *How to tackle burnout among healthcare workers*. Grattan Institute. Retrieved from: https://grattan.edu.au/news/how-to-tackle-burnout-among-healthcare-workers/

Ehrlich H., McKenney M. & Elkbuli, A. (2020). Protecting our healthcare workers during the COVID-19 pandemic. *American Journal of Emergency Medicine, 38*(7), 1527–1528. https://doi.org/10.1016/j.ajem.2020.04.024

Fernández-Aráoz, C. (2014, January 8). Creating a culture of unconditional love. *Harvard Business Review*. https://hbr.org/2014/01/creating-a-culture-of-unconditional-love

Goh, S. C., Chan, C. & Kuziemsky, C. (2013). Teamwork, organizational learning, patient safety and job outcomes. *International Journal of Health Care Quality Assurance, 26*(5), 420–432. https://doi.org/10.1108/IJHCQA-05-2011-0032

Groysberg, B., Lee, J., Price, J. & Cheng, J. Y. (2018). Changing your organization's culture can improve its performance. Here's how to do that. *The Leader's Guide to Corporate Culture*. Harvard Business Review. Retrieved 18 February 2024 from: https://egn.com/dk/wp-content/uploads/sites/3/2020/01/HBR-The-Leaders-guide-to-Corporate-Culture.pdf

Hegland, L. T., Tarcon, K. A. & Krueger, M. (2010). Building culture from the ground up in a new hospital. *Physician Executive, 36*(1), 56–60.

Jun, J., Ojemeni, M. M., Kalamani, R., Tong, J. & Crecelius, M. L. (2021). Relationship between nurse burnout, patient and organizational outcomes: Systematic review. *International Journal of Nursing Studies*, *19*, 103933. https://doi.org/10.1016/j.ijnurstu.2021.103933

Lamb, E., Burford, B. & Alberti, H. (2022). The impact of role modelling on the future general practitioner workforce: A systematic review. *Education for Primary Care*, *33*(5), 265–279. https://doi.org/10.1080/14739879.2022.2079097

Laschinger, H. K. S., Cummings, G. G., Wong, C. A. & Grau, A. L. (2014). Resonant leadership and workplace empowerment: The value of positive organizational cultures in reducing workplace incivility. *Nursing Economic$*, *32*(1), 5–15.

Leo, C. G., Saverio, S., Tumolo, M. R., Bodini, A., Ponzini, G., Sabato, E. & Mincarone, P. (2021). Burnout among healthcare workers in the COVID 19 era: A review of the existing literature. *Fronters of Public Health*, *9*. https://doi.org/10.3389/fpubh.2021.750529

Line, M. B. (1999). Types of organisational culture. *Library Management*, *20*(2), 73–75. https://doi.org/10.1108/01435129910251520

Manley, K., Sanders, K., Cardiff, S. & Webster, J. (2011). Effective workplace culture: The attributes, enabling factors and consequences of a new concept. *International Practice Development Journal*, *1*(2), Article 1.

Maslach C., Schaufeli, W. B. & Leiter, M. P. (2001). Job burnout. *Annual Review of Psychology*, *52*, 397–422. https://doi.org/10.1146/annurev.psych.52.1.397

Mid Staffordshire NHS Foundation Trust Public Inquiry. (2010). *Independent inquiry into care provided by Mid Staffordshire NHS Foundation Trust, January 2005 – March 2009: Volume 1* (Chaired by R. Francis QC). Retrieved from National Archives website: http://webarchive.nationalarchives.gov.uk/20130107105354/http://www.dh.gov.uk/prod_consum_dh/groups/dh_digitalassets/%40dh/%40en/%40ps/documents/digitalasset/dh_113447.pdf

Morrison, D. (2013). Chief of Army message regarding unacceptable behaviour [Australian Army HQ video file]. Retrieved 18 February 2024 from: https://www.youtube.com/watch?v=dRQBtDtZTGA

Murat, M., Köse, S. & Savaser, S. (2020). Determination of stress, depression and burnout levels of front-line nurses during the COVID-19 pandemic. *International Journal of Mental Health Nursing*, *30*(2), 533–543. https://doi.org/10.1111/inm.12818

Mutonyi, B. R., Slåtten, T., Lien, G. & González-Pieñero, M. (2022). The impact of organizational culture and leadership climate on organizational attractiveness and innovative behavior: a study of Norwegian hospital employees. *BMC Health Service Research*, *22*, 637. https://doi.org/10.1186/s12913-022-08042-x

Namin, B. H., Øgaard, T. & Røislien, J. (2022). Workplace incivility and turnover intention in organizations: A meta-analytic review. *International Journal of Environmental Research and Public Health*, *19*(1), 25. https://doi.org/10.3390/ijerph19010025

O'Farrell, C. & Nordstrom, C. R. (2013). Workplace bullying: Examining self-monitoring and organizational culture. *Journal of Psychological Issues in Organizational Culture*, *3*(4), 6–17. https://doi.org/10.1002/jpoc.21079

Quinn, R. E. & Rohrbaugh, J. (1983). The spatial model of effectiveness criteria: Towards a competing values approach to organizational analysis. *Management Science*, *29*(3), 363–377. https://doi.org/10.1287/mnsc.29.3.363

Rana, W., Mukhtar, S. & Mukhtar, S. (2022). Job satisfaction, performance appraisal, reinforcement and job tasks in medical healthcare professionals during the COVID-19 pandemic outbreak. *International Journal of Health Planning Management*. *37*(4), 2345–2353. https://doi.org/10.1002/hpm.3476

Rauf, A., Rook, L., Rajapakse, B., Lartey, J. K. S. & Almeida, S. (2024). Resource loss a significant issue for healthcare professionals: A case study of an Australian regional hospital. *Stress Health*, *40*(5), e3461. https://doi.org/10.1002/smi.3461

Razai, M. S., Kooner, P. & Majeed, A. (2023). Strategies and interventions to improve healthcare professionals' well-being and reduce burnout. *Journal of Primary Care and Community Health, 14.* https://doi.org/10.1177/21501319231178641

Restauri, N. & Sheridan, A. D. (2020). Burnout and posttraumatic stress disorder in the coronavirus disease 2019 (COVID-19) pandemic: Intersection, impact, and interventions. *Journal of the American College of Radiology, 17*(7), 921–926. https://doi.org/10.1016/j.jacr.2020.05.021

Royal Commission into Aged Care Quality and Safety. (2021). *Final Report: Care, dignity and respect.* Retrieved from: https://www.royalcommission.gov.au/aged-care

Safer Care Victoria. (n.d.). *Just culture guide for health services.* Retrieved 14 October 2024 from: https://www.safercare.vic.gov.au/sites/default/files/2022-08/SCV-Just-Culture-Guide-for-Health-Services.pdf

Schedlitzki, D. & Edwards, G. (2014). *Studying leadership: Traditional and critical approaches.* Sage.

Schein, E. (2010). *Organizational culture and leadership* (4th ed.). Wiley.

Scott, T., Mannion, R., Davies, H. & Marshall, M. (2003). The quantitative measurement of organizational culture in health care: A review of available instruments. *Health Services Research, 38*(3), 923–945. https://doi.org/10.1111/1475-6773.00154

Sergeant, J. & Laws-Chapman, C. (2012). Creating a positive workplace culture. *Nursing Management, 18*(9), 14–19. https://doi.org/10.7748/nm2012.02.18.9.14.c8889

Sharifi, M., Asadi-Pooya, A. A. & Mousavi-Roknabadi, R. S. (2020). Burnout among healthcare providers of COVID-19: A systematic review of epidemiology and recommendations. *Archives of Academic Emergency Medicine, 9*(1), e7. https://doi.org/10.22037/aaem.v9i1.1004

Siourouni, E., Kastanioti, C. K., Tziallas, D. & Niakas, D. (2012). Health care provider's organizational culture profile: A literature review. *Health Science Journal, 6*(2), 212–233. http://hsj.gr

Smallwood, N., Karimi, L., Bismark, M. et al. (2021). High levels of psychosocial distress among Australian frontline healthcare workers during the COVID-19 pandemic: A cross-sectional survey. *General Psychiatry, 34*, e100577. https://doi.org/10.1136/gpsych-2021-100577

Søvold, L. E., Naslund, J. A., Kousoulis, A. A., Saxena, S., Qoronfleh, M. W., Grobler, C. & Münter, L. (2021). Prioritizing the mental health and well-being of healthcare workers: An urgent global public health priority. *Frontiers of Public Health, 9.* https://doi.org/10.3389/fpubh.2021.679397

Spence, J. (2024). How leaders influence culture: The crucial role of leadership in shaping organizational culture. *Business Leadership Today.* Retrieved 18 February 2024 from: https://businessleadershiptoday.com/how-leaders-influence-culture/

Spicer, A. (2020). Organizational culture and COVID-19. *Journal of Management Studies, 57*(8). https://doi.org/10.1111/joms.12625

Sutherland, J. R. & Watters, D. A. (2024). Assessing organizational culture within Australian healthcare settings: Implications for training and accreditation. *ANZ Journal of Surgery, 94*(5), 791–794. https://doi.org/10.1111/ans.18863

Tomlinson, G. (2010). Building a culture of high employee engagement. *Strategic HR Review, 9*(3), 25–31. https://doi.org/10.1108/14754391011040046

Vizheh, M., Qorbani, M., Arzaghi, S. M., Muhidin, S., Javanmard, Z. & Esmaeili, M. (2020). The mental health of healthcare workers in the COVID-19 pandemic: A systematic review. *Journal of Diabetes and Metabolic Disorders, 19*, 1967–1978. https://doi.org/10.1007/s40200-020-00643-9

Westrum, R. (2004). A typology of organisational cultures. *Quality and Safety in Health Care, 13*(Suppl 2), ii22–ii27. https://doi.org/10.1136/qshc.2003.009522

Wolniak, R. (2013). A typology of organizational cultures in terms of improvement of the quality management. *Manager, 17*, 7–21.

Wolters Klewer (2023). Proven effective strategies to prevent and treat provider burnout. Wolters Klewer. Retrieved 18 February 2024 from: https://www.wolterskluwer.com/en/expert-insights/proven-effective-strategies-to-prevent-and-treat-provider-burnout

Leading and managing change

27

Gary E. Day
With acknowledgement to Elizabeth Shannon

Learning objectives

How do I:

- plan and lead change within a workplace?
- choose a relevant change-management framework?
- plan the change process and the human-management component of the change?
- develop my skills in leading organisational change?
- coach and mentor my staff through change?
- understand how First Nations peoples' culture can influence successful change management?

Introduction

This chapter introduces the world of change management. Firstly, it sets out the case for change – why change management matters – then looks at the theories concerning individual and organisational change. Finally, the role of the professional change manager is discussed.

Definitions

For the purposes of this chapter, change is viewed from an organisational perspective. **Organisational change** is a systematic approach to reshaping organisations in line with their future goals, aims, vision and philosophy. By its very nature, organisational change needs to be actively managed to ensure the desired outcomes. Organisational change management requires the manager to take account of the range of internal and external forces that can augment, shape, hinder or derail organisational change. Organisational change 'aims to move organisations from the current state to one that is more desirable, ranging from minor to radical changes. Change represents an opportunity that must be anticipated, prepared for, and managed. Changes in organisations are complex, continuous, iterative, and uncertain. The rate of change is dependent on the organisation's context, nature, and external events' (Lozano, 2022, p. 75). The manager should realise that any number of these internal and external events may need to be actively managed simultaneously to ensure a successful outcome.

> **Organisational change:** A systematic approach to reshaping organisations in line with their future goals, aims, vision and philosophy

Management of change

Healthcare organisations are 'constantly changing as a result of technological advancements, ageing populations, changing disease patterns, new discoveries for the treatment of diseases and political reforms and policy initiatives. Changes can be challenging because they contradict humans' basic need for a stable environment' (Nilsen, Seing, Ericsson, Birken & Schildmeijer, 2020, para 1).

Braithwaite (2018) argues that the challenge of change in health care is due to its complexity. The healthcare system is continually evolving as a complex adaptive system with the system's performance and behaviour changing over time. Therefore the healthcare system cannot be understood by simply understanding the component parts. Even if we understand the system that provides health care, each patient presents with varying health needs requiring different interventions. The various combinations of care, activities, events, interactions and outcomes are, for all intents and purposes, infinite (Braithwaite, 2018). Organisational changes in health care are 'more likely to succeed when health care professionals have the opportunity to influence the change, feel prepared for the change and recognize the value of the change, including perceiving the benefit of the change for patients' (Nilsen et al., 2020, para 4).

The Change Management Institute identifies 13 knowledge areas that change managers need to understand (Change Management Institute, 2020, p. 8); these are:

1. A change management perspective – the overarching theories behind change
2. Defining change – what is the change?

3. Managing benefits – ensuring change delivers value
4. Stakeholder strategy – how to identify and engage stakeholders
5. Communication and engagement – communicating change effectively
6. Change impact – assessing change impact and progress
7. Change readiness, planning and measurement – preparing for change
8. Project management – change initiatives, projects and programs
9. Education and learning support – training and supporting change
10. Facilitation – facilitating group events through a change process
11. Sustaining systems – ensuring that change is sustained
12. Personal and professional management – developing personal effectiveness
13. Organisational considerations – critical elements of awareness for professional change managers.

There has been unprecedented change in health care over the past few years, exacerbated by organisational and systemic change brought about by the COVID-19 pandemic. In part, it has:

> accelerated the development and use of technology solutions in health care. These technology tools were originally identified as mechanisms that would make future care easier or better; however, as a result of the pandemic technical solutions are now viewed as essential. The use of technology accelerated during the crisis because technology provided distance, safety for health care professionals and patients, faster results reporting, virtual visits, and more. (Clipper, 2020, p. 500)

The rapid changes to service provision, patient care, management of the health workforce, health research, clinical education, and management of stores and supplies during this worldwide crisis highlight the need for health managers to have the necessary skills to lead staff through change, often multiple change processes at once.

MANAGING CHANGE THROUGH A PANDEMIC

Amid the tumult of the pandemic, a large regional government hospital emerged as a beacon of resilience, showcasing an exemplary case of change management in the healthcare sector. Faced with an unprecedented surge in COVID-19 cases, the hospital's leadership swiftly initiated a multifaceted approach to adapting and navigating the evolving landscape.

Recognising the need for expanded capacity, the hospital underwent a rapid transformation, repurposing medical wards into dedicated COVID-19 units and expanding the ICU and CCU units. This architectural shift was not merely logistical; it symbolised a profound organisational pivot towards prioritising infectious disease control for both staff and patients. The seamless coordination between clinical and administrative teams ensured a swift and effective conversion process, emphasising the hospital's agility in the face of crisis.

Embracing technology became a cornerstone of change. The implementation of telehealth services revolutionised patient-care delivery, enabling healthcare professionals to maintain connection with patients while adhering to safety protocols. Training programs

> **MANAGING CHANGE THROUGH A PANDEMIC**
> Continued
>
> were swiftly deployed to bridge the digital divide among staff, highlighting the hospital's commitment to innovation amid adversity. With new drug and treatment protocols changing on almost a daily basis, hospital managers had to manage rapid change by coordinating the dissemination of new treatment regimens, updating policies and procedures, ensuring staff understood the new approaches and the pharmacy and stores departments were informed of changes and updates.
>
> Supply chain disruptions posed another formidable challenge. The hospital's procurement team demonstrated ingenuity by forging partnerships with local suppliers, ensuring a steady inflow of crucial resources. This collaborative approach not only secured essential supplies but also strengthened community ties.
>
> Communication was paramount throughout this transformative journey. Transparent updates, town-hall meetings and digital platforms became vital conduits for information flow, fostering a shared sense of purpose among the hospital's personnel. In addition, clear communication with several government agencies was paramount in providing data.
>
> The hospital's response to the pandemic stands as a testament to effective change management – a dynamic blend of adaptability, technology integration, collaborative partnerships and transparent communication, ultimately safeguarding the health and wellbeing of the patients and staff in the face of unprecedented challenges.

People and change

Actively managing the change process requires a focus on the human element of change. The negative consequences of poor change management can be seen in time and cost blowouts, false starts and failure to complete projects, as well as adverse health outcomes in staff. The literature is clear that failing to manage change effectively can have serious psychological and physiological effects on staff, and human-resource implications such as increased staff turnover and absenteeism. For example, the human effects of a poorly managed change process can lead to deterioration in employee health and wellbeing, resulting in early exit from the labour market (Vahtera & Virtanen, 2013). Some studies have reported employees experiencing disrupted sleep, depression, weight gain and high blood pressure (Ferrie, Shipley, Marmot, Stansfeld & Smith, 1998). Other negative effects reported include an increased number of sick days (Hansson, Vingard, Arnetz & Anderzen, 2008) and a significant increase in staff receiving stress-related medication (Dahl, 2011). In the context of health services, poorly managed change can also have negative patient outcomes, including increased length of stay and mortality rates (Timmers, Hulstaert & Leenen, 2014).

Transition: The personal, emotional and mental processes a person goes through to accept and adapt to change

To ensure that change is truly successful, change and **transition** are required (Bridges & Mitchell, 2000). Therefore, the manager needs to be cognisant of the two elements: change is the external process that affects the individual staff member (most organisational change could be considered external, such as policy, practice and structure), while transition is internal – the personal, emotional and mental process the staff member goes through to accept and adapt to the change. As so aptly put by Baggio, Digentiki and Varma (2019), organisations don't change, people change!

Through transition, the staff member accepts the change as personally 'safe' and perceives a personal and organisational benefit to modifying their practice or behaviour. Managers must fully engage their staff and assist them in transition from one process to another, working through all their employees' issues and concerns with them so they embrace the proposed change. To ensure a successful transition, research suggests: 1) including frontline stakeholder perspectives in move-related decisions; 2) allocating adequate time for clinician or employee training and education in the pre-change period; 3) assessing clinician or employee wellbeing throughout move implementation; and 4) increasing unit-administrator sensitivity to clinician change-fatigue (Muir, Keim-Malpass & LeBaron, 2021, para 4).

When staff experience a series of change cycles and go through the psychological stages of change repeatedly, it can lead to **change fatigue** (Bernerth, Walker & Harris, 2011). Forthcoming change can also lead to **anticipatory grief** (Kubler-Ross & Kessler, 2005), which is associated with the future stress of change, particularly if previous change was distressing to the individual. The prospect of a new round of change will stimulate grieving for the loss of the current situation, even before the change has occurred. The sense of loss can be due to perceived or actual loss: of status, previous work accomplishments, influence, power, work history or emotional investment in a project, and to changes in the team and the prevailing culture. A clear change-management plan provides a structured approach that may give some comfort to staff damaged by poorly managed processes in the past.

In many ways, particularly during large-scale change, managers need to take staff through a process much like the grief process described by Kubler-Ross and Kessler (2005). The stages of grief model has been adopted over the years to be used in the change process, as many staff feel similar levels of loss, grief and distress during organisational change.

Change fatigue: Lassitude, apathy or passive resignation by individuals or teams as a result of constant organisational changes

Anticipatory grief: Mourning that occurs before an impending or known loss

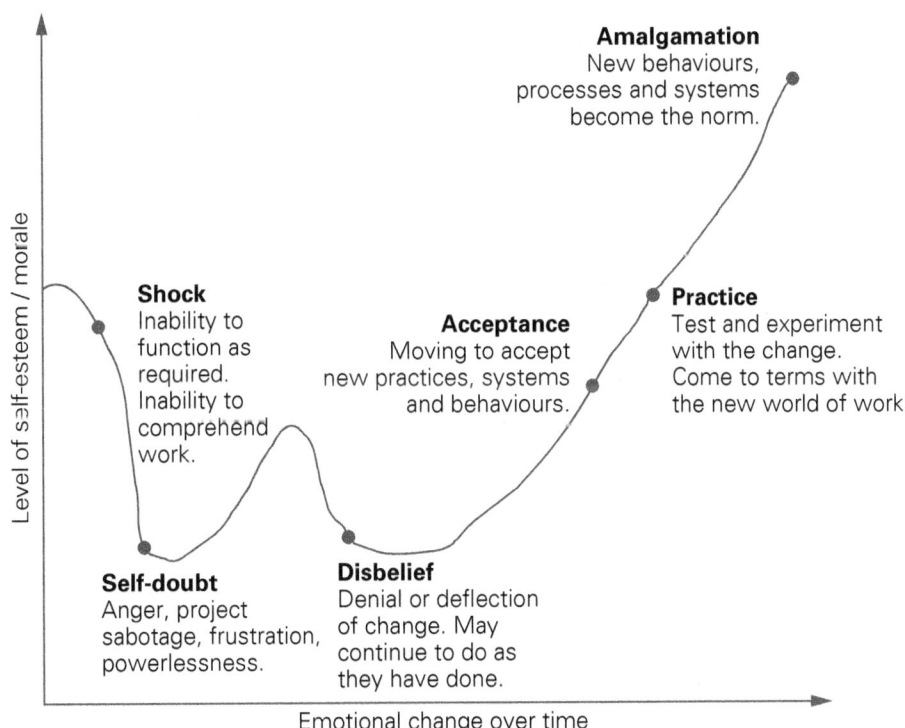

Figure 27.1 The stages of grief or change model

Managers should expect staff to go through a range of psychological stages until the change is fully integrated, including shock, disbelief, doubt in their own abilities, acceptance that the change is happening and finally practice and amalgamation. During this process, the individual and the team will experience highs and lows in self-esteem and morale as they realign themselves to the new world of work (see Figure 27.1).

Frameworks for change management

Lewin's field theory and force-field analysis

The earliest popular framework of change, developed by Kurt Lewin (1947), is the simplest. It is because of its simplicity that it is a useful starting point. Lewin introduces the idea of the change process taking three steps: 'unfreezing' the original situation, 'moving', or introducing the change, and 'refreezing' the new situation, to make the new standard permanent. He describes change as occurring through the interaction of social forces, some of which support change while others oppose it, within a 'field of action'.

However, while Lewin does describe the opposing forces as a kind of force field, he does not recommend that change managers undertake the kind of force-field analysis that commonly bears his name today. Force-field analysis lists the forces for change on one side of a page and the forces against change on the other side. It simply and graphically illustrates where arguments and stakeholders sit in relation to the change.

In the first stage, 'before commencing any change activities, time and attention should be given to conducting detailed analyses and preparatory work to establish the foundation for the implementation phase. In the second stage, a clear set of multiple implementation tactics are used to ensure the change process is effective. In the final stage, an evaluation of the success of the change is undertaken and measures are put in place to ensure it is sustained over time' (Allen, 2016, p. 58). While Lewin's change approach remains a popular tool for change managers, it is sometimes criticised as being too simplistic to be effective (Burnes & Cooke, 2013).

Kotter's theory of organisational change

Fifty years later, John Kotter (2012) took Lewin's (1947) three steps and expanded them into eight steps for successful change, as outlined in the following section. Kotter's work has been used extensively in a range of fields, including the health industry, to frame a structured approach to change management.

'Establishing a sense of urgency'

In Kotter's first step, the health manager must get enough staff to see there are challenges or opportunities that need to be addressed in the short term. Without an adequate sense of urgency, the manager will find it nearly impossible to achieve the necessary traction to get staff moving and taking the problem seriously. The manager may need to work through a range of staff emotions, such as complacency, anger, self-protection, pessimism, change fatigue, self-interest or reluctance. Each of these negative staff attitudes will need to be worked through to find the issues that unite the team to move ahead so that they might address the problem in a coordinated fashion (Kotter, 2012, pp. 37–52).

'Creating the guiding coalition'

Creating the guiding coalition relies on the manager developing a cohesive team to help drive and guide the change. Central to this stage of the process is bringing together the right people with the right skills to do the right job. The manager's roles at this stage are to ensure good two-way communication, motivate staff and create a sense of excitement, share information important to developing trust and establish team norms and protocols (Kotter, 2012, pp. 53–68).

'Developing a vision and strategy'

The manager's role in this crucial step is to help staff, and the guiding coalition, to see possibilities: what the future might be. The manager also needs to develop a solid strategy (plans and budgets) to underpin the future possibilities. They should ensure that they build on the sense of urgency and the reason staff accepted the change in the first place (Kotter, 2012, pp. 69–86).

'Communicating the change vision'

At this stage the manager needs to communicate a clear and unambiguous vision. Staff are likely to have a lot of questions by this point, and the manager should be proactively answering questions and communicating to maintain momentum. It is important to keep on-message and ensure that the message is communicated in clear language that staff can understand. It may be necessary for the manager to repackage the same message in different forms so that all staff are clear about why the change is important (Kotter, 2012, pp. 87–104).

'Empowering employees for broad-based action'

The manager needs to remove barriers and allow staff to make the necessary changes. Barriers may be restrictive policies and protocols, outdated management practices, insecure managers and negative language regarding the change (Kotter, 2012, pp. 105–120). Kotter and Cohen (2002) suggest that, at this stage, the manager should not try to do everything at once, instead breaking the solution down into smaller projects and allowing staff to act on these smaller, bite-sized objectives.

'Generating short-term wins'

At this stage, the manager should try to achieve a few small wins. This will bolster the guiding coalition and demonstrate that the overall process can be successful. Wins create confidence in the change process and help build momentum. Each win must be appropriately celebrated and communicated. The manager needs to provide constructive feedback to staff. Each win stage also provides a perfect opportunity to evaluate how the project is proceeding and what learnings can be used in other elements of the process (Kotter, 2012, pp. 121–136).

'Consolidating gains and producing more change'

There is a danger of celebrating wins too early and stopping there. In this step, the manager needs to keep up the urgency and ensure that there is continued enthusiasm for the project.

It is a good time to remind staff about how far they have come to date and how close the project is to finishing. Continuing to sell the vision is a positive way of encouraging staff to consider why they signed on in the first place and what is at stake if they finish the change prematurely (Kotter, 2012, pp. 137–152).

'Anchoring new approaches in the culture'

At this final stage, the manager is responsible for ensuring the project does not slip or the staff return to old habits, processes and approaches. New approaches and behaviours should be highlighted, recognised and rewarded. The manager needs to build the change into everyday work practices, including orientation of new staff and revised protocols and documentation. The completed change process must be communicated to staff and the improvements that have arisen from the new change emphasised (Kotter, 2012, pp. 153–166).

Kotter's change framework works well when combined with other process-improvement methodologies, such as Lean Sigma Six in order to reduce waste and raise the level of service quality (Al Owad et al., 2025).

ADKAR model

Hiatt (2006, p. 2) proposes a stepped model of change management which integrates individual change and organisational change: by changing individuals within an organisation, he claims, it is possible to change the organisation as a whole. Individual change requires the following qualities, from which the ADKAR mnemonic is taken:

- **A**wareness of the need to change
- **D**esire to support and participate in the change
- **K**nowledge of how to change
- **A**bility to implement required skills and behaviors
- **R**einforcement to sustain the change.

Awareness and desire take the individual away from the current way of doing things. Knowledge and ability guide them through the transition. Reinforcement takes the change securely into the future (Hiatt, 2006).

The amount of change management required in any circumstance is a function of the extent or scope of change required and the time in which the process must occur (Hiatt & Creasey, 2012). In other words, small-scale, incremental change requires less management than large-scale, radical change.

The amount of change management required will also depend on the organisation's history. How has change been managed previously? What outcomes have resulted from earlier change processes? If change has been managed poorly, it may be more difficult to engage people in the current change (Hiatt & Creasey, 2012).

Hiatt and Creasey (2012) describe change management as supported when certain individual roles and organisational conditions are fulfilled. In the first instance, communication about the change must be delivered by the appropriate individual. Corporate messages – the big picture – should be communicated by senior managers. Immediate supervisors should be available to discuss the personal impacts on individual staff. While senior managers have the authority to mandate and sponsor the change, immediate supervisors can help staff become more comfortable and less resistant to the change.

Mentoring and coaching staff through change: Key success factors for health managers

Organisational change is a constant in today's dynamic environment, and effective leadership strategies are crucial to navigating these transitions. Mentoring and coaching emerge as powerful tools for supporting staff through change, fostering resilience and maximising the positive outcomes of transformation.

Managers play a crucial role in successfully taking their teams or departments through change. Managers need to be 'sensitive to the culture and specifics of that organisation, because change takes place within people rather than within the organisation itself' (Cleary, West, Arthur & Kornhaber, 2019, p. 966). The key leadership skills of mentoring and coaching staff are central to engaging staff through the change-transition process.

Mentoring and coaching, while similar in many ways, have key differences, and both can be used at different stages of the change process. Coaching is often focused on specific goals and tasks, providing guidance and feedback to help individuals improve their performance. The coaching process is usually coach-driven and is focused on organisational outcomes or improved performance. Coaching staff through change may be one-on-one or in groups. On the other hand, mentoring is 'a more holistic and long-term relationship, where a mentor shares their knowledge, wisdom, and experience to guide the mentee's personal and professional growth' (Mundey, 2023, n.p.). In this relationship, the agenda is largely mentee-driven and is usually one-on-one (Mundey, 2023).

Mentoring

Mentoring staff through change is largely about professional and personal growth. In this one-on-one mentoring relationship, trust and confidentiality are paramount. In this relationship the mentee often draws on the skills and experience of the mentor to help them understand their own feelings and stress related to the organisational change. It is often the case that the mentor comes from another part or is external to the organisation, rather than as a line manager or supervisor. The goal of the mentoring relationship is that the mentee progresses in terms of personal and professional development, self-reflection and self-awareness. Some of the benefits to the mentee, particularly when it comes to change, can include:

- helping to 'foster an understanding of the enduring elements of practice within the organisation' (Burgess, van Diggele & Mellis, 2018, p. 197)
- increasing skills and knowledge
- improving understanding of their roles
- providing insights into the culture and unwritten rules of the health industry
- creating a supportive environment in which successes and failures can be evaluated
- using a powerful learning tool to acquire competencies and professional experience
- developing professional and self-confidence
- empowerment (ACHSM, 2018, p. 7).

Much like coaching, the approach to mentoring staff through change includes having empathy, setting goals and action planning, and having emotional intelligence and communication skills (reflective listening, powerful questioning, feedback and constructive challenging). For mentoring, 'these skills are commonly held by senior leaders' (HETI,

2020, p. 14). When the mentoring relationship is working well, positive behaviours include aligning expectations, building rapport, maintaining open communication and facilitating mentee agency.

As mentoring relationships can go on for some time, it is important that the mentor and mentee set out clear expectations and boundaries at the start to avoid any form of professional overdependence or manipulation (Mentoring Complete, 2023), conflict of interest, imbalance of power and unrealistic expectations (Burgess et al., 2018).

Coaching

Coaching is a powerful tool to help staff understand and embrace change. Managers in healthcare organisations are in a perfect position to play an active and positive role in the change and transition processes. The hospital executive looks to middle managers to lead the change process at the local level, while at the same time staff look to the same managers to give them support and guidance during this often stressful time. Managers need to move from a directing style of leadership to one that is more aligned with supporting and coaching staff.

Coaching is a great technique if used effectively and can:

- Encourage people to see change as an opportunity rather than a threat
- Help staff understand and embrace change
- Build a stronger and more communicative team, where everyone knows their role and their value to the organisation
- Identify training needs and develop talent
- Prevent negative perceptions of change from getting out of control and spreading across a team (MindTools, 2024)
- Encourage staff to experiment, make mistakes and learn

In the coaching role, managers need to ensure they communicate effectively and frequently to ensure staff understand what is happening or is about to happen. This will help allay fears and concern and can reduce anxiety. Equally, as part of communicating effectively, health leaders need to develop the art of storytelling. Leaders need to tell a compelling story that explains the 'why' for change, which in turn will lead naturally to the 'how'. One of the key goals in this part of the coaching process is to give people a context of meaning and purpose for the change (Daskal, 2019).

Another of the key coaching skills for change management is active listening. Listening is the act of deeply hearing what the other person is saying and having positive regard for the other while taking in their tone of voice, body language and other verbal and non-verbal cues. Listening is not thinking of things to say as soon as the other person has stopped talking. Keys to active listening include:

- Asking questions: Asking open-ended questions.
- Affirming: Affirming the speaker's thoughts and feelings.
- Reflection: Reflecting what you heard.
- Summary: Summarising the conversation (Elliott, 2024, n.p.).

Support listening by asking open-ended questions. Questions will help the coach to understand how the change is affecting the staff member, their key concerns and how well they are transitioning to the new way of working. The range of open-ended coaching questions that can be asked is almost endless; however, the following are a good start for managers wanting to ask questions about staff member attitudes and fears about change:

- What did you like about that? What didn't you like?
- What do you think went well? What didn't?
- Are there any other options available to you?
- Who can help you with that?
- What else?
- What's the best-case scenario?
- What's the worst-case scenario?
- Can you tell me more? (Elliott, 2024, n.p.)

Things to remember as a manager coaching staff through change:

- Don't get frustrated if you already agree with the change and the person you're coaching doesn't 'get it' straight away.
- Take time to understand why people feel the way they do. Don't rush this – some people may not want to talk about their feelings at work. Others may be confused about their many emotions. As a coach, you'll need to take an individual approach (MindTools, 2024, n.p.).
- Make sure that the person you're coaching knows why you are doing it.
- Explain why the organisation is changing and the benefits of the change. You must explain this from everyone's perspective, including those whose jobs or current work roles might be at risk.
- People must understand how the future will look and how this will affect them. Then focus on how the person's goals fit with the organisation's goals following the change (MindTools, 2024, n.p.).

Mentoring and coaching emerge as indispensable tools in the leader's toolkit during organisational change. Their ability to provide personalised guidance, foster resilience and enhance skills positions them as key components of successful change-management strategies.

Cultural considerations in managing change with First Nations peoples

Health managers will face a range of cultural issues and challenges when it comes to organisational change. Cultural consideration of First Nations peoples during change promotes inclusivity, respect and identity. To ensure a successful change process, managers need to consider these matters where change directly or indirectly affects these groups, or where immigrant or Indigenous staff are part of the change agenda.

There are several approaches that have shown to have a positive effect in ensuring success in the change-management process when working with First Nations people or staff. These approaches include:

- the creation of a 'collective responsibility' to achieve the vision for change, utilising participatory change-management processes, both internally and externally (Coombe, 2008, p. 639)
- achieving consensus through meetings (Mika & O'Sullivan, 2012)

- understanding that 'any health intervention strategies for Aboriginal and Torres Strait Islander communities need to be based on participatory change management processes and a fundamental systems change management approach that recognises change as an inherent quality of a living system, not an imposed driving force, in order to ensure that the interventions will be sustainable' (Coombe, 2008, p. 639)
- ensuring managers avoid assuming roles of power and authority, rather than treating staff inclusively in the process. Resentment to change can occur due to 'historical events of oppression by a western system or have had family members victims of historical trauma, will naturally resent a dictatorial change management style' (Coombe, 2008, p. 643)
- deeply engage First Nations people in the change process rather than doing the change to them or for them. Create a sense of agency in the change process. 'Seeing oneself as an agent rather than an object is empowering' (McEwan, Tsey, McCalman & Travers, 2010, p. 365)
- building extra time into the change-management timeline. The change process may take longer to achieve. It has been noted that organisational change with First Nations peoples may not follow a clear, linear trajectory, due in part to the struggles individuals may encounter as part of personal growth and development (McEwan et al., 2010)
- asking Aboriginal and/or Torres Strait Islander staff about how it is to work there. Listen to what you are told with an open heart, however uncomfortable this may be
- ensuring any Aboriginal and/or Torres Strait Islander-related work is led and informed by Indigenous people. This means engaging with Indigenous people both inside and outside your organisation
- developing specific principles for your own organisation that guide how Indigenous community engagement and employment should work in practice
- consulting with Indigenous staff on how to minimise the **cultural load** while increasing **cultural safety**. This will take honest discussion and probably the commitment of resources (Young & Ragg, 2020, n.p.).

Cultural load: 'Cultural load is the extra burden carried by Aboriginal and/or Torres Strait Islander people in workplaces where there are few or no other Indigenous people' (Young & Ragg, 2020, n.p.)

Cultural safety: '[C]reating an environment that is safe for Aboriginal and Torres Strait Islander people. This means there is no assault, challenge or denial of their identity and experience' (Department of Health, 2023, n.p.)

Summary

- Change management is an important emerging discipline.
- Managers must consider both the external process of change and the internal process of transition for change to be successful.
- Several change models can be applied to organisational change.
- Change managers must possess skills in areas such as education and training, communication and engagement, and facilitation, as well as a detailed understanding of change and change processes.
- Mentoring and coaching are effective skills for health managers transitioning staff through change.
- Managers may need a nuanced approach to change management that incorporates consultation with First Nations peoples and staff.

Reflective questions

1. What is the most recent change process you have experienced? Was it successful in achieving its goals? What impact did it have on you and your team?
2. Can you describe what is meant by 'organisational change'?
3. What do you think is the relationship between individual and organisational change?
4. Have you ever experienced the six psychological stages of grief in relation to a change? How long did it take from start to finish?
5. Can you describe how change was communicated or implemented during the COVID-19 pandemic? Was it different than before the pandemic? What role did you play and how did it make you feel?

Self-analysis questions

Think about a time when you were intensely involved in a significant change – either leading or being affected by it. How effective was the change? Did it achieve what it set out to do? How did you feel about it? Which one of the change-management frameworks presented in this chapter best describes that change process? If you knew then what you know now about change and change management, might you have acted any differently?

References

Allen, B. (2016). Effective design, implementation and management of change in healthcare. *Nursing Standard*, *31*(3), 58–71. https://doi.org/10.7748/ns.2016.e10375

Al Owad, A., Yadav, N., Kumar, V., Swarnakar, V., Jayakrishna, K., Haridy, S. & Yadav, V. (2025). Integrated Lean Six Sigma and Kotter change management framework for emergency healthcare services in Saudi Arabia. *Benchmarking: An International Journal*, *32*(1), 299–331. https://doi.org/10.1108/BIJ-05-2023-0335

Australasian College of Health of Health Service Management (ACHSM). (2018). *ACHSM mentoring program. Mentor guide*. ACHSM. Retrieved 17 February 2024 from: https://achsmmembers.memnet.com.au/Portals/15/Mentor-Guide.pdf

Baggio, A., Digentiki, E. & Varma, R. (2019). Organizations don't change. People change! McKinsey & Associates. Retrieved 14 February 2024 from https://www.mckinsey.com/capabilities/people-and-organizational-performance/our-insights/the-organization-blog/organizations-do-not-change-people-change#

Bernerth, J. B., Walker, H. J. & Harris, S. G. (2011). Change fatigue: Development and initial validation of a new measure. *Work and Stress*, *25*(4), 321–337. https://doi.org/10.1080/02678373.2011.634280

Braithwaite, J. (2018). Changing how we think about healthcare improvement. *BMJ*, *361*. https://doi.org/10.1136/bmj.k2014

Bridges, W. & Mitchell, S. (2000). Leading transition: A new model for change. *Leader to Leader*, *16*(Spring), 30–36.

Burgess, A., van Diggele, C. & Mellis, C. (2018) Mentorship in the health professions: A review. *The Clinical Teacher*, *15*(3), 197–202. https://doi.org/10.1111/tct.12756

Burnes, B. & Cooke, B. (2013). Kurt Lewin's field theory: A review and re-evaluation. *International Journal of Management Reviews*, *15*, 408–425. https://doi.org/10.1111/j.1468-2370.2012.00348.x

Change Management Institute. (2020). *Accreditation handbook*. Change Management Institute.

Cleary, M., West, S., Arthur, D. & Kornhaber, R. (2019). Change management in health care and mental health nursing. *Issues in Mental Health Nursing*, *40*(11), 966–972. https://doi.org/10.1080/01612840.2019.1609633

Clipper, B. (2020). The influence of the COVID-19 pandemic on technology: Adoption in health care. *Nurse Leader*, *18*(5), 500–503. https://doi.org/10.1016/j.mnl.2020.06.008

Coombe, L. L. (2008). The challenges of change management in Aboriginal community-controlled health organisations. Are there learnings for Cape York health reform? *Australian Health Review*, *32*(4), 639–647. https://doi.org/10.1071/AH080639

Dahl, M. S. (2011). Organizational change and employee stress. *Management Science*, *57*(2), 240–256. https://doi.org/10.1287/mnsc.1100.1273

Daskal, L. (2019). This is how the best leaders coach through change. *Lolly Daskal*. Retrieved 16 February 2024 from: https://www.lollydaskal.com/leadership/this-is-how-the-best-leaders-coach-through-change/

Department of Health, State of Victoria. (2023). *Aboriginal and Torres Strait Islander cultural safety*. Retrieved from: https://www.health.vic.gov.au/health-strategies/aboriginal-and-torres-strait-islander-cultural-safety

Elliott, K. (2024). 5 coaching skills every leader needs during times of change. *People Managing People*. Retrieved 16 February 2024 from: https://peoplemanagingpeople.com/personal-development/coaching-skills-change/

Ferrie, J. E., Shipley, M. J., Marmot, M. G., Stansfeld, S. & Smith, G. D. (1998). The health effects of major organisational change and job insecurity. *Social Science and Medicine*, *46*(2), 243–254. https://doi.org/10.1016/S0277-9536(97)00158-5

Hansson, A.-S., Vingard, E., Arnetz, B. B. & Anderzen, I. (2008). Organizational change, health and sick leave among health care employees: A longitudinal study measuring stress markers, individuals and work site factors. *Work and Stress*, *22*(1), 69–80. https://doi.org/10.1080/02678370801996236

HETI. (2020). *Mentoring for leadership and management development. A guide for mentees*. NSW Government.

Hiatt, J. M. (2006). *ADKAR: A model of change in business, government and our community*. Prosci Learning Center.

Hiatt, J. M. & Creasey, T. J. (2012). *Change management: The people side of change* (2nd ed.). Prosci Learning Center.

Kotter, J. P. (2012). *Leading change* (2nd ed.). Harvard Business.

Kotter, J. P. & Cohen, D. S. (2002). *The heart of change*. Harvard Business.

Kubler-Ross, E. & Kessler, D. (2005). *On grief and grieving: Finding the meaning of grief through the five stages of loss*. Scribner.

Lewin, K. (1947). Frontiers in group dynamics: Concept, method and reality in social science; Social equilibria and social change. *Human Relations*, *1*(5), 5–41. https://doi.org/10.1177/001872674700100103

Lozano, R. (2022). Organisational change management for sustainability. *Toward sustainable organisations. Strategies for sustainability*. Springer. https://doi.org/10.1007/978-3-030-99676-5_5

McEwan, A. B., Tsey, K., McCalman, J. & Travers, H. J. (2010). Empowerment and change management in Aboriginal organisations: A case study. *Australian Health Review*, *34*, 360–367. https://doi.org/10.1071/ah08696

Mentoring Complete. (2023). 7 common challenges in mentoring relationships. Retrieved 17 February 2023 from: https://www.mentoringcomplete.com/7-common-challenges-in-mentoring-relationships/

Mika, J. P. & O'Sullivan, J. G. (2012). A Māori approach to management: Contrasting traditional and modern Māori management practices in Aotearoa New Zealand. *Journal of Management & Organization*, *20*(5).

MindTools. (2024). Coaching through change. Retrieved 16 February 2024 from: https://www.mindtools.com/agjj594/coaching-through-change

Muir, K. J., Keim-Malpass, J. & LeBAron, V. T. (2021). Examining the cultural impacts of an emergency department move using ethnography. *International Emergency Nursing*, *59*. https://doi.org/10.1016/j.ienj.2021.101082

Mundey, M. (2023). Mentoring vs coaching: The key differences and benefits. *Think Learning*. Retrieved 16 February 2024 from: https://www.think-learning.com/employee-engagement/mentoring-vs-coaching/

Nilsen, P., Seing, I., Ericsson, C. Birken, K. & Schildmeijer, S. A. (2020). Characteristics of successful changes in health care organizations: an interview study with physicians, registered nurses and assistant nurses. *BMC Health Services Research*, *20*(147). https://doi.org/10.1186/s12913-020-4999-8

Timmers, T. K., Hulstaert, P. F. & Leenen, L. P. H. (2014). Patient outcomes can be associated with organizational changes: A quality improvement case study. *Critical Care Nursing Quarterly*, *37*(1), 125–134. https://doi.org/10.1097/CNQ.0000000000000011

Vahtera, J. & Virtanen, M. (2013). The health effects of major organisational changes. *Occupational Environmental Medicine*, *70*, 677–678. https://doi.org/10.1136/oemed-2013-101635

Young, N. & Ragg, M. (2020). 10 ways employers can include Indigenous Australians. *The Conversation*. Retrieved 16 February 2024 from: https://theconversation.com/10-ways-employers-can-include-indigenous-australians-149741

28 Healthcare quality and service improvement

Mohamed Khalifa
With acknowledgement to Martin Connor

Learning objectives

How do I:

- implement a comprehensive healthcare quality framework covering the 12 key dimensions, including patient-centeredness and evidence-based practice?
- explore service-improvement strategies to enhance healthcare efficiency, effectiveness and quality?
- leverage technology and patient-centred care to improve healthcare access, personalise patient care and enhance service quality?
- address healthcare equity and accessibility to ensure equitable care for individuals, regardless of background or circumstance?
- develop sustainability in healthcare systems for long-term effectiveness, efficiency and resilience?

Introduction

In the evolving landscape of healthcare, quality and service improvement are at the forefront, driving the shift towards more efficient, effective and patient-centred care. Quality in healthcare includes not only the excellence of medical interventions but also extends to the patient experience and ensuring safe, effective care. The importance of quality is highlighted by the Institute of Medicine's (IOM) six dimensions: safety, effectiveness, patient-centredness, timeliness, efficiency and equity. These dimensions provide a comprehensive framework for evaluating and enhancing healthcare quality and services (Agency for Healthcare Research and Quality (AHRQ), 2022). This chapter seeks to broaden the comprehensiveness of the healthcare quality and service-improvement model suggested by the IOM and provides real-life case studies in which each of the 12 dimensions is examined and discussed.

History of healthcare quality and improvement

The history of **healthcare quality** and **service improvement** went through a fascinating journey that has evolved significantly over the past century. This journey is marked by groundbreaking contributions from pioneering figures such as Walter Shewhart and Edward Deming, and extends through transformative movements and the integration of systemic philosophies into healthcare management.

The early twentieth century: Statistical process control emerges

The origins of modern healthcare quality improvement can be traced to the early twentieth century, particularly to 1924, when Walter Shewhart, working at the Western Electric Company, introduced the concept of statistical process control. Shewhart's revolutionary ideas proposed a shift in focus from inspecting finished products to improving production processes and applying statistical methods to the management of process variations to improve quality and enhance outcomes (Dahlgaard, Reyes, Chen & Dahlgaard-Park, 2019).

Mid-twentieth century: Deming's philosophical expansion

Edward Deming, mentored by Shewhart, further developed these ideas, integrating a philosophical dimension into the concept of quality improvement. Deming introduced four principles that expanded on Shewhart's work, highlighting the systemic nature of work, the importance of understanding process variations, the role of psychology in change management and the necessity of a theoretical framework for knowledge development. Deming's work emphasised the holistic approach to quality improvement, considering not just the statistical aspects but also the human and systemic factors (Harrison et al., 2021).

Late twentieth century: Quality improvement in health care

The latter part of the 20th century saw the application of these quality improvement philosophies to health care. Pioneers including Dr Brent James at Intermountain Healthcare adopted Deming's principles and initiated significant improvements in healthcare delivery

> **Healthcare quality:** The degree to which health services for individuals and populations increase the likelihood of desired health outcomes and are consistent with current professional knowledge (WHO, 2024)
>
> **Service improvement:** Systematic efforts to increase the efficiency, effectiveness and quality of healthcare services. This involves identifying areas of service delivery that require enhancement and implementing strategies to improve outcomes, patient satisfaction and access to care (Hill, Stephani, Sapple & Clegg, 2020)

and outcomes. James's work, alongside that of others, demonstrated the potential of quality improvement methods to enhance patient care, reduce costs and improve overall healthcare system performance (Bowen, 2016).

Crossing the quality chasm: A new healthcare paradigm

The publication of 'Crossing the Quality Chasm' by the Institute of Medicine (IOM, 2001) marked a pivotal moment in healthcare quality improvement. This seminal text advocated for a systemic approach to healthcare improvement, emphasising the need for a fundamental redesign of the healthcare system. The report highlighted six aims for improvement: safety, effectiveness, patient-centredness, timeliness, efficiency and equity, which have guided much of the healthcare quality improvement efforts since (AHRQ, 2022). The report also emphasises the crucial role of leadership and management accountability in establishing a culture of quality and safety in healthcare. Effective leaders set expectations, promote open communication and ensure teams are held accountable for maintaining high standards. They must actively foster and sustain safety oriented practices, highlighting leadership's key role in driving lasting improvements in healthcare quality and safety (Sfantou et al., 2017).

The 21st century: Integrating technology and patient-centred care

Value-based care: An evidence-based, person-centred approach to support healthcare decision-making and system transformation, with the aim of improving both health outcomes and the experience of care across a full care pathway for people, service providers, communities; health professionals and populations (Queensland Health, 2022)

Continuous quality improvement (CQI): A structured organisational process of improvement of healthcare services and outcomes through systematic, data-driven approaches. CQI involves identifying benchmarks of excellence, measuring performance and implementing changes to close gaps between current and desired performance (McCalman et al., 2018)

In the 21st century, healthcare quality and service improvement continue to evolve, with a growing emphasis on technology integration, patient-centred care and the use of data analytics for decision-making. Healthcare systems worldwide are increasingly adopting electronic health records (EHRs), telehealth and mobile health technologies to improve access to care, enhance the quality of service and facilitate personalised patient care (Stoumpos, Kitsios & Talias, 2023). Moreover, the concept of **value-based care** has gained prominence, focusing on outcomes and patient satisfaction as key metrics for evaluating healthcare quality (Teisberg, Wallace & O'Hara, 2020).

Challenges and future directions

Despite significant progress, healthcare quality and service improvement face continuing challenges, including social determinants of health, disparities in access and the complexity of healthcare systems. Leadership plays a critical role in overcoming these challenges by fostering a culture of **continuous quality improvement (CQI)**. Leaders must also manage resistance to change, engage interdisciplinary teams and ensure that CQI processes are embedded into daily healthcare operations for lasting success. Effective leaders utilise practical tools such as Fishbone diagrams to identify root causes of issues and run charts to monitor performance (Latino, Latino & Latino, 2019). Data-driven decision-making is essential for evaluating interventions and ensuring sustained improvement. Future directions in healthcare quality improvement will likely involve leveraging advanced technologies, such as artificial intelligence and machine learning, to predict patient needs, personalise care and optimise healthcare processes (Bajwa, Munir, Nori & Williams, 2021).

The modified 12-domains model for healthcare quality and improvement

The development of this modified 12-domains model is inspired by the foundational six domains of the IOM. Recognising the need for a more comprehensive approach and actionable framework for improving healthcare quality and outcomes, the authors sought to expand upon the IOM model by integrating current literature and emerging best practices. This led to the inclusion of six additional domains to address critical aspects of healthcare that were not emphasised in the original model. The 12 dimensions now include:

1. patient-centredness
2. evidence-based practice
3. safety
4. effectiveness
5. efficiency
6. timeliness
7. integration
8. information-rich
9. equity
10. accessibility
11. consistency
12. sustainability.

This sequence starts with the core principle of patient-centred care, progresses through the necessary conditions for high-quality care (safety, effectiveness, efficiency), addresses how care is delivered (timely, integrated, informed) and concludes with broader system goals (accessibility, equity, consistency and sustainability). This progression logically builds from the individual patient focus to systemic improvements, ensuring that each dimension supports and enhances the others for comprehensive healthcare quality and improvement. Figure 28.1 shows the 12 dimensions of healthcare quality and improvement.

1. Patient-centredness

Patient-centred care emphasises respect and responsiveness to individual patient preferences, needs and values. It positions patients as active participants in their care, fostering decisions made in partnership with healthcare providers (O'Neill, 2022). This approach centres on effective communication, empathy and respecting patients' values and needs. Enhancing patient-centeredness involves training for healthcare providers in communication and empathy, shared decision-making practices and integration of patient feedback into care planning. Technological aids such as patient portals offer access to medical information, improve communication and support self-management, exemplified by shared decision-making tools in cancer care that enable informed, value-aligned patient choices (ElKefi & Asan, 2021). This not only boosts patient satisfaction and engagement but also optimises health outcomes through personalised treatment (Kwame & Petrucka, 2021). In Victoria, Australia, the Department of Health emphasises patient-centred care to boost healthcare quality, focusing on dignity, involvement in health decisions, and a safe, private environment.

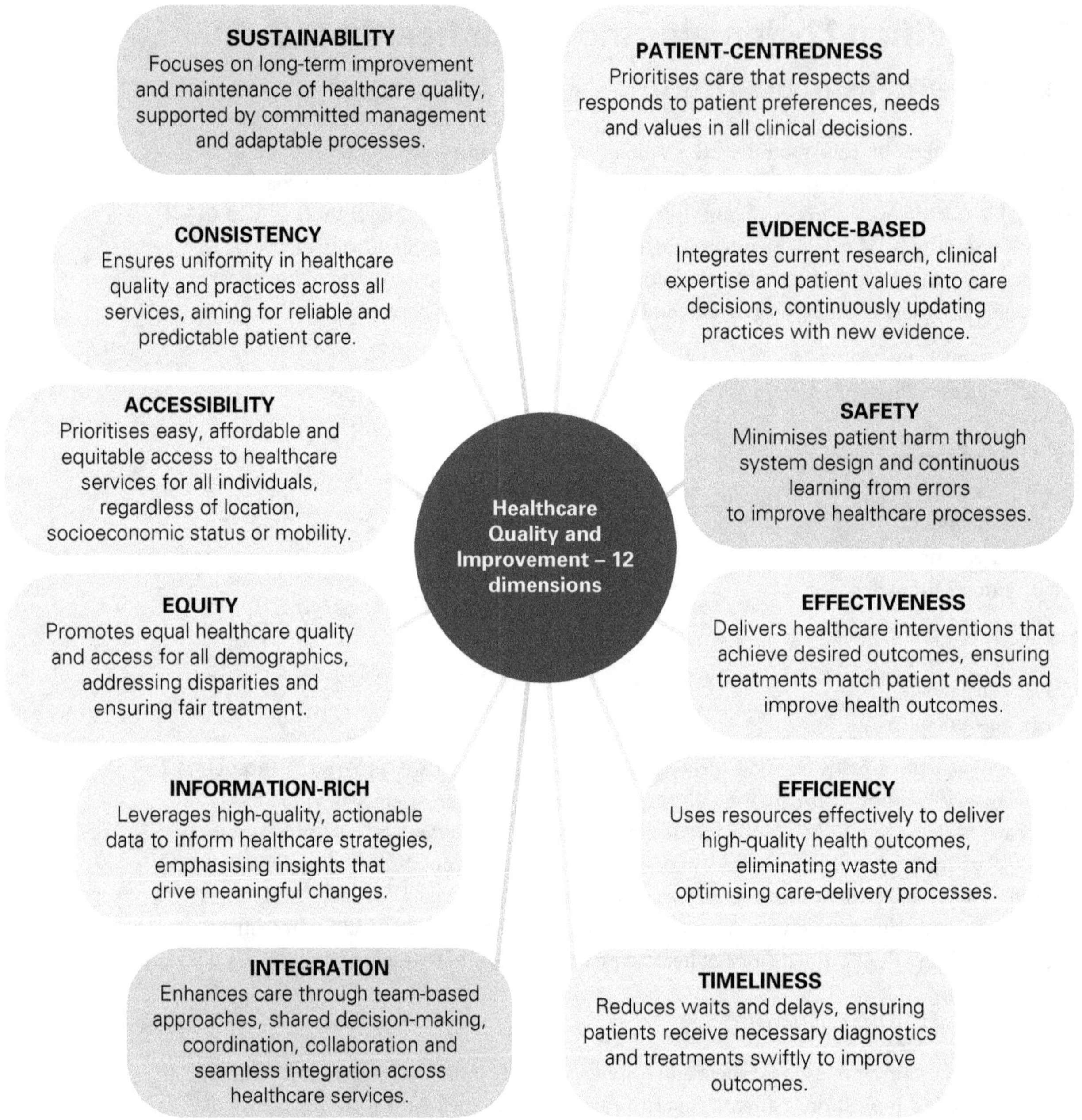

SUSTAINABILITY
Focuses on long-term improvement and maintenance of healthcare quality, supported by committed management and adaptable processes.

PATIENT-CENTREDNESS
Prioritises care that respects and responds to patient preferences, needs and values in all clinical decisions.

CONSISTENCY
Ensures uniformity in healthcare quality and practices across all services, aiming for reliable and predictable patient care.

EVIDENCE-BASED
Integrates current research, clinical expertise and patient values into care decisions, continuously updating practices with new evidence.

ACCESSIBILITY
Prioritises easy, affordable and equitable access to healthcare services for all individuals, regardless of location, socioeconomic status or mobility.

SAFETY
Minimises patient harm through system design and continuous learning from errors to improve healthcare processes.

Healthcare Quality and Improvement – 12 dimensions

EQUITY
Promotes equal healthcare quality and access for all demographics, addressing disparities and ensuring fair treatment.

EFFECTIVENESS
Delivers healthcare interventions that achieve desired outcomes, ensuring treatments match patient needs and improve health outcomes.

INFORMATION-RICH
Leverages high-quality, actionable data to inform healthcare strategies, emphasising insights that drive meaningful changes.

EFFICIENCY
Uses resources effectively to deliver high-quality health outcomes, eliminating waste and optimising care-delivery processes.

INTEGRATION
Enhances care through team-based approaches, shared decision-making, coordination, collaboration and seamless integration across healthcare services.

TIMELINESS
Reduces waits and delays, ensuring patients receive necessary diagnostics and treatments swiftly to improve outcomes.

Figure 28.1 The modified 12-dimensions model of healthcare quality and improvement

Strategies include effective communication, respecting decision-making rights and organisational integration of patient-centred principles through staff training and leadership (Department of Health, 2015).

2. Evidence-based practice

Implementing evidence-based practice (EBP) involves questioning clinical practices, searching for and appraising evidence, applying findings and evaluating outcomes, facilitated by online databases, clinical-decision support systems and guidelines for accessible evidence. Education in research literacy and critical appraisal is vital for healthcare professionals to implement EBP effectively, thereby overcoming the existing EBP gap (Li, Cao & Zhu, 2019; Department of Health, 2021). The application of protocols based on current evidence in stroke care has significantly reduced the time to treatment for patients, resulting in better outcomes and reduced long-term disability. EBP not only improves patient care but also promotes a culture of inquiry and lifelong learning among healthcare professionals, ensuring that healthcare evolves in line with scientific advancements (Juckett, Wengerd, Faieta & Griffin, 2020). Additionally, the Allied Health Leadership in Value-Based Health Care initiative by Queensland Health demonstrates EBP in Australia through case studies focusing on person-centred, sustainable care. These include value-based approaches to radiation therapy, lymphoedema screening, audiology care, COVID-19 vaccination rollouts and culturally responsive care with Aboriginal communities; they illustrate EBP's role in enhancing patient outcomes and promoting a culture of inquiry and lifelong learning among healthcare professionals (Queensland Health, 2023).

3. Safety

Safety in healthcare encompasses a wide range of practices designed to protect patients from errors, injuries, accidents, adverse events and infections. This involves multidisciplinary efforts and a culture of safety to develop protocols, guidelines and systems that prevent harm (Emanuel et al., 2009). Tools including EHRs and barcode medication-administration systems play crucial roles in ensuring accurate patient information and medication delivery, and reduce the likelihood of errors (Mulac, Mathieson, Taxis & Granås, 2021). One example is the use of surgical safety checklists, which have been shown to significantly reduce complications and deaths associated with surgery. These checklists ensure that all team members confirm the patient's identity, surgical site and procedure, and that all necessary equipment and medications are prepared and available (Chhabra et al., 2019). Reducing patient falls in the older population is another example. An Australian study highlighted five strategies: educating patients and staff, promoting patient exercise, diagnosing and treating relevant medical conditions, improving the environment and using information technology for monitoring (Khalifa, 2019). The *State of patient safety and quality in Australian hospitals* report by the Australian Commission on Safety and Quality in Health Care (ACSQHC, 2019) outlines Australia's achievements in enhancing patient safety and healthcare quality through standards, promoting the culture of safety and continuous improvement.

4. Effectiveness

Effectiveness within healthcare prioritises the achievement of positive outcomes for patients, concentrating on the tangible improvements in health that result from healthcare interventions. This dimension emphasises the delivery of services that are directly aligned with the actual health needs of patients, ensuring treatments are not just theoretically sound but practically successful in enhancing patient wellbeing (Hannawa, Wu, Kolyada, Potemkina & Donaldson, 2022; Kruk et al., 2018). The basis of improving effectiveness relies on the careful selection and application of interventions that have demonstrated real-world success in improving patient health. For instance, in the management of chronic conditions such as asthma, the focus is on optimising medication regimens and lifestyle adjustments that have been shown to effectively control symptoms and prevent exacerbations, regardless of the theoretical underpinnings (Castillo, Peters & Busse, 2017). The Australian Centre for Value-Based Healthcare presented a case study on the implementation of a value-based healthcare approach to improve the effectiveness of radiation therapy for adolescents and young adults in Brisbane. This initiative focused on developing and embedding a new model of care to improve outcomes that matter to patients and their families (Australian Centre for Value-Based Healthcare, 2023).

5. Efficiency

Efficiency involves maximising resource use to achieve the best possible patient outcomes. It means minimising waste, not just of materials, but also of time, energy and finances, while maintaining or improving the quality of care (Kerasidou, 2019; Kruk et al., 2018). Efficiency requires an understanding of the flow of processes within healthcare delivery, the identification of bottlenecks and the implementation of solutions that streamline operations. Strategies to enhance efficiency include process re-engineering, adopting lean management techniques and leveraging technology such as health-information technology systems, telemedicine and EHR. These tools and methodologies reduce unnecessary steps, automate routine tasks and facilitate smoother patient transitions through the care continuum. Efficient healthcare systems reduce wait times, prevent duplicate tests and optimise resources, thus improving patient satisfaction and outcomes. By integrating systems, they save time and reduce harm, enhance care access and experiences, and contribute to system sustainability (Pakdil, Harwood & Isin, 2020). A case study in Queensland, Australia, demonstrated that Hospital in the Home services using a public–private partnership model achieved shorter average lengths of stay without compromising patient outcomes, when compared to traditional public models. This study highlighted the effectiveness of governance strategies, criteria-led discharge and financial incentives in supporting efficient healthcare delivery (Kivic & Hines, 2020).

6. Timeliness

Timeliness is critical in ensuring that patients receive the care they need when they need it. This dimension addresses the reduction of waiting times and harmful delays, both in receiving and providing care. Timeliness affects not only patient satisfaction and experience but also the effectiveness of treatments and interventions (Hannawa et al., 2022; Sreeramoju et al., 2020). Strategies to improve timeliness include optimising appointment scheduling systems, reducing bottlenecks in care delivery through process re-engineering to improve patient flow and leveraging technology to streamline operations using alerts and reminders (Boone, Celhay, Gertler, Gracner & Rodriguez, 2022). For instance, an emergency department that re-engineers its triage process can significantly reduce wait times for patients requiring urgent care, thereby improving outcomes and patient satisfaction (Khalifa, 2016). Improving timeliness requires a systematic approach to identifying and addressing the root causes of delays, ensuring that patients have timely access to diagnostic services, treatments and care coordination (Khan, Khalid, Almorsy & Khalifa, 2016). A case study from Canada shows that an otolaryngology department's quality initiative doubled the rate of surgical discharge summaries issued within 48 hours following discharge to more than 50 per cent, using auto-authentication, education and audits. This improved patient-care transitions and healthcare quality without added workload or frequent revisions (You, Liu, Moist, Fung & Strychowsky, 2022). Another good example is the introduction of telehealth in rural and remote locations to improve timely access to assessment, diagnosis and treatment, which were previously compromised by geographic isolation and workforce shortages (Haleem, Javaid, Singh & Suman, 2021).

7. Integration

Integration is essential for provision of comprehensive, patient-centred care, particularly in complex cases that involve various specialists and services. It encapsulates both the coordination and collaboration aspects of healthcare delivery, ensuring that all elements of a patient's care journey are seamlessly interconnected through effective communication (NSW Health, 2023). Strategies for successful integration involve employing care coordinators, using shared EHRs and forming multidisciplinary teams. These approaches enable comprehensive care plans for chronic diseases such as diabetes, thereby enhancing condition management, patient engagement and satisfaction. Integration also incorporates community and social services, addressing broader health determinants for a holistic patient-care approach, fostering a culture of teamwork and shared goals, leading to more personalised, efficient and effective care (Taberna et al., 2020). One case study from Australia shows that the Western Sydney Integrated Care Program aimed to improve healthcare for chronic illnesses by integrating primary and secondary care. The program enhanced care coordination and access, connecting patients with services and facilitating general practice–specialist communication. The study highlights the need for long-term investment in information-sharing to fully realise the benefits of integrated care (Trankle et al., 2019). Moreover, better integration will also enable effective management in the community, thus preventing unnecessary hospitalisations (Australian Institute of Health and Welfare, 2020).

8. Information-rich

Being information-rich means leveraging comprehensive, accurate and timely data to inform decisions at all levels of care delivery. This dimension underscores the importance of actionable insights derived from data analytics, patient records and evidence based research to improve health outcomes, enhance patient safety and optimise the efficiency of healthcare services (Khalifa & Househ, 2021). For example, a telehealth program leveraging real-time data analytics to monitor patients with chronic diseases can proactively manage health conditions, thereby reducing hospital readmissions and emergency department visits. By effectively using health data, especially through artificial intelligence, healthcare providers can tailor interventions to individual patient needs, predict and prevent adverse events, and continuously monitor and improve the quality of care (Alowais et al., 2023). A case study from Australia involves the development of an automated decision-support system for community mental health services using Australia's national electronic health records. This project aimed to enhance mental health service delivery through data-driven insights. It highlights the value of leveraging national health data to support mental health services, illustrating the potential of data analytics in transforming the quality of healthcare delivery (van Kasteren, Strobel, Bastiampillai, Linedale & Bidargaddi, 2022).

9. Equity

Equity is the fair and just provision of care to all individuals, regardless of their backgrounds, socioeconomic statuses, geographic locations or other characteristics that might lead to health disparities. Equity ensures that everyone has access to the same high-quality care and opportunities to achieve optimal health outcomes (O'Kane et al., 2021). Improving healthcare equity involves addressing social determinants, launching outreach to underserved populations and providing culturally competent care. Utilising geographic information systems and telehealth extends healthcare services to remote areas by improving geographical access and overcoming physical barriers to care. These technologies ensure that patients in underserved locations can receive timely and essential medical attention. However, ensuring the acceptability of services is equally important. Training in cultural competency enhances providers' understanding of diverse patient needs, preferences and values, fostering trust and respect (Anawade, Sharma & Gahane, 2024; Haleem et al., 2021). Initiatives such as mobile health clinics and community health workers in marginalised communities have shown significant improvements in health outcomes and reduced disparities (Budhwani et al., 2022). Research from the University of Technology Sydney reveals that high out-of-pocket fees for specialist medical services disproportionately affect those in lower socioeconomic groups, limiting their access to necessary care. Despite some providers offering reduced fees, the overall financial barrier remains significant, leading to delayed or avoided treatments. The study emphasises the need for improved healthcare pathways by considering costs, waiting times and medical recommendations (Australian Healthcare and Hospitals Association, 2022).

10. Accessibility

Healthcare accessibility refers to the ease with which individuals can obtain needed medical services (Dhar, Sharma, Chakraborty, Khanna & Ali, 2024). It encompasses factors such as the geographical distribution of healthcare facilities, availability of healthcare providers, affordability of care and the adequacy of health information (Reilly, 2021). A critical aspect of accessibility is the elimination of barriers that prevent people from seeking or receiving care. These barriers can be physical, such as distance from healthcare facilities; financial, including high costs of services or lack of insurance coverage; and informational, such as unawareness of available services or rights to care (Nolan-Isles et al., 2021). Improving healthcare accessibility, especially for residents of rural and remote areas, involves strategies such as expanding insurance coverage, increasing the number of healthcare providers in underserved areas and implementing telemedicine services to reach remote populations (Mathew et al., 2023). For example, Australia is allocating more than $9 million from the National Health and Medical Research Council for seven research projects to improve healthcare accessibility and equity. These projects, from blood donation screening to HIV prevention, involve collaboration among health researchers, governments and not-for-profits organisations, emphasising the role of partnerships in enhancing health services and developing policies for broad health benefits across the country (Kearney, 2023).

11. Consistency

Consistency in health care refers to the provision of care that maintains high standards of quality across all services and over time. It ensures that patients receive the same level of care regardless of when or where they access services. Achieving consistency involves implementing standardised care protocols, guidelines and pathways to guide healthcare delivery, ensuring every patient encounter adheres to the best practices established by clinical evidence (ACSQHC, 2017). Continuous quality improvement efforts are crucial in maintaining consistency; they involve regular review of clinical outcomes, patient feedback and process efficiency to identify areas for improvement. Tools such as quality management systems play a pivotal role in monitoring care delivery and facilitating the identification and correction of variations in care. Consistent health care improves patient outcomes by reducing variability, ensuring that all patients have access to care that meets established standards of excellence, thereby enhancing patient trust and satisfaction. This can be achieved through implementing clinical practice guidelines and key performance indicators (Hill et al., 2020; McCalman et al., 2018).

12. Sustainability

Healthcare sustainability is fundamentally about crafting health systems that are resilient and capable of enduring over the long term, and that ensure future generations have access to necessary high-quality care. This concept extends beyond achieving short-term objectives to maintaining long-term gains and focusing on creating a healthcare infrastructure that supports community health and wellbeing sustainably (Kruk et al., 2018). Moreover, incorporating environmental sustainability into health care involves adopting green practices such as energy conservation, waste reduction and sustainable procurement. These strategies aim to reduce health care's environmental impact while maintaining quality care, contributing to resource preservation, reducing pollution and improving community health, thereby enhancing the healthcare system's long-term resilience and effectiveness (Smith & Severn, 2023). For example, the Sunshine Coast Hospital and Health Service (SCHHS) in Queensland, Australia, has taken significant steps to enhance sustainability through a collaborative pilot project focused on transitioning to low-carbon, climate-resilient healthcare services. SCHHS highlights the importance of sustainable health care by prioritising staff education, implementing environmentally sustainable practices and using innovative tools such as the Environmental Sustainability Checklist to promote sustainable operations throughout the organisation (Climate and Health Alliance, 2023).

DATA-DRIVEN INSIGHTS FOR CONTINUOUS IMPROVEMENT

A critical component of the success in Australia's community mental health services was their commitment to data sharing and utilisation across the care continuum. This initiative required the establishment of secure and efficient mechanisms for exchanging patient information among primary care providers, mental health specialists and community services. The creation of integrated patient records enabled a comprehensive view of each individual's mental health journey, allowing for more informed decision-making and personalised care adjustments. Additionally, the systematic collection and analysis of data were vital in monitoring the effectiveness of this integrated care model. Evaluative measures focused on clinical outcomes, patient and provider satisfaction, and the cost-effectiveness of the approach, offering valuable insights for continuous improvement and future enhancements in community mental health services across Australia.

Summary

- The modified 12-domains model for healthcare quality and improvement emphasises the complex and multifaceted nature of enhancing healthcare services.
- It addresses the evolving needs of patients and the broader community.
- This comprehensive approach to quality improvement can drive significant advancements in healthcare delivery.
- By implementing this model, the standard of care can be elevated across healthcare systems.

Recommendations for future practice

- Prioritise patient-centred care by involving patients in decision-making, respecting their preferences and ensuring care is tailored to their needs.
- Accelerate the adoption of health information technology, telehealth and data analytics to enhance care coordination, improve accessibility and facilitate real-time decision-making.
- Embed continuous quality improvement processes within operations, using feedback loops, performance metrics and evidence-based practices.
- Promote interdisciplinary collaboration and integration across healthcare services to ensure comprehensive care delivery that addresses all aspects of patient health.
- Address disparities in healthcare access and outcomes, focusing on underserved populations to ensure equitable care for all individuals.
- Embrace sustainability practices within healthcare settings to minimise environmental impact and promote a healthy community, ensuring the long-term viability of healthcare systems.

Reflective questions

1. How does integrating patient-centred care improve health outcomes?
2. What role does EBP play in quality improvement?
3. How can healthcare safety be enhanced through quality improvement efforts?
4. In what ways does efficiency affect patient satisfaction and care delivery?
5. Why is equity important in achieving high-quality healthcare for all?

Self-analysis question

Reflect on the 12 dimensions of healthcare quality and improvement discussed in the chapter. Which dimension do you think is the most challenging to implement in your healthcare setting, and why?

References

Agency for Healthcare Research and Quality (AHRQ). (2022). *Agency for Healthcare Research and Quality: Six domains of healthcare quality*. Retrieved from: https://www.ahrq.gov/talkingquality/measures/six-domains.html

Alowais, S. A., Alghamdi, S. S., Alsuhebany, N., Alqahtani, T., Alshaya, A. I., Almohareb, S. N., Aldairem, A., Alrashed, M., Bin Saleh, K. & Badreldin, H. A. (2023). Revolutionizing healthcare: The role of artificial intelligence in clinical practice. *BMC Medical Education, 23*(1), 689.

Anawade, P. A., Sharma, D. & Gahane, S. (2024). A comprehensive review on exploring the impact of telemedicine on healthcare accessibility. *Cureus, 16*(3).

Australian Centre for Value-Based Healthcare. (2023). *Adopting a VBHC approach in providing radiation therapy to adolescent and young adults*. Retrieved from: https://valuebasedcareaustralia.com.au/publications/case-studies/

Australian Commission on Safety and Quality in Health Care (ACSQHC). (2019). *The Australian Commission on Safety and Quality in Health Care: The state of patient safety and quality in Australian hospitals 2019*. Retrieved from: https://www.safetyandquality.gov.au/sites/default/files/2019-07/the-state-of-patient-safety-and-quality-in-australian-hospitals-2019.pdf

——— (2017). *The Australian Commission on Safety and Quality in Health Care: National safety and quality health service standards*. Retrieved from: https://www.safetyandquality.gov.au/sites/default/files/migrated/National-Safety-and-Quality-Health-Service-Standards-second-edition.pdf

Australian Healthcare and Hospitals Association. (2022). *Improving equity and access to healthcare in Australia*. Retrieved from: https://ahha.asn.au/improving-equity-and-access-to-healthcare-in-australia

Australian Institute of Health and Welfare (AIHW). (2020). *1 in 15 hospitalisations could be prevented through early health interventions*. Retrieved from: https://www.aihw.gov.au/news-media/media-releases/2020/february/1-in-15-hospitalisations-could-be-prevented-throug

Bajwa, J., Munir, U., Nori, A. & Williams, B. (2021). Artificial intelligence in healthcare: Transforming the practice of medicine. *Future healthcare journal, 8*(2), e188.

Boone, C. E., Celhay, P., Gertler, P., Gracner, T. & Rodriguez, J. (2022). How scheduling systems with automated appointment reminders improve health clinic efficiency. *Journal of Health Economics, 82*, 102598.

Bowen, E. O. (2016). Quality Improvement Programs' Contribution to Successful Clinical Practice Changes (PhD thesis, University of the Incarnate Word). Retrieved from: https://athenaeum.uiw.edu/uiw_etds/15

Budhwani, S., Fujioka, J., Thomas-Jacques, T., De Vera, K., Challa, P., De Silva, R., Fuller, K., Shahid, S., Hogeveen, S. & Chandra, S. (2022). Challenges and strategies for promoting health equity in virtual care: Findings and policy directions from a scoping review of reviews. *Journal of the American Medical Informatics Association, 29*(5), 990–999.

Castillo, J. R., Peters, S. P. & Busse, W. W. (2017). Asthma exacerbations: Pathogenesis, prevention, and treatment. *The Journal of Allergy and Clinical Immunology: In Practice, 5*(4), 918–27.

Chhabra, A., Singh, A., Kuka, P. S., Kaur, H., Kuka, A. S. & Chahal, H. (2019). Role of perioperative surgical safety checklist in reducing morbidity and mortality among patients: An observational study. *Nigerian Journal of Surgery, 25*(2), 192–197.

Climate and Health Alliance. (2023). *Sustainable healthcare case study: Collaborating for sustainable and climate resilient healthcare*. Retrieved from: https://www.caha.org.au/sh5

Dahlgaard, J. J., Reyes, L., Chen, C.-K. & Dahlgaard-Park, S. M. (2019). Evolution and future of total quality management: Management control and organisational learning. *Total quality management & business excellence, 30*(sup1), S1–S16.

Department of Health, State of Victoria. (2021). *Implementing evidence-based practice*. Retrieved from: https://www.health.vic.gov.au/patient-care/implementing-evidence-based-practice

——— (2015). *Implementing person centred practice*. Retrieved from: https://www.health.vic.gov.au/older-people-in-hospital/person-centred-practice

Dhar, B., Sharma, P., Chakraborty, R., Khanna, T. & Ali, S. H. (2024). Improving health equity through digital healthcare. In L. Chatterjee & N. Gani (eds), *Multi-sector analysis of the digital healthcare industry* (pp. 80–109). IGI Global.

ElKefi, S. & Asan, O. (2021). How technology impacts communication between cancer patients and their health care providers: A systematic literature review. *International Journal of Medical Informatics, 149*, 104430.

Emanuel, L., Berwick, D., Conway, J., Combes, J., Hatlie, M., Leape, L., Reason, J., Schyve, P., Vincent, C. & Walton, M. (2009). What exactly is patient safety? *Journal of Medical Regulation*, *95*(1), 13–24.

Haleem, A., Javaid, M., Singh, R. P. & Suman, R. (2021). Telemedicine for healthcare: Capabilities, features, barriers, and applications. *Sensors International*, *2*, 100117.

Hannawa, A. F., Wu, A. W., Kolyada, A., Potemkina, A. & Donaldson, L. J. (2022). The aspects of healthcare quality that are important to health professionals and patients: A qualitative study. *Patient education and counseling*, *105*(6), 1561–1570.

Harrison, R., Fischer, S., Walpola, R. L., Chauhan, A., Babalola, T., Mears, S. & Le-Dao, H. (2021). Where do models for change management, improvement and implementation meet? A systematic review of the applications of change management models in healthcare. *Journal of Healthcare Leadership*, *13*, 85–108.

Hill, J. E., Stephani, A.-M., Sapple, P. & Clegg, A. J. (2020). The effectiveness of continuous quality improvement for developing professional practice and improving health care outcomes: A systematic review. *Implementation Science*, *15*(1), 1–14.

Juckett, L. A., Wengerd, L. R., Faieta, J. & Griffin, C. E. (2020). Evidence-based practice implementation in stroke rehabilitation: A scoping review of barriers and facilitators. *The American Journal of Occupational Therapy*, *74*(1).

Kearney, G. (2023). Activating collaboration to improve healthcare access and equity. Retrieved from: https://www.health.gov.au/ministers/the-hon-ged-kearney-mp/media/activating-collaboration-to-improve-healthcare-access-and-equity

Kerasidou, A. (2019). Empathy and efficiency in healthcare at times of austerity. *Health Care Analysis*, *27*(3), 171–184.

Khalifa, M. (2019). Improving patient safety by reducing falls in hospitals among the elderly: A review of successful strategies. *ICIMTH*, *262*, 340–343.

——— (2016). Utilizing health analytics in improving emergency room performance. In W. Sermeus et al. (eds), *Nursing Informatics 2016* (pp. 138–142). IMIA and IOS Press. https://doi.org/10.3233/978-1-61499-658-3-138

Khalifa, M. & Househ, M. (2021). Utilizing health analytics in improving the performance of hospitals and healthcare services: Promises and challenges (pp. 23–39). In M. Househ, E. Borycki & A. Kushniruk (eds), *Multiple perspectives on artificial intelligence in healthcare: Opportunities and challenges*. Springer.

Khan, M., Khalid, P., Almorsy, L. & Khalifa, M. (2016). *Improving timeliness of diagnostic healthcare services: Effective strategies and recommendations*. ICIMTH.

Kivic, A. & Hines, L. (2020). Using governance and patient flow strategies to improve healthcare service efficiency. *Australian Health Review*, *45*(1), 22–27.

Kruk, M. E., Gage, A. D., Arsenault, C., Jordan, K., Leslie, H. H., Roder-DeWan, S., Adeyi, O., Barker, P., Daelmans, B. & Doubova, S. V. (2018). High-quality health systems in the Sustainable Development Goals era: Time for a revolution. *The Lancet Global Health*, *6*(11), e1196–e1252.

Kwame, A. & Petrucka, P. M. (2021). A literature-based study of patient-centered care and communication in nurse-patient interactions: Barriers, facilitators, and the way forward. *BMC Nursing*, *20*(1), 1–10.

Latino, M. A., Latino, R. J. & Latino, K. C. (2019). *Root cause analysis: Improving performance for bottom-line results*. CRC Press.

Li, S., Cao, M. & Zhu, X. (2019). Evidence-based practice: Knowledge, attitudes, implementation, facilitators, and barriers among community nurses—systematic review. *Medicine*, *98*(39).

Mathew, S., Fitts, M. S., Liddle, Z., Bourke, L., Campbell, N., Murakami-Gold, L., Russell, D. J., Humphreys, J. S., Mullholand, E. & Zhao, Y. (2023). Telehealth in remote Australia: A supplementary tool or an alternative model of care replacing face-to-face consultations? *BMC Health Services Research*, *23*(1), 1–10.

McCalman, J., Bailie, R., Bainbridge, R., McPhail-Bell, K., Percival, N., Askew, D., Fagan, R. & Tsey, K. (2018). Continuous quality improvement and comprehensive primary health care: A systems framework to improve service quality and health outcomes. *Frontiers in Public Health*, 76.

Mulac, A., Mathiesen, L., Taxis, K. & Granås, A. G. (2021). Barcode medication administration technology use in hospital practice: A mixed-methods observational study of policy deviations. *BMJ Quality & Safety*, *30*(12), 1021–1030.

Nolan-Isles, D., Macniven, R., Hunter, K., Gwynn, J., Lincoln, M., Moir, R., Dimitropoulos, Y., Taylor, D., Agius, T. & Finlayson, H. (2021). Enablers and barriers to accessing healthcare services for Aboriginal people in New South Wales, Australia. *International Journal of Environmental Research and Public Health*, *18*(6), 3014.

NSW Health. (2023). *What is integrated care?* Retrieved from: https://www.health.nsw.gov.au/integratedcare/Pages/what-is-integrated-care.aspx

O'Kane, M., Agrawal, S., Binder, L., Dzau, V., Gandhi, T. K., Harrington, R., Mate, K., McGann, P., Meyers, D., Rosen, P., Schreiber, M. & Schummers, D. (2021). An equity agenda for the field of health care quality improvement. *NAM Perspectives*, *2021*. Retrieved from: https://nam.edu/an-equity-agenda-for-the-field-of-health-care-quality-improvement/

O'Neill, N. (2022). *The eight principles of patient-centered care*. Retrieved from: https://www.oneviewhealthcare.com/blog/the-eight-principles-of-patient-centered-care/

Pakdil, F., Harwood, T. N. & Isin, F. B. (2020). Implementing lean principles in the healthcare industry: A theoretical and practical overview. *Delivering Superior Health and Wellness Management with IoT and Analytics* (pp. 383–413). Springer.

Queensland Health. (2023). *Queensland Health: Allied health leadership in value-based health care*. Retrieved from: https://valuebasedcareaustralia.com.au/publications/case-studies/

——— (2022). *Value-based health care*. Retrieved from: https://www.health.qld.gov.au/ahwac/html/allied-health-workforce/VBHC

Reilly, M. (2021). Health disparities and access to healthcare in rural vs. urban areas. *Theory in Action*, *14*(2).

Sfantou, D. F., Laliotis, A., Patelarou, A. E., Sifaki-Pistolla, D., Matalliotakis, M. & Patelarou, E. (2017). Importance of leadership style towards quality of care measures in healthcare settings: A systematic review. *Healthcare*, *5*(4), 73. https://doi.org/10.3390/healthcare5040073

Smith, A. & Severn, M. (2023). *Reducing the environmental impact of clinical care*. CADTH Horizon Scan.

Sreeramoju, P. V., Weber, S. G., Snyder, A. A., Kirk, L. M., Reed, W. G. & Hardy-Decuir, B. A. (2020). *The patient and health care system: Perspectives on high-quality care*. Springer.

Stoumpos, A. I., Kitsios, F. & Talias, M. A. (2023). Digital transformation in healthcare: Technology acceptance and its applications. *International Journal of Environmental Research and Public Health*, *20*(4), 3407.

Taberna, M., Gil Moncayo, F., Jané-Salas, E., Antonio, M., Arribas, L., Vilajosana, E., Peralvez Torres, E. & Mesía, R. (2020). The multidisciplinary team (MDT) approach and quality of care. *Frontiers in Oncology*, *10*, 85.

Teisberg, E., Wallace, S. & O'Hara, S. (2020). Defining and implementing value-based health care: A strategic framework. *Academic Medicine*, *95*(5), 682.

Trankle, S. A., Usherwood, T., Abbott, P., Roberts, M., Crampton, M., Girgis, C. M., Riskallah, J., Chang, Y., Saini, J. & Reath, J. (2019). Integrating health care in Australia: A qualitative evaluation. *BMC Health Services Research*, *19*(1), 1–12.

van Kasteren, Y., Strobel, J., Bastiampillai, T., Linedale, E. & Bidargaddi, N. (2022). Automated decision support for community mental health services using national electronic health records: Qualitative implementation case study. *JMIR Human Factors*, *9*(3), e35403.

WHO (World Health Organization). (2024). *Quality of care*. Retrieved from: https://www.who.int/health-topics/quality-of-care

You, P., Liu, J., Moist, L., Fung, K. & Strychowsky, J. E. (2022). Improving timeliness in surgical discharge summary distribution: A quality improvement initiative. *OTO Open*, *6*(4), 2473974X221134106.

29 Leading and managing in the digital age

Mark Keough and James Boyd

Learning objectives

How do I:

- explain the key concepts of digital health, including big data, artificial intelligence and telehealth?
- identify the benefits and challenges associated with digital health implementation?
- describe the role of data analytics in health care, including its applications for population-health interventions?
- discuss the importance of data governance and security measures in protecting patient privacy in the digital healthcare system?
- evaluate the potential of artificial intelligence and machine learning to transform healthcare delivery, considering both opportunities and potential risks?
- identify the main principles associated with the emergence of telehealth and virtual teams?

Introduction

The advent of the digital age has brought about significant changes in how information is created, disseminated and consumed. Recent developments in the use of big **data** and artificial intelligence (AI) have brought all things digital into sharp focus.

Big data and AI have played pivotal roles in shaping the digital landscape. The term 'big data' describes the vast amounts of structured and unstructured data generated every day. Advanced analytics on big data enable businesses and organisations to extract valuable insights, make informed decisions and enhance various processes. AI, on the other hand, has brought about a paradigm shift in how machines learn, reason and perform tasks traditionally associated with human intelligence. Machine-learning algorithms, a subset of AI, process vast datasets to identify patterns and make predictions. This has applications across diverse fields, including health care, finance, marketing and more. The combination of big data and AI has fuelled advancements in areas such as personalised recommendations, predictive analytics and automation in all aspects of our day-to-day lives.

Digital innovation and technological advances within the health and care industries have been transformative, offering new opportunities to enhance patient care, streamline processes and improve overall efficiency within the industry. Within the realm of health-service management, digital innovation is categorised in three ways: **technology** based enhancements in *health administration*, in *clinical practice* and in *health therapy*. In this chapter we introduce these distinct domains and provide definitions and an overview to encourage further investigation.

The emphasis is on pathways for continuing investigation rather than immediate, critical innovations, and on considering the long-term trajectories that can shape the future. As an initial reflection, it is important that you consider your own situation and reflect on the impact of technological innovations within your current view of the world. There have been several critical and high-level technological innovations that inform all others. The development in the early 1990s of the worldwide web (Mosaic) and hypertext language were the key innovations that made knowledge universally available. The development of the smartphone from about 2007 brought about a paradigm shift in how we interact with technology. The combination of powerful computing capabilities, internet connectivity and a user-friendly interface in a portable device has made information omnipresent. The ability to access information, communicate with others and perform a myriad of tasks on a device that fits in the palm of the hand has fundamentally changed the way we navigate and engage with the world. These two developments have enabled the collection, collation, verification and application of data and information into a powerful engine for innovation.

The interface between technology and health care has become colloquially known as 'digital health'. The term is broad and encompasses a wide range of technologies, applications and initiatives that leverage digital tools to enhance healthcare delivery, management and outcomes. However, it is simply too large a concept to think about as one whole thing; it can be confusing because all health authorities and many universities and research centres use this term as a catch-all for high-level planning and management purposes.

Data: Digital health relies heavily on data generated from various sources, including medical record systems, wearable devices, medical devices and patient-reported information. Analysing this data can lead to valuable insights and personalised care decisions

Technology: The scope of technologies that sit under the digital-health umbrella include software, hardware and platforms that enable data collection, analysis and communication. Examples include electronic medical records (EMR), wearable devices, mobile health apps, telehealth platforms and AI tools

What is clear is that advances in technology based innovations are occurring at unimaginable speeds, and so in the interest of patient outcomes it is important for every health clinician, manager and administrator to maintain a close eye on innovations that affect them in the immediate and near future.

Key benefits

Better patient engagement

Patients can access self-management tools such as health record portals and phone- and tablet-based applications (apps). Through more active participation there is improved health self-management and more informed decision-making. Improving patient engagement through digital technology has become a key focus in health care, aiming to enhance communication, empower patients and optimise health outcomes.

Personalised and accessible care

Health services can be provided to regional and underserved areas and audiences. Therapeutic services are more easily personalised, tailored and targeted. By combining personalisation and accessibility through digital technology, healthcare can become more patient-centric, thereby improving outcomes, enhancing preventive care and promoting overall wellness.

Efficiency

Streamlined administrative processes are possible through electronic medical records (EMR) and the use of traceable communications such as SMS text messages and email. By leveraging various digital tools and solutions, healthcare organisations can streamline processes, improve communication, optimise resource allocation and ultimately deliver better patient care.

Better communication

By leveraging digital communication technologies, healthcare organisations can overcome traditional communication barriers, improve care coordination, enhance patient engagement and ultimately contribute to better healthcare outcomes. Aside from being traceable, communication across professions and between different points of service provision is much more efficient and accurate. This can have a significant impact on the costs of service provision.

Definitions

Electronic medical records

Also known as the electronic health record (EHS), EMR systems are used by large hospital systems and multi-site health services to manage patient administration and clinical records in a consistent and secure manner. The Australian government also maintains a national public system called My Health Record. My Health Record is an optional, or opt-out, system, meaning the patient is automatically signed up to the national system by the general practitioner unless they state otherwise. My Health Record is available to any patient at any time as well as their doctor, irrespective of where they are in Australia. Most state/territory and regional health systems have chosen a single EMR system so that records can be shared by clinicals and health service providers that have a common patient list or clientele. Popular EMR and patient health management systems used in Australia and internationally include Cerner Millennium and EPIC.

Clinical management

The interface between patient administration and medical and therapeutic management is often described as clinical management. It describes the point-in-time, and the continuing management, of the health of a patient from a clinical perspective.

Big data

Big data refers to exceptionally large datasets that exceed the capacity of traditional data-processing systems. This data can come from various sources, including social media, sensors, transaction records and more. The volume of data is so massive that it requires specialised tools and techniques for storage, processing and analysis. Big data includes both structured and unstructured data. Structured data is organised in a tabular format with clear relationships between fields (e.g. databases), while unstructured data lacks a predefined data model and include text, images, videos and other formats. Big-data technologies can handle both types of data, thus providing a comprehensive view of information.

Artificial intelligence

AI is the replication of human intelligence in machines designed to execute tasks that traditionally require human intelligence. These tasks involve learning, reasoning, problem-solving, natural language comprehension and perception. AI is a multidisciplinary field that draws on computer science, mathematics, psychology, linguistics, neuroscience and other disciplines.

Machine learning

Machine learning (ML) is a field within AI that involves creating algorithms and models that enable computers to learn from data and make predictions or decisions without explicit instructions. The key principle of machine learning is to enable systems to automatically learn and improve from experience or data.

Telehealth

Telehealth refers to the delivery of healthcare services or related activities using technology as an alternative for in-person consultations. This includes, but is not limited to, videoconferencing, internet and telephone. It does not encompass the use of technology during a face-to-face encounter. It is important to note that not all healthcare services are suitable for telehealth.

Challenges of health care in the digital age

The digital transformation of health care comes with significant benefits, but it also poses various challenges that demand attention and resolution. A primary concern is the security and privacy of patient data. The increasing digitisation of health records raises the risk of data breaches and unauthorised access. Balancing the utilisation of health data for improved care with the imperative to safeguard patient privacy is a continuing challenge, necessitating robust security measures and adherence to regulatory standards.

Interoperability and data silos are additional hurdles. Inconsistent standards for data formats and communication protocols can impede the seamless exchange of information between different healthcare systems. Integrating diverse health information technology systems, EMRs and medical devices proves complex and can obstruct the flow of information across the healthcare ecosystem.

Digital literacy and accessibility present challenges, since not all patients have equal access to digital health tools, and potentially create healthcare disparities. Similarly, healthcare professionals may encounter difficulties adapting to new technologies; this highlights the importance of adequate workforce training.

Regulatory compliance adds another layer of complexity. Evolving regulations and compliance requirements, particularly in areas such as data protection and telehealth, challenge healthcare organisations to maintain compliance and adapt to regulatory changes. The cross-border flow of healthcare data further complicates compliance with data management and privacy provisions.

The ethical use of AI introduces concerns regarding bias in AI algorithms and the explainability of AI decisions. Ensuring fairness and transparency in AI applications within health care is crucial.

Patient engagement and behavioural change are ongoing concerns despite the availability of digital health tools. Encouraging sustained patient engagement and motivating behavioural change based on digital health insights are complex tasks.

The integration of wearables and remote monitoring tools generates vast amounts of data, thereby posing challenges for healthcare providers in effectively incorporating this information into clinical workflows. Ensuring the accuracy and reliability of data from these devices is critical in making informed healthcare decisions.

Stakeholders: Include patients, carers, healthcare providers, researchers, information technologists, hardware engineers, entrepreneurs, inventors and policy-makers. Collaboration and integration among these groups are crucial for successful implementation of digital health innovations

Resistance to change within healthcare organisations and among healthcare professionals can hinder the adoption of digital technologies. Overcoming cultural and organisational barriers is crucial for successful implementation.

Addressing these challenges requires collaborative efforts from policy-makers, healthcare providers, technology developers and other **stakeholders**. Continuous attention to these issues is essential for maximising the benefits of digital technology in healthcare while minimising potential risks as the digital landscape continues to evolve. A crucial emphasis lies in effectively harnessing health systems data to enhance system efficiency and population-level planning. Additionally, leveraging this data is paramount to improving the experiences and outcomes of individual patients.

Data analytics in health care

Analytics is a multifaceted process that involves collecting, processing, analysing and interpreting data to extract meaningful insights. The practice of analytics seeks to make sense of available data and then to form contextual information that assists in making strategic decisions about trends, planning and resource use. The goal is to provide decision-makers with the information they need to make informed and strategic choices, whether it is identifying opportunities, mitigating risks or optimising resource allocation. The use of business, clinical and medical analytics as a health service manager often calls for new skills to understand the place of analytics in decision-making and ensure your confidence in the veracity of the data used as a basis for management.

Big data: Implications for population health interventions

Big data has emerged as a transformative force in supporting population-health interventions, offering avenues to refine understanding of systems, optimise decision-making and enhance health outcomes. It has many uses and spans various domains, beginning with enhanced monitoring that enables rapid responses to emerging health threats.

Predictive analytics facilitates early risk identification and the design of targeted interventions, including lifestyle modifications and preventative care. In the realm of precision medicine, big-data integration of genomic and health data enables personalised health plans and improved treatment outcomes.

An example in the latter situation is the need to increase staff in periods that are predicted to be busy, or in a health service setting a survey of patients might indicate improvements that can be made in service provision.

Predictive analytics interrogates information from past activity to predict future outcomes. Predictive analytics about the mutation of the COVID-19 virus were used by epidemiologists to support decisions designed to avoid catastrophic risks for communities and governments – and continue to do so. Predictive analytics is often a specialist field; examples of roles in society that use predictive analytics include economists, epidemiologists, insurance actuaries and stock market analysts.

The benefit of sound descriptive analytics is that a dashboard of past performance can be created; for example, 'average time to answer phone calls' from a telephone system, or financial performance based on hourly patterns across a day in a health facility such as a hospital ward. Accounting and financial management are common examples of reporting based on descriptive analytics. Descriptive analytics is useful in providing a clear description of what happened in past events, whereas predictive analytics seeks to forecast future outcomes or scenarios.

The analysis of social determinants of health contributes to a more comprehensive understanding, informing interventions that address the root causes of health disparities. Behavioural insights benefit from big data analytics, guiding the crafting of personalised behavioural change programs. Social media and sentiment analysis within big data analytics enhance community engagement and public health messaging.

Collaboration and data sharing across sectors are critical, presenting opportunities for global insights. Despite the immense potential, challenges related to data governance, ethics and equitable access demand attention, with policy-makers, healthcare professionals and data scientists playing pivotal roles in navigating these complexities for the optimal advancement of population-health interventions.

Integrity of health data: Privacy, confidentiality and security

It seems self-evident that privacy and confidentiality are key and core requirements in management in the digital age, and with such advances in accessible information technologies. However, in recent times the prevalence of criminal actors accessing and interrogating large data sources has made the establishment of sophisticated detection and protection mechanisms essential. Several key considerations and measures contribute to maintaining the security of health data:

- Secure data collection, transmission and curation require robust data governance policies, including clear guidelines on handling, storing and accessing health data, and continuous employee training on data privacy and security, to create a robust organisational framework.
- Data-minimisation and the need-to-know principle emphasise the need to collect health data only as necessary for specific purposes, thereby reducing risks associated with unnecessary storage. Implementing comprehensive audit trails, logging and monitoring access, and setting up alert systems contribute to detecting and investigating unauthorised activities promptly.
- Legal and regulatory compliance, such as adhering to appropriate legal and governance frameworks, is essential, with a specific focus on developing a data-breach response plan. This includes establishing an incident response team and clear procedures for notification of affected individuals and regulatory authorities.
- Access controls, including role-based access control and two-factor authentication, play a crucial role in restricting access to health data based on individuals' roles and enhancing access security. Additional security can involve using secure application programming interfaces (APIs) for data exchange and implementing encryption when utilising cloud services.
- Third-party security assessments ensure that vendors and service providers meet high standards of data protection, backed by contractual agreements outlining their responsibilities. Obtaining informed consent from individuals before collecting and processing their health data, coupled with transparent communication about data use and security measures, supports ethical data practices.
- Regular security audits and assessments, including penetration-testing and comprehensive security audits, are vital for identifying vulnerabilities and ensuring overall compliance with regulation and policies. By implementing this comprehensive approach, healthcare organisations can maintain a robust data protection framework and adapt to emerging threats and evolving regulatory requirements through regular reassessment and updates to security measures.
- Patient modesty and religious and cultural needs have become additional dimensions in the privacy and confidentiality domain.

Leveraging data to improve health management decisions

The Australian healthcare system has large volumes of digital data capable of revolutionising healthcare delivery on a personalised, real-time basis. However, despite the overall quality of healthcare at the population level, the system suffers from acute data fragmentation. This fragmentation hinders individuals, their caregivers and service providers, as well as policy-makers, in making informed decisions. Key factors contributing to this fragmentation include the diverse array of healthcare settings, providers, funding sources and regulatory frameworks.

Efforts to improve health data collection have been made over the past two decades, but they often result in fragmented datasets lacking comprehensive information. Initiatives like My Health Record have struggled to gain widespread acceptance. Contrastingly, tapping into comprehensive, real-time healthcare datasets could provide richer insights for consumers, caregivers and system planners.

EMRs provide the greatest benefits when they are fully implemented and consistently adopted and used by every stakeholder in a health system. While that is always the goal, it is also one of the greatest challenges facing health systems.

As we enter the fifth decade of the digital era, the reluctance to integrate personal health data contrasts with consumer demands for instant, personalised services. Other countries have boldly leveraged health data for preventive and curative care. However, the effective utilisation of healthcare data and care data in Australia, whether for care delivery or clinical research, faces obstacles due to the absence of standardised data governance frameworks and their interpretation, as well as different legislation at state and federal levels for health data-sharing (Connor, Day & Meston, 2015).

In the future, decision-support tools will play an integral role in all facets of health and social care. Therefore, having robust, transparent and universally understood data-governance mechanisms for employing such tools in care delivery and population health research will be crucial for their timely, safe and cost-effective adoption.

Paradoxically, the absence of a standardised approach to data governance has spurred the development of tools and techniques to compensate for inconsistencies in data sharing, especially with electronic health records. In the research ecosystem, safe and secure record-linkage methods, including privacy preserving record linkage, have emerged as a way to integrate data from across the entire health system. These linked datasets enable researchers to gain a comprehensive understanding of the evolving needs of individuals, families and communities. This approach facilitates a deeper insight into the complexities of healthcare systems and enables more targeted interventions and support mechanisms.

Artificial intelligence and machine learning: Implications for health service delivery

AI and ML are revolutionising health service delivery. In clinical decision support, AI and ML algorithms analyse diagnostic data, aiding healthcare professionals in making more accurate and timely diagnoses while also suggesting personalised treatment plans. Predictive analytics and risk stratification facilitate early disease detection and population health management, enabling proactive interventions and resource allocation. Remote patient monitoring, powered by AI, enables continuous tracking of vital signs, thus facilitating early intervention and preventing complications, particularly for those with chronic conditions.

Telehealth benefits from AI-driven virtual health assistants to optimise initial assessments and scheduling, while integration with remote monitoring provides a comprehensive view of patients' health. Personalised medicine advances are occurring through AI and ML analysing genomic data for precision treatment options and tailoring treatment plans based on individual characteristics. Operational efficiency sees improvements as AI streamlines administrative processes, automates tasks and optimises workflows, thus reducing burdens on healthcare professionals. Natural language processing automates clinical documentation and supports research by extracting insights from vast amounts of clinical text.

Medication management benefits from ML that predicts adherence and recommends personalised plans, while fraud detection and cyber security employ AI for enhanced security and prevention of billing fraud. Continuous learning and improvement are inherent in adaptive ML algorithms that evolve, thereby incorporating feedback from healthcare professionals and patients.

However, challenges such as securing data privacy, ethical considerations and the need for transparent and explainable AI systems must be addressed for responsible and effective deployment. Collaborative efforts from healthcare providers, policy-makers and technology developers are crucial in harnessing the full potential of AI and ML for the benefit of patients and the healthcare ecosystem.

Telemedicine

The terms 'telemedicine' and 'telehealth' are often used interchangeably to describe clinical or therapeutic practices delivered remotely using voice, voice and video, or remote-monitoring devices, which are the key elements that define a telemedicine service. In its purest form, telemedicine is a subset of telehealth, in that telehealth includes telemedicine, remote monitoring and health education, while telemedicine focuses on remote clinical services and medical care.

The COVID-19 pandemic saw a significant growth in the use and scope of telemedicine. In the years following, significant commentary has ensued about the benefits and limitations of telehealth.

The Australian Society for Telehealth declared October 2023 as 'Telehealth Awareness Month' and promoted the following principles:

> October 2023 is Telehealth Awareness Month where telehealth and virtual care campaigns will be scheduled across the various states.
>
> For a unified voice, jurisdictions are encouraged to embrace the theme of Telehealth: enabling sustainable health care – highlighting the role of telehealth in:
>
> - Enabling equitable consumer access to high quality health services closer to home … meaning less time away from community, work and school.
> - Supporting clinicians to access peer support and upskilling … to increase skill, reduce isolation and increase workforce retention.
> - Enabling healthcare providers to collaborate to deliver high quality, integrated care … regardless of where the consumer in located.

- Improving health system efficiency by optimising workforce capability to deliver care virtually ... from or to any location.
- Reducing the environmental footprint of providing health care ... reduced clinician and consumer travel means fuel savings and less carbon emissions. (Telehealth Victoria, 2020)

The wider adoption of Telehealth has led to significant benefits in terms of access to care and efficient use of resources.

VICTORIAN VIRTUAL EMERGENCY DEPARTMENT

The Victorian Virtual Emergency Department, established in October 2020, stands out as a pioneering initiative designed to alleviate challenges related to emergency department overcrowding by providing non-urgent patients with remote access to emergency care throughout Victoria, 24/7.

The collaborative effort involves Northern Health, La Trobe University and the Victorian Department of Health, aiming to safely triage self-presenting emergency patients, streamline patient care to bypass the waiting room and provide an acceptable alternative model for the public. The overall aim is to use telehealth services to manage a proportion of emergency patients in the community.

Using telehealth services to manage a proportion of emergency patients in the community reflects a patient-centred and technology driven approach to healthcare delivery. Operational around the clock, the Virtual Emergency Department addresses issues such as prolonged waiting times, resource diversion and overall dissatisfaction in both patients and staff associated with overcrowded traditional emergency departments. Regular evaluation and refinement of telehealth strategies will contribute to continuing improvements in community based emergency care.

Dr Loren Sher, Clinical Director of the Victorian Virtual Emergency Department, emphasises the global concern of emergency department overcrowding, attributing it to factors such as the ageing population and a rise in chronic and complex diseases. The uniqueness of the Virtual Emergency Department lies in its direct-care approach, distinguishing it from traditional telehealth models, and aims to reduce the need for patient transfers, thereby optimising resource utilisation.

The service targets various challenges linked to emergency department overcrowding, including resource diversion from critical cases, prolonged waiting times, adverse health outcomes, staff stress, bed blockages, and patient and staff dissatisfaction.

Implications for health managers in a digital age

Significant changes in communications and information technologies have led to an ever-burgeoning scope of new challenges for managers. The idea that change is constant is not new; however, it is the overwhelming nature of the pace of technological change that offers the greatest challenge.

Leading virtual teams

The 'virtual' office has been possible for many years, and has been used as a way of operating small businesses and enterprises from home and from shared office spaces since the mid-1990s. However, the COVID-19 pandemic saw the exponential growth of people working from home. For many reasons this trend has continued, with many people in health organisations working virtually for at least some of the week.

Flexible working arrangements have brought with them the ability for organisations to access human resources across large distances in an effective and efficient manner. The features and functions of teleconferencing software have improved to meet demands, and many of us have become highly accustomed to the protocols of participating in online meetings.

What is accentuated when working with virtual teams is the need to communicate clearly and respectfully. Working and meeting virtually can accentuate a sense of isolation and it can lead to mistrust about productivity. Non-verbal cues, usually experienced face to face, are largely absent. Teleconferencing software accommodates these changes with the use of gestures and emoticons to enable some semblance of normal human interaction.

As a leader of a virtual team, a manager has an even greater requirement for proactive communication. When working remotely, it is possible for people to feel isolated and less connected to their team. It is also likely that some people will find difficulty with a lack of work–life separation that undermines balance. The use of email also creates an asynchronous effect in communications, whereby email can be used in a transactional manner, not enabling the normal adjustments in task management that come from a synchronous interaction.

With flexible working arrangements it is also common for the lines to be blurred regarding when people are on shift and off shift. Emailing at midnight someone who normally works from nine to five, can be disruptive in an unfair manner.

These risks can lead to issues in workplace health and safety, and problematic psychosocial behaviours between team members and with leadership.

Despite these risks, the benefits of operating virtual teams are well documented. This is true in both health-service management and telemedicine settings. Recently, significant improvements have occurred in accessibility for disadvantaged groups, and well as efficiency in communication due, in part, to reductions in the pricing of technology, the use of smartphones and improvements in online communication software. There are many indicators that patient outcomes benefit from the greater veracity of information being obtained and shared by monitoring systems and clinicians alike.

When managing virtual teams, regular and short meetings tend to provide more benefit than longer, drawn-out sessions. Adopting the principles of agile project management, including weekly or daily 'stand up' meetings, is often beneficial.

Summary

- Digital innovation has transformed health care, enhancing patient care, streamlining processes and improving efficiency.
- Digital health technologies (e.g. EMRs, wearables, AI) have improved patient engagement, personalised care, efficiency and communication.
- Challenges include data security, interoperability, digital literacy, regulatory compliance, ethical AI use and resistance to change.
- Analytics (especially big data) is crucial for population-health interventions, enabling monitoring, risk prediction, targeted interventions and analysis of social determinants of health.
- Data integrity requires robust governance, legal compliance, access controls, security assessments and audits.
- Health managers face challenges due to rapid technological change. They need agility, adaptability and understanding of the implications of digital innovation.
- Workforce training is essential in leveraging new technologies and workflows.
- In navigating these multifaceted challenges, health managers require not only technical expertise but also an understanding of the broader implications of digital innovation on healthcare delivery and patient outcomes. Those capable of navigating these complexities with agility and foresight are poised to lead their organisations into the future of healthcare.

Reflective questions

1. How has your perspective on digital health and its role in healthcare delivery changed? Consider any personal experiences you might have had with telehealth or other digital health tools.
2. What are the potential challenges associated with digital health implementation, such as data security and privacy, and what strategies or solutions do you think are most important to consider for successful implementation?
3. Imagine you are a healthcare professional. How could data analytics be most effectively used in your field to improve patient care or population-health outcomes?
4. As digital health continues to evolve and rely heavily on sensitive patient data, how can we ensure a balance between innovation and ethical data-handling practices? What are your biggest concerns regarding data privacy and security?
5. Considering the potential of AI in health care, what specific applications do you find most exciting? On the other hand, what potential risks associated with AI in health care do you think warrant the most attention?

Self-analysis questions

How has your experience of health systems changed with the increased use of digital tools and systems? What professional development might you consider in this field?

References

Connor, M., Day, G. & Meston, D. (2015). Successful linking of patient records between hospital services and general practice to facilitate integrated care in a hospital and health service in south-east Queensland. *Australian Health Review*, *40*(1), 78–81. https://doi.org/10.1071/AH15048

Telehealth Victoria. (2020). Telehealth awareness month. Retrieved from: https://web.archive.org/web/20240306232136/https://telehealthvictoria.org.au/resources/telehealth-awareness-month-2020/

Part 6
Shapes Systems

30 Workforce planning

Ged Williams and Ben Archdall

Learning objectives

How do I:

- improve my skills in workforce planning?
- assimilate the principles of workforce planning?
- consider the Australian health workforce in relation to the structures, processes and trends in the global healthcare context?
- consider workforce demand and supply factors in the Australian healthcare sector that may affect workforce planning?

Introduction

Workforce planning in the healthcare system continues to be a politically charged issue in many countries due to the continuing shortage of various health professional groups and the subsequent costs and liabilities to governments hoping to generate improvements and efficiencies.

In 2016, the World Health Organization (WHO) released the *Global strategy on human resources for health: Workforce 2030*, whose overall goal was to improve health, social and economic development outcomes by ensuring universal availability, accessibility, acceptability, coverage and quality of the health workforce through adequate investment to strengthen health systems and the implementation of effective policies at national, regional and global levels (WHO, 2016). The Strategy reaffirms the importance of the WHO Global Code of Practice on the International Recruitment of Health Personnel (World Health Assembly, 2010), which recommends countries, including Australia and Aotearoa New Zealand, aim for workforce self-sufficiency with regard to workforce planning.

Governments around the world require detailed data and robust systems to effectively plan the healthcare workforce. The government of Canada, for example, has established a dedicated health workforce agency aimed at improving workforce planning through digital tools and health-workforce data, in addition to training and sustainability strategies for retention and recruitment (Health Canada, 2023).

The movement of trained health professionals between countries can be influenced by governments or individual motivating factors such as career development and quality of life. Countries that recruit or receive migrant healthcare workers have a responsibility to maximise these workers' experience and skills to improve long-term retention and contribute to a supported, stable, well-educated and resilient workforce (Pressley, Newton, Garside, Stephenson & Mejia-Olivares, 2023).

At the time of writing, Australia has a new national medical workforce strategy (Commonwealth of Australia DoHA, 2021a), and is developing a new national nursing workforce strategy (Commonwealth of Australia DoHA, 2024a), the intention being that they will provide a road map to encourage collaboration between states and territories to support a national approach to health workforce planning and sustainability. Additionally, the significant challenges of attracting health workers to rural and remote locations has been a perennial problem for communities throughout Australia and is being addressed through the Stronger Rural Health Strategy, which aims to provide an additional 3000 doctors and 3000 nurses by 2028 (Commonwealth of Australia DoHA, 2021b).

This chapter discusses the principles, processes and pitfalls of workforce planning in the healthcare sector, giving particular emphasis to the Australian perspective.

Definitions

Workforce planning is an ongoing business process aimed at ensuring the right people with the right skills are in the right place at the right time and at the right cost. It is an active and continuous process used to 'generate business intelligence to inform business of the current and future impact of the external and internal environment on the business, enabling the business to be resilient to structural and cultural changes to better position itself for the future' (International Organisation of Standardization (ISO), 2015; Australian Public Service Commission, 2023).

Workforce planning is not a rigid, linear process. Many considerations are needed to inform the plan, and yet the future is never static, so the plan must remain dynamic if it is to serve the purpose for which it has been designed. Furthermore, health services are forever being asked to curtail costs, thus workforce planners are forced to find innovations and reforms that can improve productivity and reduce ever-growing workforce costs. Healthcare planners must consider, now and into the future, workforce productivity opportunities such as service redesign or model of care changes as part of the workforce planning process (Birch, Gibson & McBride, 2020).

Australia's healthcare workforce: Demand and supply

There are many demand and supply factors that can affect Australia's ability to plan for its healthcare workforce. In terms of size, the 2021 Australian Census estimated that more than 1.7 million people worked in the health care and social assistance industry, with hospital settings accounting for 31.4 per cent of this number (Australian Bureau of Statistics (ABS), 2022). Employment in health care and social assistance is projected to grow by 301 000 (or 15.8%) over the five years to November 2026 (Commonwealth of Australia, Jobs and Skills, 2024), with projected population changes a significant demand driver as Australia grows from 27 million in 2024 to as high as 36 million by 2050, along with an ageing population as the percentage of those aged 65 years and older grow from 13 per cent of the population in 2010 to 23 per cent in 2050 (Commonwealth of Australia DoHA, 2010).

This ongoing demand for healthcare workers comes at a significant cost for both government and non-government organisations. In 2021–22, health spending accounted for 10.5 per cent of gross domestic product in Australia, which is comparatively higher than the OECD average of 38 countries at 9.7 per cent. Of the $241 billion spent on healthcare in Australia that year, government funded $176 billion (72.9%) with non-government sources funding the remaining $65.3 billion (27.1%); approximately 70 per cent of healthcare expenditure is related to workforce costs (AIHW, 2023).

In addition to population-driven health workforce demand, government policy factors such as the National Disability Insurance Scheme (NDIS), introduced in 2013, he created significant challenges to supply the consequent disability workforce, with a 31 per cent expected growth in the period 2020–24 (Commonwealth of Australia, 2021c). During the period 2016 to 2021, healthcare occupations such as those listed in Table 30.1 had grown by as much as 43 per cent in response to government policies and priorities such as the NDIS, while the national growth in jobs was around 3 per cent. This makes some healthcare roles among the fastest-growing occupational groups in the country (AIHW, 2022).

Impermanent demand factors can also affect certain health workforce cohorts, resulting in the need for rapid workforce redeployment within existing supply pools. This was apparent during the COVID-19 pandemic when international skilled migration was restricted and there was a significant spike in demand for intensive care beds and intensive

Table 30.1 Key workforce statistics by health profession 2015–20

Profession	Measure	2015	2020	% change
Allied health	Number of practitioners	118 418	166 048	40.2
	FTE total	106 500	152 559	43.2
	FTE per 100 000 population	447	594	32.9
Dental practitioners	Number of practitioners	19 051	21 549	13.1
	FTE total	17 613	19 450	10.4
	FTE per 100 000 population	74	76	2.7
Medical practitioners	Number of practitioners	87 999	105 293	19.7
	FTE total	93 356	107 777	15.4
	FTE per 100 000 population	392	420	7.0
Nurses and midwives	Number of practitioners	306 487	349 589	14.1
	FTE total	270 368	305 855	13.1
	FTE per 100 000 population	1135	1191	4.9
All professions	Number of practitioners	531 955	642 479	20.8
	FTE total	487 837	585 642	20.0
	FTE per 100 000 population	2048	2280	11.3

Source: AIHW (2022).

care-trained nurses. The lack of skilled workers and supply options resulted in adjusted models of care and increasing reliance on less-experienced staff from local supply pools (Topple et al., 2023).

The healthcare industry's response to managing these varied workforce demands has resulted in many anomalies in the profile of the Australian health workforce, which possibly represent the consequences of poor workforce planning. For instance, the number of registered nurses and aged and disabled carers born overseas is 40 per cent (ABS, 2022), while the percentage of Australian general practitioners (GPs) who are international medical graduates is 29 per cent, with the proportion of GPs who graduated from an international university being greatest among registrars (43%) (Royal Australian College of General Practitioners, 2023). While an overseas-born workforce is an expedient solution to Australia's needs, it is not clear from the literature whether unintended consequences are harming the industry in those countries from where this workforce originates. Australia's reliance on international workforce supply sources may pose a long-term risk to addressing future population changes, government policy and impermanent demands if investment into self-sustainable local solutions does not also continue, not to mention the ethical considerations of the 'brain drain' from lower-income countries that can ill afford to lose health professionals (Kamarulzaman, Ramnarayan & Mocumbi, 2022).

While globalisation trends in the health workforce vary from country to country, there are ongoing efforts by the Australian healthcare industry to increase the supply of Australian graduating healthcare professionals. In response to workforce-demand projections, the number of medical schools across Australia continues to grow, accommodating 18 359 medical practitioner students in 2023, up from around 17 000 in 2016. However, the graduating number peaked at 3805 in 2022 and has hovered around 3600 in the period 2018–23 (Medical Deans Australia and New Zealand, 2024). The proportion of medical student enrolments completed by international students remains relatively constant, at around 15 per cent during the same period.

Students commencing and completing general nursing courses in Australia in the period 2015–18 grew 20 and 26 per cent, respectively (Commonwealth of Australia DoH, 2020); however, the challenge of securing clinical placements in the health system can restrict the ability of Australian universities to meet enrolment demands. Australian government-supported clinical placement programs, such as the Aged Care Nursing Clinical Placements program, assist students with high-quality clinical placements and raise awareness of opportunities in specific healthcare sectors (Commonwealth of Australia DoHA, 2023). After many years of lobbying by health professions' advocacy groups, the Australian government has announced the establishment of a Commonwealth Prac Payment to support students undertaking mandatory workplace placements required for university and vocational education and training qualifications, including nursing, midwifery and social work, commencing in July 2025 (Clare, 2024).

Measures have been introduced to improve local workforce supply and graduate retention, and to maximise productivity of the existing workforce by removing barriers to health professionals working to their full scope of practice; this contributes to greater capacity and resilience within the health system (Commonwealth of Australia DoHA, 2024b).

Doleman and colleagues (2023) provide a retrospective analysis of graduate nurse employment, showing a 26 per cent reduction in the number still working at 6 months, yet beyond this point 91 per cent of those who were working at 6 months were still working in nursing at 36 months. The ability of non-medical graduates to secure work in their chosen health profession is variable and can lead to boom-and-bust workforce supply.

The irony of this bizarre situation is not lost on policy advisors in the Australian health system, who on the one hand state that the country cannot afford to support the current numbers of healthcare graduates from the nation's universities, and on the other must concede that all of them (and more) are needed if Australia is to achieve **health workforce sustainability** into the future.

Health workforce sustainability: Maintenance of the specific staff (doctors, nurses, allied health professionals, specialist support staff) required to meet the health needs of the given area or population

Framework for workforce planning

Organisations that do not follow a structured and integrated framework for workforce planning are exposed to reactive activities such as international recruitment campaigns, which may become necessary in response to acute increases in service demand or shortages in workforce supply.

Such as framework should incorporate and align with organisational governance structures, policies, data standards and digital tools to enable the delivery of quality planning outcomes. Many conceptual models with commonly themed phases have been developed throughout the past decades in Australia and internationally to provide a framework through which workforce planning can be understood and followed, and several are easy to find online (see Figure 30.1.)

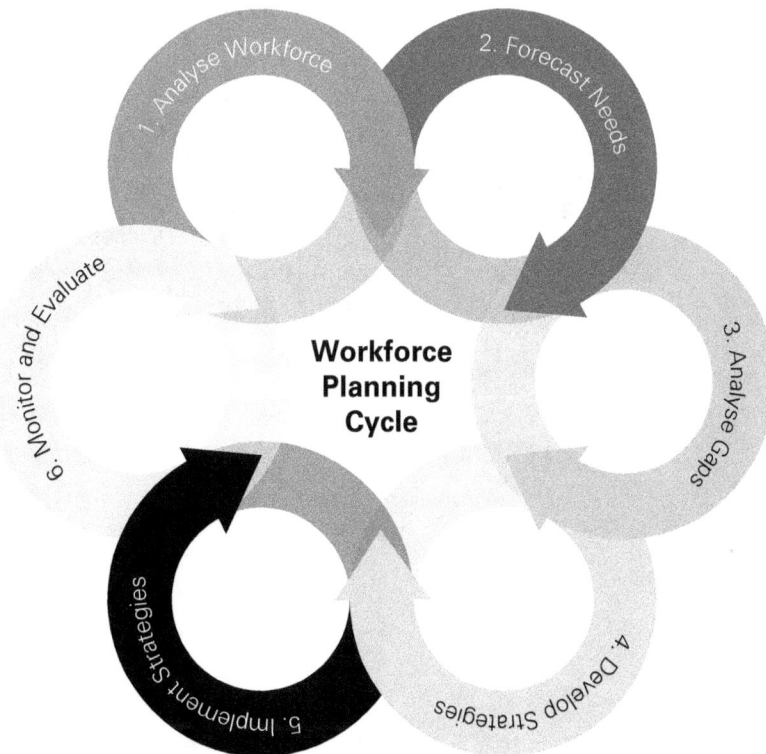

Figure 30.1 Workforce planning cycle

Source: Australian Public Service Commission (2023).

The World Health Assembly (2010) and several partners developed the Human Resources for Health (HRH) Action Framework (Figure 30.2), which includes six action fields (human resources management systems, leadership, partnership, finance, education and policy) and a four-phase action cycle, which illustrates the phases to follow in applying the framework (situational analysis, planning, implementation, and monitoring and evaluation). To ensure a comprehensive approach to a given challenge, users of the framework are advised to address all action fields and phases of the action cycle, paying particular attention to the set of critical success factors. (For more detailed analysis and background information, see the HRH Action Framework website: http://www.capacityproject.org/framework.)

By merging the many conceptual models, we have developed a workforce planning framework that represents the core phases for a foundation to successful planning outcomes (see Figure 30.3). The workforce planning framework can be applied universally when conducting operational (0–18 months) or strategic (2–5 years) workforce planning activities.

Before being discussed in detail, the five phases in the workforce planning framework are listed, followed in parentheses by the corresponding language used in the example HRH action framework phases:

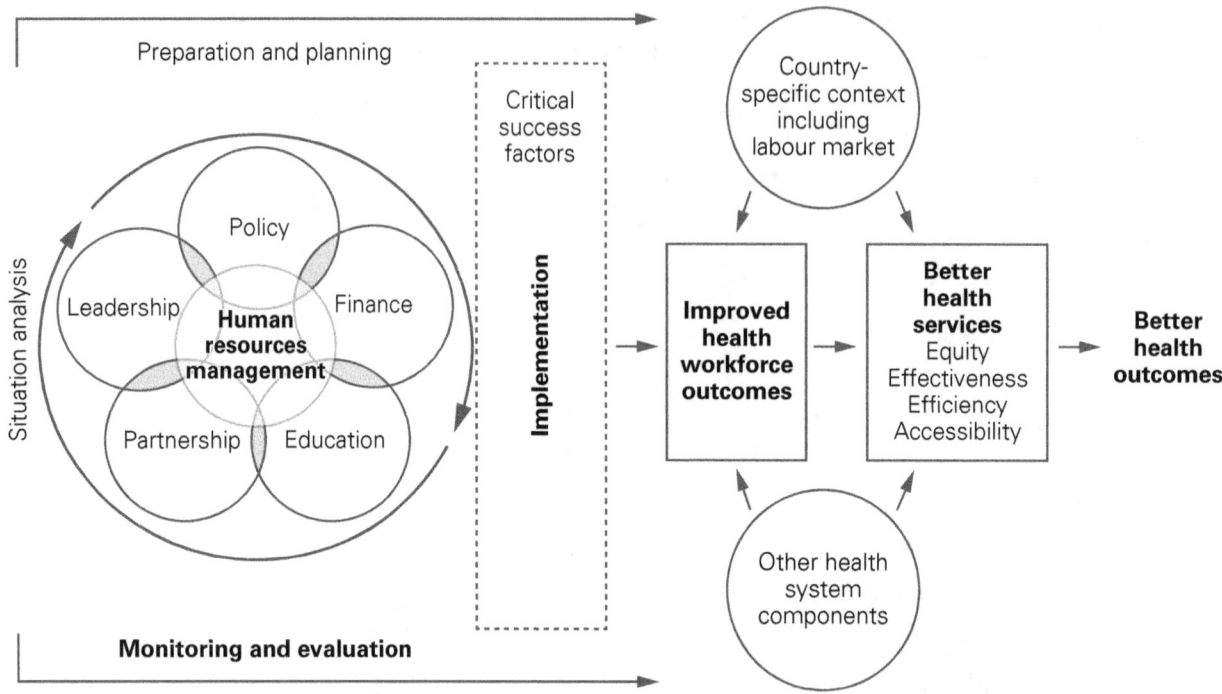

Figure 30.2 Human Resources for Health action framework
Source: World Health Assembly (2010).

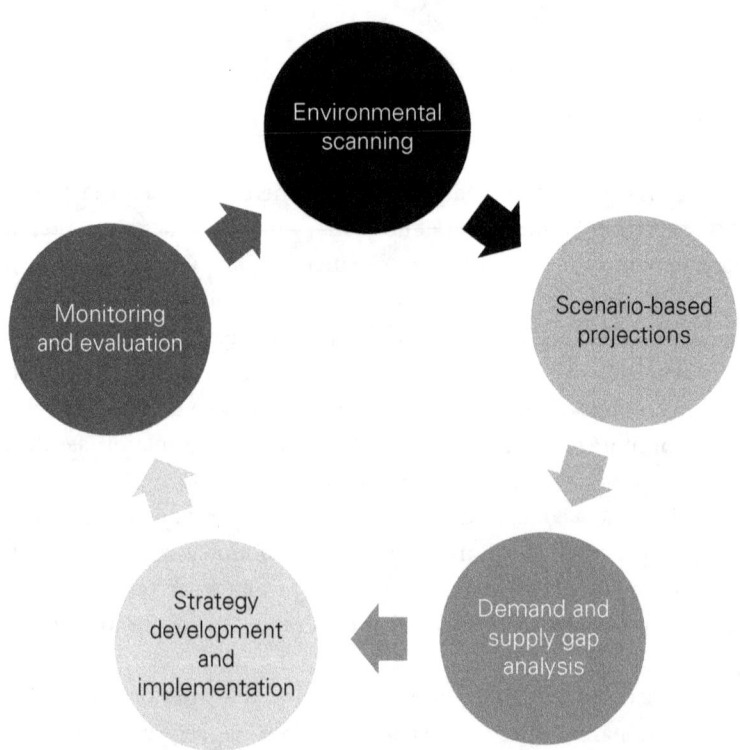

Figure 30.3 Workforce planning framework involving an ongoing, sequenced process

- environmental scanning (situational analysis)
- scenario-based **workforce projections** (preparation and planning)
- demand and supply gap analysis (preparation and planning)
- strategy development and implementation (implementation)
- monitoring and evaluation (monitoring and evaluation).

Workforce projection: A forecast or estimate of what the workforce delivering health services may look like in the future

The number or breakdown of phases and time spent on each planning activity is dependent on the capacity of the resources allocated to perform the task within the defined timeline. Workforce planning capability such as skill or access to digital or artificial intelligence tools will also influence the volume and quality of outputs from each phase. While the phases are typically cyclical in nature, the sequence can be variable and may need to occur concurrently due to the volatility of health system changes.

Environmental scanning

Also known as situational analysis, environmental scanning requires planners to understand the existing workforce and the factors (internal and external) that will affect the organisation and its workforce needs. Analysis of the existing workforce should consider the following elements:

- **demographics**: age, sex, length of tenure and location
- **health context**: service, hospital, district, state or territory and country
- **human capital**: key people, core positions and job satisfaction
- **critical role**: types of new or emerging roles
- **capability**: education and training, qualifications and general wellbeing
- **capacity**: productivity, skill mix, role or service redesign.

Environmental scanning can be used in developing assumptions for future workforce attrition and can inform staff development, recruitment or retention strategies. A review of factors that will affect the workforce in the future should also consider the following:

- organisational strategic priorities
- service demands
- capital infrastructure
- technology
- fiscal constraints
- industrial awards, policy and legislative reform
- other strengths, weaknesses, opportunities and threats (a SWOT analysis).

These factors, associated assumptions and validated existing workforce data can form the metric drivers for future, scenario-based projections.

Scenario-based workforce projection

This phase involves using the results of environmental scanning to generate realistic, scenario-based workforce projections for both the existing workforce and the supply chain. When deciding which factors to include as drivers in workforce projections, both their likelihood of occurring and their potential effects should be considered.

In their simplest form, workforce projections can be produced by linking the existing workforce profiles, head count and/or full-time equivalents with future service demands in a linear algorithm; for example, if demand increases by 50 per cent, so will the workforce.

This demand-driven model is then adjusted on the basis of further assumptions and scenarios identified in the environmental-scanning process. Attrition and supply calculations are based on similar principles but use different drivers; for example, attrition can be driven by several factors, such as finding a better job, for cause, retirement, restructuring, cost-cutting, mergers and divestitures (Mendonsa, Stolberg, Viswanathan & Crum, 2020), while supply can come from several different sources, including increased training, migration and incentives (WHO, 2017).

Demand and supply gap analysis

The objective of this phase is to provide a set of findings around which strategies and implementation plans can be based. Considering both head count and full-time equivalent variations, some critical gaps to explore and report may include:

- workforce versus budget
- attrition versus new graduates and external recruitment (including overseas)
- education pathways versus critical roles or specialties
- minimum number of staff required to operate a service (critical mass) versus service-demand volume and ability to respond to peaks and troughs in demand.

Furthermore, the profile of the workforce projection should be articulated and refined, especially in terms of occupation types, broad skill sets and specialist skill sets. This analysis can inform the education sector to be targeted, or to partner with, to fill the identified gap — for example, schools, universities and TAFEs.

Strategy development and implementation

Strategic workforce planning initiatives should link with and support the organisation's objectives. Strategies may need to address:

- workforce development
- workforce re-engineering and substitution
- recruitment and retention
- service redesign, research and innovation
- financial constraints
- industrial or policy reform.

All strategies require consultation and must be documented, understandable, specific, measurable, affordable, accountable and timely (DUSMAAT). Documented and in an accessible place, preferably online, the strategy must be understandable, meaning that employees and all other stakeholders can read it and understand the intention. It should identify specific tasks and actions that are clear and linked directly to the goal; measures must also link to the goal and be easy to obtain, update and review to inform progress and performance. As with any business strategy, the plan must be affordable and integrated with the organisation's operating structure so each action can have an accountable officer — that is, a specific person or position named as responsible for the completion of the task within a certain timeframe. This may involve representatives from multiple departments not traditionally involved in the strategic or operational planning process. Essentially, strategic workforce planning initiatives involve change-management theory applied to workforce planning, and it relies on good leadership and systems for execution.

Monitoring and evaluation

Once clear measures and accountabilities are documented, staff, unions, managers and other stakeholders can monitor and review progress. If available, organisations should use an integrated electronic software platform to provide a shared level of ownership and transparency, and enable dialogue on performance metrics as required. It is during this phase that adjustments can be made to respond to changing dynamics, needs and projections. This will contribute to improvements in future workforce planning iterations and provide a basis to evaluate the return on investment.

GOLD COAST UNIVERSITY HOSPITAL WORKFORCE PLANNING

Background

Gold Coast University Hospital is a $1.75 billion, 750-bed, tertiary level public healthcare facility co-located with Griffith University. It opened in 2013 to service a population of more than 600 000 people located within the greater Gold Coast region. The hospital was built on a greenfield site to replace the 500-bed Gold Coast Hospital, which was decommissioned following the transfer of beds and services to the new site. Today, Gold Coast Health Service continues to apply workforce planning frameworks and strategies established during the workforce planning project for the Gold Coast University Hospital and associated services.

Workforce planning framework

The framework applied by the workforce project conducted in 2009 involved environmental scanning of 270 services, workforce projections over a 5-year commissioning period, workforce demand and supply gap analysis by clinical professionals, and provision of strategic recommendations.

Findings

The execution of the workforce planning activities was generally constrained by the scale and volume of services involved. New systems and processes were developed to improve service-planning coordination across clinical professions and to identify erroneous baseline data.

The workforce planning framework resulted in a projected workforce growth of 83 per cent during the proposed 5-year commissioning period for the Gold Coast University Hospital. The demand drivers for this growth identified by the environmental scanning included a projected increase in clinical activity, associated with expanded and new services; the effects of new capital infrastructure, including the design and scale of the new facility; and an increase in patient acuity, resulting from new and expanded tertiary level services being offered.

The gap analysis between workforce demand and supply found that the supply chains within the regional education network were inadequate to meet the projected growth for

> ### GOLD COAST UNIVERSITY HOSPITAL
> ### WORKFORCE PLANNING Continued
>
> some clinical professions, such as nursing. This supply shortage would be compounded by retention issues related to an ageing workforce.
>
> Several recommendations were made and strategies implemented in 2009 that remain today, including the development of partnerships with the local education sector to 'grow our own' sustainable workforce to meet the projected workforce demand and the sustained use of planning tools to manage scale and volume involved.

Management and workforce planning

Automation

An automated electronic digital tool able to receive detailed data from numerous integrated sources to inform assumptions and algorithms is critical in the workforce planning process. Queensland Health developed the WorkMAPP system, which is used to manage and forecast workforce planning data for the entire public health workforce across the state of Queensland – almost 100 000 staff. Through this tool, Queensland Health can continuously review various scenario projections and speculate on the possible outcomes from an almost infinite series of scenarios – provided the raw data sources supplied by services are reliable and accurate.

Retention and satisfaction

In addressing retention and staff-satisfaction needs, it is critical to identify strategies that have been proven to make a difference (Wakerman et al., 2019; Beccaria et al., 2021), as well as those that are most affordable, and then use a knowledgeable stakeholder group to decide how and when to implement such strategies.

Retention strategies may be organisation-wide, such as the establishment of employer-of-choice programs to build reputation, or targeted strategies, such as the Bonded Medical Program scheme funded by the Australian government, which provides financial incentives in exchange for a commitment to work 3 years after the student completes their course in a rural or remote area of Australia (Commonwealth of Australia DoHA, 2024c).

Working smarter

To work smarter means to produce more outputs per unit of time – that is, to bring about the same or better outputs with the same or less workforce. This can be achieved through increased training and skills development (to improve quality, efficiency, safety and breadth of work per employee), better work organisation (such as a reduction in time spent on administrative work and more time spent on clinical work) and technological progress (such as a reduction in operating time and a move to day surgery, brought about by more effective techniques) (Ono, Lafortune & Schoenstein, 2013).

Working longer

More working hours means that workers can produce more outputs over a certain period of time (a day, a week or a year). For example, a GP may be able to see three or four more patients in every additional hour of work added to the current working day, which would create a marginal cost for the business but an improvement in productivity.

Workforce plasticity

Workforce plasticity means that the workforce is encouraged to constantly review the traditional boundaries of set roles and to be flexible in the tasks they can do within their scope of practice. For example, an assistant in nursing can take on some of the tasks of the enrolled nurse, who can take on some of the tasks of the registered nurse, who may then pick up tasks of the doctor, who if necessary may complete tasks of all those employees if they have the capacity; for example, the doctor can clean the dressing trolley while the nurse assists the patient to dress and leave the room. A workforce that embraces workforce plasticity can improve productivity and resilience when faced with impermanent fluctuations in demand.

Summary

- Australia has more than 1.7 million people working in the healthcare and social assistance industry, with 301 000 (or 15.8%) projected growth over the 5 years to November 2026.
- To ensure an efficient and effective health workforce, the right people with the right skills must be in the right place at the right time and at the right cost.
- Workforce planning is a complex process requiring robust data and digital systems supported by integrated partnerships with service planning, human resource management, leadership, finance, education and policy.
- An effective workforce planning framework involves a continuous action cycle of environmental scanning, scenario-based projections, demand and supply gap analysis, strategy development and implementation, and monitoring and evaluation.
- Strategies to increase the capacity, resilience and capability of the health workforce include automation of monitoring and evaluation systems, working smarter, working longer, working more flexibly, and improving recruitment, retention and satisfaction in the workplace.

Reflective questions

1. What are the greatest threats to your organisation's workforce requirements in the next 5 years?
2. Conduct a brief environmental scan of your organisation and identify the five key measures you would want to know to inform a workforce plan.
3. If you were able to influence your organisation to improve its readiness for the future in terms of workforce, what two specific strategies would you recommend?

4. Consider your own profession. Based on what you have studied so far, conduct a strength, weakness, opportunity and threat (SWOT) analysis of the workforce.
5. Consider the arguments for and against a deliberate strategy to recruit part of your workforce from a developing country.

Self-analysis questions

Imagine you are the chief executive officer or professional head of your organisation and you are required to maintain your current productivity but reduce costs by 5 per cent. Where in the workforce would be the most likely opportunity for reductions, and why? Consider the steps you would take to lead such a change.

References

Australian Bureau of Statistics. (2022). A caring nation – 15 per cent of Australia's workforce in health care and social assistance industry. [Media release 12 October]. Retrieved 10 March 2024 from: https://www.abs.gov.au/media-centre/media-releases/caring-nation-15-cent-australias-workforce-health-care-and-social-assistance-industry#:~:text=Census%20data%20that%20we%27ve,are%20employed%20in%20our%20hospitals

Australian Institute of Health and Welfare (AIHW). (2022). Health workforce. [7 July]. Retrieved 10 March 2024 from: https://www.aihw.gov.au/reports/workforce/health-workforce

——— (2023). Health expenditure. Retrieved 25 October 2023 from: https://www.aihw.gov.au/reports/health-welfare-expenditure/health-expenditure

Australian Public Service Commission (APSC). (2023). Workforce planning guide, 2023 edition. Retrieved 10 March 2024 from: https://www.apsc.gov.au/initiatives-and-programs/aps-workforce-strategy-2025/workforce planning-resources

Beccaria, L., McIlveen, P., Fein, E. C., Kelly, T., McGregor, R. & Rezwanul, R. (2021). The importance of attachment to place in growing a sustainable Australian rural health workforce: A rapid review. *Australian Journal of Rural Health*, *29*(5), 620–642. https://doi.org/10.1111/ajr.12799

Birch, S., Gibson, J. & McBride, A. (2020). Opportunities for, and implications of, skill mix changes in health care pathways: Pay, productivity and practice variations in a needs-based planning framework. *Social Science & Medicine*, *250*, 112863. https://doi.org/10.1016/j.socscimed.2020.112863

Clare, J. (2024). Cost-of-living support for teaching, nursing and social work students. [Press release 6 May 2024]. Retrieved 5 October 2024 from: https://ministers.education.gov.au/clare/cost-living-support-teaching-nursing-and-social-work-students

Commonwealth of Australia, Department of Health. (2020). 2019 Nurses and midwives. Retrieved from: https://hwd.health.gov.au/resources/publications/factsheet-nrmw-2019.pdf

Commonwealth of Australia, Department of Health and Aged Care. (2024a). National Nursing Workforce Strategy. Retrieved 18 January 2024 from: https://www.health.gov.au/our-work/national-nursing-workforce-strategy#about-the-strategy

——— (2024b). Unleashing the potential of our health workforce – scope of practice review. Retrieved 10 March 2024 from: https://www.health.gov.au/our-work/scope-of-practice-review?language=en

——— (2024c). About the bonded medical program. Retrieved 10 March 2024 from: https://www.health.gov.au/our-work/bonded-medical-program/about

——— (2023). Aged care nursing clinical placement program. Retrieved 10 March 2024 from: https://www.health.gov.au/our-work/aged-care-nursing-clinical-placements-program

——— (2021a). National medical workforce strategy 2021–2031. Retrieved 10 March 2024 from: https://www.health.gov.au/our-work/national-medical-workforce-strategy-2021-2031

——— (2021b). Stronger rural health strategy. Retrieved 10 March 2024 from: https://www.health.gov.au/topics/rural-health-workforce/stronger-rural-health-strategy#:~:text=The%20Stronger%20Rural%20Health%20Strategy,3%2C000%20extra%20nurses%20by%202028

——— (2021c). NDIS national workforce plan: 2021–2025.

——— (2010). Australia in 2050: Future challenges. Retrieved 10 March 2024 from: https://treasury.gov.au/sites/default/files/2019-03/IGR_2010_Overview.pdf

Commonwealth of Australia, Jobs and Skills. (2024). Health care and social assistance. Retrieved 10 March 2024 from: https://labourmarketinsights.gov.au/industries/industry-details?industryCode=Q

Doleman, G., Duffield, C., Li, I. W. & Watts, R. (2022). Employment of the Australian graduate nursing workforce: A retrospective analysis. *Collegian, 29*(2), 228–235. https://doi.org/10.1016/j.colegn.2021.12.002

Health Canada. (2023). Health Workforce Canada established to improve health workforce data and planning. [News release 6 Dec 2023]. Retrieved 10 March 2024 from: https://www.canada.ca/en/health-canada/news/2023/12/health-workforce-canada-established-to-improve-health-workforce-data-and-planning.html

International Organisation of Standardization (ISO). (2015). Human resource management – workforce planning. ISO/DIS 30409(en). Retrieved 10 March 2024 from: https://www.iso.org/obp/ui/#iso:std:iso:30409:dis:ed-1:v1:en

Kamarulzaman, A., Ramnarayan, K. & Mocumbi, A. O. (2022). Plugging the medical brain drain. *Lancet, 400*(10362), 1492–1494. https://doi.org/10.1016/S0140-6736(22)02087-6

Medical Deans Australia and New Zealand. (2024). Medical school graduates (data – power BI). Retrieved 10 March 2024 from: https://medicaldeans.org.au/

Mendonsa, K., Stolberg, M., Viswanathan, V. & Crum, S. (2020). Predicting attrition – A driver for creating value, realizing strategy, and refining key HR processes. *SMU Data Science Review, 3*(2), Article 2. https://scholar.smu.edu/datasciencereview/vol3/iss2/2

Ono, T., Lafortune, G. & Schoenstein, M. (2013). Health workforce planning in OECD countries: A review of 26 projection models from 18 countries. *OECD Health Working Papers*, No. 62. OECD Publishing. https://doi.org/10.1787/5k44t787zcwb-en

Pressley, C., Newton, D., Garside, J., Stephenson, J. & Mejia-Olivares, J. (2023). Internationally recruited nurses and their initial integration into the healthcare workforce: A mixed methods study. *International Journal of Nursing Studies Advances, 5*, 100154. https://doi.org/10.1016/j.ijnsa.2023.100154.

Royal Australian College of General Practitioners. (2023). *General practice health of the nation 2023: An annual insight into the state of Australian general practice.* Retrieved from: https://www.racgp.org.au/getmedia/122d4119-a779-41c0-bc67-a8914be52561/Health-of-the-Nation-2023.pdf.aspx

Topple, M., Jaspers, R., Watterson, J., McClure, J., Rosenow, M., Pollock, W. & Pilcher, D. (2022). Nursing workforce deployment and intensive care unit strain during the COVID-19 pandemic in Victoria, Australia. *Australian Critical Care, 36*(1), 84–91. https://doi.org/10.1016/j.aucc.2022.12.001

Wakerman, J., Humphreys, J., Russell, D., Guthridge, S., Bourke, L., Dunbar, T., Zhao, Y., Ramjan, M., Murakami-Gold, L. & Jones, M. P. (2019). Remote health workforce turnover and retention: What are the policy and practice priorities? *Hum Resour Health, 17*(99). https://doi.org/10.1186/s12960-019-0432-y

World Health Assembly. (2010). WHO global code of practice on the international recruitment of health personnel [63rd World Health Assembly, Agenda item 11.5, WHA63.16]. Retrieved from: http://apps.who.int/gb/ebwha/pdf_files/WHA63/A63_R16-en.pdf

World Health Organization (WHO). (2017). *Health workforce and labor market dynamics in OECD high-income countries: A synthesis of recent analyses and simulations of future supply and requirements.* [Human Resources for Health Observer, 20, Licence: CC BY-NC-SA 3.0 IGO]. Retrieved from: https://iris.who.int/bitstream/handle/10665/259361/9789241512282-eng.pdf

——— (2016). *Global strategy on human resources for health: Workforce 2030.*

31 Strategic planning and sustainability

Sandra G. Leggat

Learning objectives

How do I:

- complete a strategic plan?
- adopt strategic management for sustainability in my position?
- improve the strategic planning and management processes within my organisation?
- plan the implementation of my organisation's strategic plan for my area?

Introduction

Effective strategic planning, implementation and management drive organisational performance (Rudd, Greenley, Beatson & Lings, 2008). Healthcare managers have recognised the increasing importance of strategic planning and management as the healthcare industry has become more dynamic and complex (Subramanian, Kumar & Yauger, 2011). However, development of feasible strategy can be difficult, and implementation of even well-developed strategy is often challenging. This has become increasingly complex as healthcare organisations aim to implement triple bottom-line (TBL) reporting to better ensure sustainability (Vergunst et al., 2020). This chapter provides advice on leading and improving strategic planning and management for sustainability in health-service organisations.

Use of strategic planning

Strategic planning was identified decades ago as essential for organisations competing in a variety of industries, with most of the seminal literature arising in the 1980s. Strategic planning has been linked to successful operations in public sector healthcare organisations when applying previously developed concepts (Ekiz Kavukoğlu & İşci, 2023).

The Australian Commission on Safety and Quality in Health Care (2011) defines safety and quality standards for health services. Standard 1, which is concerned with governance, leadership and culture, requires the governing body to establish the strategic direction for the organisation and endorse a strategic and policy framework. This is consistent with the *Australian standard: Good governance principles* (Standards Australia, 2003), which indicates that governing bodies are responsible for ensuring the strategic direction of their organisations, and *Governance of organizations – Governance maturity model* (Standards Australia, 2023).

While there are differences in operations between public and private health services, researchers have found that for-profit and not-for-profit hospitals tend to have similar strategic capabilities (Reeves & Ford, 2004). Therefore, this chapter does not distinguish between these types of health services; the tools and techniques discussed can be used in both public and private sector strategic planning and management.

Forward-looking organisations have evolved from episodic strategic planning to **strategic management**, which effectively links the identified strategies with daily operations (Zuckerman, 2006). The intention of strategic management is that the managers assist their staff to understand the strategic direction and how their positions and job responsibilities are essential to achieving the organisation's strategies. This suggests the need for communication to, and involvement of, staff throughout the strategic-planning process, as well as during the implementation and monitoring of the strategic plan. Jasper and Crossan (2012) say that nurse managers have tremendous influence over the success or failure of a strategic plan, and emphasise the need for nurse managers to translate the strategies into outcomes that will deliver high-quality care. This is true for all healthcare managers.

> **Strategic planning:** 'A disciplined effort to produce fundamental decisions and actions shaping the nature and direction of an organisation's activities within legal bounds' (Olsen & Eadie, 1982, p. 4)

> **Strategic management:** 'An externally-oriented philosophy of managing an organisation that links strategic thinking and analysis to organisation action' (Ginter, Swayne & Duncan, 2002, p. 13)

Framework for strategic planning

Despite the many strategic planning models available, all strategic planning follows the simple 10-step iterative process outlined in Figure 31.1 and discussed in detail in the following sections.

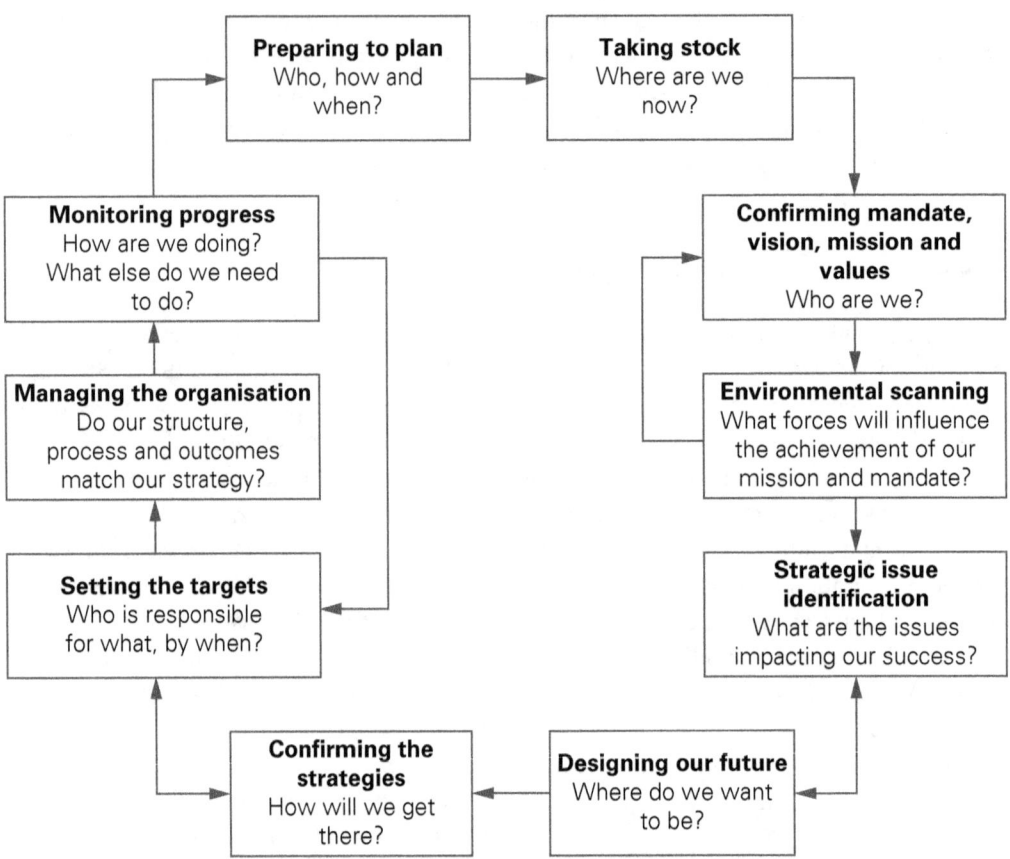

Figure 31.1 The strategic planning process

Preparing to plan

The first step requires agreement regarding the planning process. This includes identifying who will be involved, when the planning will take place, what the process will look like and the resources required. The literature suggests the need for governing board involvement in strategic planning (Nadler, 2004; Standards Australia, 2003) and for the staff responsible for the implementation to be involved (Baldwin & McConnell, 1988). In addition, as outlined, the Australian national standards require consumer involvement (Australian Commission on Safety and Quality in Health Care, 2011). There are many recent examples of planning for new hospitals and other healthcare services in which consumers have been involved in all phases of the planning and development process.

Successful strategic planning requires a champion in a position of power in the organisation to legitimise the process; a planning team that has the time, energy and support to complete the process; willingness within the team to construct and consider a variety of arguments for the future for the benefit of the organisation; and the ability to pull information and people together at key points for important discussions and decisions (Bryson, 1988). It has been recognised that spending time at the beginning of the process to outline who should participate and how – that is, defining roles and responsibilities – leads to a strategic planning process that results in a more feasible strategic plan (Zuckerman, 2006).

Taking stock

This planning step requires an honest appraisal of the current position of the organisation relative to similar organisations, with identification of its existing strengths and weaknesses. This appraisal contributes to the **SWOT analysis**, one of the most useful strategic planning tools identified by managers (Wright, Paroutis & Blettner, 2012). The participants consider the effects of the organisational strengths and weaknesses on the achievement of current plans. (The later environmental scanning step enables the external opportunities and threats that contribute to the SWOT to be identified.)

SWOT analysis: Strengths, Weaknesses, Opportunities and Threats – a technique used to identify the internal and external aspects of the organisation that need to be addressed in the strategic plan

Confirming mandate, vision, mission and values

This step requires the confirmation of the externally imposed formal **mandate** and the mission, vision and values. Organisational annual reports usually contain a **mission statement** and a **vision statement**. The mission and mandate need to be consistent and support each other, describing the purpose of the organisation. Many mission statements also include a **statement of values**. Organisational employees are expected to uphold the documented values in their role responsibilities.

The vision statement is forward-looking and is meant to answer the question of what the organisation is striving to become in the larger environment in which it functions (Bryson, 1988). Leggat and Holmes (2015) stress that an organisational vision needs to include both a guiding philosophy and a tangible image. The guiding philosophy should communicate the organisation's core values and beliefs, such as a religious or other foundation. The tangible image communicates the contribution the organisation will make to society if it is successful in achieving its mission.

Mandate: The formal, externally authorised organisational purpose that is usually outlined in legislation, articles of incorporation, charters or regulations

Mission statement: A translation of the mandate into the immediate purpose of the organisation

Vision statement: A description of how the organisation will contribute to society through its mission

Statement of values: An outline of how the purpose or mission will be achieved; the set of principles and beliefs that guide the operations

Environmental scanning

The strategic plan should provide direction for the organisation over a timeframe of 3 to 5 years. Therefore, it is important that the process includes consideration of factors likely to affect the organisation during this period. A strategic plan will be most successful if it is designed with consideration of changes in the environment; this requires collection, analysis and discussion of information gained through **environmental scanning**. Researchers have found an association between more sophisticated environmental scanning and improved organisational performance (Subramanian et al., 2011).

The literature distinguishes between the micro-environment, or task environment, which includes direct organisational contacts such as customers and suppliers, and the macro-environment, or general environment, which includes the political, economic, ecological, societal and technological forces that surround the organisation (Subramanian et al., 2011; Vecchiato, 2012). Both must be considered in an environmental scan (see e.g. Friesen & Bell, 2007).

Environmental scanning: Monitoring, evaluating and disseminating information from outside the organisation to key managers within the organisation (Snyder, 1981)

Organisations use a variety of environmental scanning techniques. They may be as simple as generating a list of current and future drivers of change using the framework of 'politics, economics, ecology, society and technology' to ensure all aspects are identified. The planning team reviews the list for completeness and uses it to foster discussion of the likelihood and potential impact of various changes on the organisation.

Scenario-building: Constructing future scenarios that propose how the identified changes are likely to affect the organisation

Scenario-building has been used since the 1970s in industries looking for ways to ensure that strategic planning captures future trends that may be difficult to identify. Various future scenarios are constructed that propose how the identified changes are likely to affect the organisation. Constructing scenarios involves defining the issues, confirming the major stakeholders, describing trends, identifying uncertainties and writing alternative scenarios (Schoemaker, 1995).

Strategic-issue identification

Strategic issues: Areas critical to the sustainability of the organisation requiring decisions to be made and communicated in the strategic plan

Strategic issues are fundamental choices to be made by an organisation when there is no obvious best solution. If the solution were known, it could be operationalised and would not therefore be considered a strategic decision.

Bryson (1988) suggests that strategic issues should be identified using three elements, the first of which is a single-paragraph question used to describe the issue. For example, a strategic issue relating to the service-delivery model might generate the following question: 'Economic analysis suggests that the current acute-care service volumes are not sufficient to capitalise on economies of scale in resource utilisation and staff expertise. We cannot afford to expand the capacity of all of our acute services, yet all have high need. Which ones should we focus on?'

Sustainable healthcare: 'A complex system of interacting approaches to the restoration, management and optimisation of human health that has an ecological base, that is environmentally, economically and socially viable indefinitely, that functions harmoniously both with the human body and the non-human environment, and which does not result in unfair or disproportionate impacts on any significant contributory element of the healthcare system' (Alliance for Natural Health International, 2010, p. 9)

The second element is a list of the factors that make this an important question for the future of the organisation. This might include proposed changes to casemix funding models, changing demographics of the service population, consumers' perspectives and constraints imposed by outdated facilities. The final element is an outline of the consequences of failure to address the strategic issue (such as, 'the hospital is likely to report a $15 million deficit by 2026 and may be unable to attract leading medical staff').

Ensuring sustainability

Sustainability has become a focus for health-sector planning and management. Unfortunately, 'sustainability remains a multi-dimensional, multi-factorial notion that is used somewhat inconsistently or ambiguously and takes on different meanings at different times in different contexts … .' (Fleiszer, Semenic, Ritchie, Richer & Denis, 2015 p. 1494). A literature review suggests that three aspects to sustainability comprising benefit, persistence/continuation and development are important (Fleiszer et al., 2015). The definition proposed by the Alliance for Natural Health International (2010) seems to best describe sustainability in healthcare.

Triple bottom line reporting: As originally suggested by Elkington (1997), organisational reporting should be expanded beyond just profit to include people and the planet

Triple bottom line (TBL) reporting was proposed to assist organisations to measure and achieve sustainability. That is, an organisation must move beyond solely considering a profit/loss financial bottom line and focus on societal and environmental impacts (Vergunst et al., 2020). To be sustainable, an organisation must balance its financial books, measure and manage its environmental impacts, such as pollution, and consider its impact on the social determinants of health.

TRIPLE BOTTOM LINE REPORTING FOR SUSTAINABILITY

Alim and Sulley (2024) suggest the COVID-19 pandemic best illustrates the need to consider TBL for sustainability. The pandemic severely affected the financial sustainability of healthcare organisations as demands outstripped supply, as well as the sustainability of local and global economies during lockdowns, and staff shortages. The pandemic affected normal societal operations and illustrated disparities and inequity in access to healthcare within societies. Environmental concerns were raised in relation to the production and disposal of medical waste. How might you consider financial or economic, societal and environmental aspects of future pandemics when planning for your health service?

Designing our future

While sometimes forgotten, this is an important exercise that enables the participants to be clear about how the organisation will look when the strategic plan has been successfully implemented. In this stage, the participants confirm the goals and desired outcomes for the future organisation. It is difficult to envision how an organisation will look upon successful completion of the strategic plan, but creativity is required in this step. The participants should be able to predict what the organisation will be doing differently at the end of the strategic planning period – for example, 'The hospital will have increased its volume in cardiac services to 200 cases a year, have consumer representatives serving on all hospital committees and have achieved a Met with Merit rating for all 10 national standards'. This assists in the choice of strategy to achieve the desired outcomes.

Confirming the strategies

Various authors have attempted to classify strategies to assist managers in their deliberations. Three such classifications are provided here. Miles and Snow (1978) suggest that organisations adopt prospector, defender, analyser or reactor strategic stances. Prospectors search for market opportunities, tending to be the first to offer new products and services. Defenders are more conservative, competing on price and service quality; they are concerned with continually improving the efficiency of existing operations. Analysers have aspects of both prospector and defender, watching their competitors closely for new ideas and rapidly adopting the most promising. Finally, reactors lack a consistent strategy and respond to external changes only when required to do so by regulation, legislation or financial position. While there have been many studies supporting this typology, there is also concern that it does not capture all possible strategies for public and not-for-profit sector organisations (DeSarbo, Di Benedetto, Song & Sinha, 2005).

Porter (1985) identifies three generic strategies that drive competitive advantage within an industry: cost leadership, differentiation (unique products or services) and focus (or niche). More recent strategy researchers suggest that differentiation and cost leadership together can be a fourth strategy in this list (Kumar, Subramanian & Strandholm, 2001). However, competition does not operate in the same way among public-sector services as it does among those in the private sector, which may limit the applicability of Porter's strategies to public-sector healthcare organisations (Hodgkinson & Hughes, 2014), as these are more likely to pursue a mix of strategies, aiming to address conflicting goals (Boyne & Walker, 2004).

Hodgkinson and Hughes (2014) provide empirical support for a public-sector strategy typology. Their categories comprise organisations without a coherent strategy (chaotic) and three strategy stances: value differentiation, equilibrial and socially responsible. As the name suggests, those organisations without a strategy, like reactors (Miles & Snow, 1978), are disorganised, without an overall sense of direction. Value differentiators tailor services to the needs of specific groups, focusing on delivering high customer value. In contrast, the equilibrial service providers aim to meet all population needs, attempting to achieve the best service at the lowest cost. Finally, the socially responsible providers aim for the lowest costs overall.

The study results suggest that organisations with a value-differentiation approach tend to demonstrate better performance than those with the other strategy stances. Overall, it seems that having a defined strategy results in better performance than having no strategy, and a strategy that focuses on responding to customer needs, such as differentiation, is likely to be the most successful (Hodgkinson & Hughes, 2014).

Setting the targets

This step is linked with the preceding step of confirming strategies. Once the participants have confirmed how they wish the organisation to look at the end of the strategic plan implementation, they can reasonably assign feasible targets to each of the strategies. The **SMART** and **SMARTT** acronyms are often used to ensure that effective goals and targets have been outlined (Doran, 1981). Stating: 'We will provide excellent care' is not a SMARTT target, yet this is the type of target most often found in strategic plans. Reframing the statement as: 'Of all discharged patients or their families, 85 per cent will rate the overall quality of the acute care that has been provided as good, very good or excellent by 2015' provides better information for understanding the focus of the strategy and enabling progress to be effectively measured.

SMART: Targets that are Specific, Measurable, Achievable, Reasonable and Time-bound

SMARTT: Targets that are Specific, Measurable, Achievable, Realistic, Timely and Tangible

Managing the organisation

There is substantial evidence suggesting that organisations that can align their internal processes with their chosen strategies are better performers than those that cannot (Garcia & de Val Pardo, 2004; Kumar & Subramanian, 2011). It is essential that the strategic plan is backed up with internal annual operating (or business) plans that outline priority actions and support resource allocation (Baldwin & McConnell, 1988).

7-S Framework: A system designed to assist managers to consider all of the organisational factors (Structure, Systems, Style, Staff, Skills, Subordinate goals and the organisational Strategy) that may need to be modified to implement the chosen strategy (Waterman, 1982)

Two implementation frameworks are provided in this section. The first is the **7-S Framework**, designed to assist managers to consider all of the organisational factors that may need to be modified to implement the chosen strategy (Waterman, 1982). The framework suggests that there is a need for consistency between the *strategy* of the organisation and the following six organisational factors: structure, systems, style, staff, skills, subordinate goals. For example, if the strategy focuses on improving customer service and satisfaction, the staff will need to be chosen and rewarded for their skills in customer service. The organisation's systems will need to be able to measure what customers think of the service, and the internal system will have departments for direct service and support, focused on the needs of customers.

While a cost leadership strategy, aiming for the lowest costs, would not totally negate the need for customer service, the system and staff expectations would be different from those relating to the customer-service strategy. While this framework has face validity and has been used by management consultants for years, it is difficult to understand the interactions between the factors and it has not been empirically tested (Okumus, 2003).

Okumus (2003) has developed a detailed implementation framework that comprises strategic content, strategic context (including organisational structure and culture), operational processes (including planning, resources, communication, people and control) and intended outcomes. The suggestion is for managers to document the current and the required aspects of the context and processes to enable identification of needs to be addressed in implementation in order to achieve the desired outcomes of the chosen strategy.

Monitoring progress

While there are many ways to measure progress on the implementation of a strategic plan, in recent years the **balanced scorecard**, a strategic management system that enables organisations to monitor the processes needed to implement their strategies (Kaplan & Norton, 1996b), has been confirmed as an effective approach in healthcare (Zelman, Pink & Matthias, 2003). In general, the scorecard tracks performance measures in relation to the targets set in the strategic plan within four or more perspectives. These perspectives include financial, customer, business and clinical processes, learning and growth, with the intent that the financial measures focused on the shorter term are balanced with the perspectives that force a longer-term, more strategic focus (Kaplan & Norton, 1996a). More recently the creators of the balanced scorecard recognised the impact of TBL reporting. They suggest that the 'Financial perspective is replaced by "Outcomes" to encompass financial, environmental, and societal metrics; Customer becomes "Stakeholders" to reflect multiple participants in the ecosystem; and Learning & Growth becomes "Enablers" to include the new capabilities for collaboration and alignment' (Kaplan & McMillan 2020, p. 1).

Balanced scorecard: A strategic management system that enables organisations to monitor the organisational processes needed to implement the organisational strategies (Kaplan & Norton, 1996b)

Summary

- There are 10 steps that are usually completed as part of any strategic-planning process. These steps comprise a generic process that includes setting the scene, gathering and analysing the data, outlining the strategies, and implementing and evaluating the plan.
- All healthcare managers need to fully understand the strategic plan of their organisation and how their department or service contributes to the plan, as it is their job in strategic management to interpret the plan for their employees.
- Without SMART or SMARTT goals and effective monitoring systems, strategic plans are often not successfully implemented.
- Sustainability can be achieved through considering the TBL in organisational planning processes.

Reflective questions

1. How could the planning team detect strategic opportunities and strategic threats for your organisation?
2. Complete a SWOT analysis for your department.
3. What are the differences between a strategic plan and operating or business plans?
4. Using the three strategy classifications provided in this chapter, describe your organisation's strategy.
5. What departmental performance indicators would you use to cover the environmental and social aspects of TBL reporting?

Self-analysis question

Drawing upon your understanding of mission and vision as described in this chapter, write a personal mission statement in two or three sentences. It should reflect your purpose, beliefs, personal values and approaches to your life and your job. Clarifying your personal mission is a continuing process and should be regularly revisited and updated.

References

Alim, M. & Sulley, S. (2024). Beyond healing: Embracing the triple bottom line approach in post-pandemic healthcare. *Cureus*, *16*(2).

Alliance for Natural Health International (ANHI). (2010). *Sustainable healthcare: Working towards a paradigm shift*. ANHI.

Australian Commission on Safety and Quality in Health Care (ACSQHC). (2011). *National safety and quality health service standards*. ACSQHC.

Baldwin, S. R. & McConnell, M. (1988). Strategic planning: Process and plan go hand in hand. *Management Solutions*, (June), 29–36.

Boyne, G. A. & Walker, R. M. (2004). Strategy content and public service organizations. *Journal of Public Administration Research and Theory*, *14*(2), 231–252. https://doi.org/10.1093/jopart/muh015

Bryson, J. M. (1988). A strategic planning process for public and non-profit organizations. *Long Range Planning*, *21*(1), 73–81. https://doi.org/10.1016/0024-6301(88)90061-1

DeSarbo, W. S., Di Benedetto, A. C., Song, M. & Sinha, I. (2005). Revisiting the Miles and Snow strategic framework: Uncovering interrelationships between strategic types, capabilities, environmental uncertainties, and firm performance. *Strategic Management Journal*, *26*(1), 47–74. https://doi.org/10.1002/smj.431

Doran, G. T. (1981). There's a SMART way to write management's goals and objectives. *Management Review*, *70*(11), 35–36.

Ekiz Kavukoğlu, T. & İşci, E. (2023). The mediating role of strategic planning awareness in the impact of organizational innovation on business excellence in hospitals. *The TQM Journal*, 36(8), 2527–2550.

Elkington, J. (1997). *Cannibals with forks – Triple bottom line of 21st century business*. New Society Publishers.

Fleiszer, A. R., Semenic, S. E., Ritchie, J. A., Richie, M-C. & Denis, J-L. (2015). The sustainability of healthcare innovations: A concept analysis. *Journal of Advanced Nursing*, *71*(7): 1484–1498.

Friesen, K. & Bell, D. (2007). Regional health authorities, disaster management, and geomatics: Opportunities and barriers. *International Journal of Emergency Management*, *4*(2), 141–165. https://doi.org/10.1504/IJEM.2007.013987

Garcia, C. M. & de Val Pardo, I. (2004). Strategies and performance in hospitals. *Health Policy, 67*, 1–13. https://doi.org/10.1016/S0168-8510(03)00102-7

Ginter, P. M., Swayne, L. E. & Duncan, W. J. (2002). *Strategic management of health care organizations* (4th ed.). Jossey-Bass.

Hodgkinson, I. & Hughes, P. (2014). Strategy content and public service provider performance in the UK: An alternative approach. *Public Administration, 92*(3), 707–726. https://doi.org/10.1111/padm.12090

Jasper, M. & Crossan, F. (2012). What is strategic management? *Journal of Nursing Management, 20*, 838–846. https://doi.org/10.1111/jonm.12001

Kaplan, R. S. & McMillan, D. (2020). Updating the balanced scorecard for triple bottom line strategies. Harvard Business School Accounting & Management Unit Working Paper.

Kaplan, R. S. & Norton, D. P. (1996a). *The balanced scorecard*. Harvard Business.

——— (1996b) Using the balanced scorecard as a strategic management system. *Harvard Business Review*, (January–February), 75–85.

Kumar, K. & Subramanian, R. (2011). Porter's strategic types: Differences in internal processes and their impact on performance. *Journal of Applied Business Research, 14*(1), 107–124.

Kumar, K., Subramanian, R. & Strandholm, K. (2001). Competitive strategy, environmental scanning and performance: A context specific analysis of their relationship. *International Journal of Commerce and Management, 11*(1), 1–33. https://doi.org/10.1108/eb047413

Leggat, S. G. & Holmes, M. (2015). Content analysis of mission, vision and value statements in Australian public and private hospitals: Implications for healthcare management. *Asia Pacific Journal of Health Management, 10*(1), 46–55.

Miles, R. E. & Snow, C. C. (1978). *Organizational strategy, structure, and process*. McGraw-Hill.

Nadler, D. A. (2004). What's the board's role in strategy development? Engaging the board in corporate strategy. *Strategy & Leadership, 32*(5), 25–33. https://doi.org/10.1108/10878570410557633

Okumus, F. (2003). A framework to implement strategies in organizations. *Management Decision, 41*(9), 871–882. https://doi.org/10.1108/00251740310499555

Olsen, J. B. & Eadie, D. C. (1982). *The game plan: Governance with foresight*. Council of State Planning Agencies.

Porter, M. E. (1985). *Competitive advantage: Creating and sustaining superior performance*. MacMillan.

Reeves, T. C. & Ford, E. W. (2004). Strategic management and performance differences: Nonprofit versus for-profit health organizations. *Health Care Management Review, 29*(4), 298–308.

Rudd, J. M., Greenley, G. E., Beatson, A. T. & Lings, I. N. (2008). Strategic planning and performance: Extending the debate. *Journal of Business Research, 61*(2), 99–108. https://doi.org/10.1016/j.jbusres.2007.06.014

Schoemaker, P. J. H. (1995). Scenario planning: A tool for strategic thinking. *Sloan Management Review*, (Winter), 25–39.

Snyder, N. (1981). Environmental volatility, scanning intensity, and organizational performance. *Journal of Contemporary Business, 10*, 5–17.

Standards Australia. (2023). Governance of organizations: Governance maturity model (AS 37004: 2023).

——— (2003). Australian standard: Good governance principles (AS 8000–2003).

Subramanian, R., Kumar, K. & Yauger, C. (2011). The scanning of task environments in hospitals: An empirical study. *Journal of Applied Business Research, 10*(4), 104–115.

Vecchiato, R. (2012). Environmental uncertainty, foresight and strategic decision making: An integrated study. *Technological Forecasting and Social Change, 79*(3), 436–447. https://doi.org/10.1016/j.techfore.2011.07.010

Vergunst, F., Berry, H. L., Rugkåsa, J., Burns, T., Molodynski, A. & Maughan, D. L. (2020). Applying the triple bottom line of sustainability to healthcare research—A feasibility study. *International Journal for Quality in Health Care, 32*(1), 48–53.

Waterman, R. H. J. (1982). The seven elements of strategic fit. *Journal of Business Strategy*, *2*(3), 69–73.

Wright, R. P., Paroutis, S. E. & Blettner, D. P. (2012). How useful are the strategic tools we teach in business schools? *Journal of Management Studies*, *50*(1), 92–125. https://doi.org/10.1111/j.1467-6486.2012.01082.x

Zelman, W. N., Pink, G. H. & Matthias, C. B. (2003). Use of the balanced scorecard in health care. *Journal of Health Care Finance*, *29*(4), 1–16.

Zuckerman, A. M. (2006). Advancing the state of the art in healthcare strategic planning. *Frontiers of Health Services Management*, *23*(2), 3–15.

Health service planning

Chaojie Liu and John Adamm Ferrier

32

Learning objectives

How do I:

- understand when and why health service planning is required and initiated?
- identify important stakeholders and consider how they may be engaged in health service planning?
- develop critical thinking regarding the implications of various approaches and instruments used in health service planning?
- improve my skills in effective health service planning?

Introduction

Matching available health resources to consumer needs is challenging. Governments and health bureaucracies with finite resources face increasing demands from their client populations, which often have complex health issues. No country prioritises resources to meet every single health need of every citizen; consequently, effective health service planning is critical to maximising population health outcomes and ensuring value for the available money.

Due to the inherent contradictions existing between the high demand and the limited responsive supply capacity by health services, health service planning is often characterised by negotiation, lobbying and compromise among various interest groups. A consensus can best be achieved if stakeholders agree upon a set of core values, and all involved in the process endorse principles and the procedures of planning. This chapter focuses on the practice of health service planning.

Definitions

Health service planning: The planned process of aligning current and future health services and resources to the changing health patterns and demographics of a given area or region

Health service planning may stem from the perspective of consumers (population-based) or from the perspective of providers (institutional-based) (Eagar, Garrett & Lin, 2001). The ultimate choice between these two options often depends on who is responsible for performing the planning and the rationale.

Population-based planning

Population-based planning: A bottom-up planning approach that considers the current and future health resource utilisation of a given population

Population-based planning claims to adopt a bottom-up approach and usually involves multiple organisations. Such an approach requires authority and ability from planners to achieve cross-boundary cooperation. Resources ought to be allocated to health facilities in a way that can best meet consumer need. Planners – usually government agencies or joint councils – must develop a good understanding of the competency, capacity and willingness of various providers and consumers to execute the plan (Klaic et al., 2022). Population-based planning tends to regard health promotion and disease prevention as priorities rather than focusing on treatment of diseases (Issel, Wells & Williams, 2021).

Health service planning: Considerations for Indigenous populations

Significant disparities in health and health services occur all over the world, which the COVID-19 pandemic further exacerbated (Kullar et al., 2020). Health service planning seeks to address such inequities. Indigenous populations have on average shorter life expectancy when compared with non-Indigenous counterparts, which can be exacerbated by socioeconomic disadvantage and lack of access to health services that tend to be concentrated in urban areas (Australian Institute of Health and Welfare (AIHW), 2023). There is often a lack of cultural appropriateness in the delivery of healthcare services dominated by modern Western medicine (Brach & Fraserirector, 2000). Interventions that improve overall population health may unintentionally enlarge health disparities within the population: for example, digital technologies may lead to the so-called 'digital divide' (Saeed & Masters, 2021).

Cooper, Hill and Powe (2002) suggest use of the Institute of Medicine's (IOM) model of access to health services in designing interventions reducing health inequity. Strategies for reducing disparities proposed by them target both healthcare providers and users, emphasising a systems approach involving multidisciplinary teams and user engagement in (co-production of) care. In line with those strategies, a rapid evidence review (Loutfi et al., 2018) confirmed four key elements for successful health planning for Indigenous populations:

- good understanding of Indigenous health needs and their related costs
- addressing cultural safety in health planning
- proper management of organisations serving Indigenous clientele, such as Aboriginal Community Controlled Health Services (ACCHSs)
- stakeholder participation in health planning.

To enable effective planning and execution of health plans for Indigenous populations, a more equitable governance empowering Indigenous communities across the governance structure and processes is also needed (Kelaher et al., 2014). Prior experience shows that a co-design approach based on empowerment, trust and mutual respect is critical in health service planning for Indigenous peoples (Anderson et al., 2022). In the recent National Aboriginal and Torres Strait Islander Health Plan (2021–2031), the Australian government claims a real partnership with Indigenous peoples, addressing their priorities in recognition of the social determinants of health (Commonwealth of Australia DoHA, 2021). The plan puts prevention first and aims to empower Indigenous people to make healthy decisions and effectively nagivate the health system. While the plan recognises the vital role of ACCHSs in providing care and prioritises support to ACCHSs, it also maintains the accountability of governments and the responsibility of the mainstream health sector for providing culturally safe and responsive care.

Institutional-based planning

By contrast, **institutional-based planning** adopts a top-down approach and is often anchored in a single organisation or group of organisations aiming to maximise gains (in terms of finance or health outcomes or both) from the invested resources. Such planning usually focuses on the extent to which a difference is made to those who receive or would receive the services (Issel, Wells & Williams, 2021) and tends to ignore those who are not covered by the services. Therefore, the benefit to overall population health may be limited and dependent on the scope of services that may be able to be delivered by the organisation. Many health organisations perform institutional-based planning for reasons of efficiency and/or cost-effectiveness (Eagar et al., 2001).

Institutional-based planning: A top-down planning approach that is often anchored in a single organisation or group of organisations, aiming to maximise gains (in terms of finance or health outcomes or both) from the invested resources

> ### HEALTH PLANNING CONDUCTED BY AUSTRALIAN PRIMARY HEALTHCARE ORGANISATIONS AND LOCAL GOVERNMENT
>
> In an ideal world, a synergy between population-based planning and institution-based planning should be sought. In Australia, the Commonwealth government set up Primary Health Networks (previously Medicare Locals) to develop a partnership approach in addressing local population health needs. Although planning for comprehensiveness and coordination of health services is important, it is insufficient for improving local population health, which depends on a wide variety of factors and requires a continuum of action ranging from prevention and treatment of disease to action on social determinants of health.
>
> Local governments have been widely recognised in leading local community planning, including in public health. In the states of Victoria, Western Australia and South Australia, local councils have been mandated to develop municipal public health plans, identifying the risk factors affecting the health of their populations and to develop strategies to prevent and minimise the identified risks. Because health service provision is largely the responsibility of state governments, emphases have been placed on establishing partnerships between the state, the market and civil society, on building social capital and on enhancing health promotion (Edwards, 2012). A recent study shows that Primary Health Networks have committed limited time and financial support to collaboration with local government, representing a lost opportunity (Windle, Javanparast, Freeman & Baum, 2023).

Reasons for planning

There are many reasons health managers perform health service planning. Firstly, the health market is easily manipulated and distorted, and population health is simply too important to be left unplanned (Gage, 1979). The human population is characterised by rapidly changing morbidity and health needs due to prolonged life expectancy and scientific advancements, often attributable to public health initiatives that address risk factors that previously contributed to avoidable premature death (Buxbaum, Chernew, Fendrick & Cutler, 2020). Despite this, many health technologies and products brought to the market lack support from scientific evidence in terms of their efficacy (Vayda, 1977). Health provision is an example of a free-market approach being problematic, because there is a distinct power and knowledge imbalance between consumers (patients) and suppliers (health professionals). Consumers often feel disempowered in health-consumption decisions, as they often do not have a complete understanding of the issues. Suppliers have significant power, not only because of their inherent specialist knowledge, but also because they act as gatekeepers to treatments and drugs (Timmermans, 2020).

Secondly, a society can only offer services it can afford, and governments often must meet competing demands from other services, such as defence and social welfare (Semple, 1977). Escalating health expenditure has become a public concern in Western countries, regardless of whether the method of financing is socialised or privatised, or a mixture of the two. Health service planning enables people within the system to collect anecdotal evidence of program effectiveness (Issel et al., 2021) and rationalise health expenditure.

Thirdly, there are several control measures growing out of planning, 'from a centralized and directed kind to a decentralized, negotiating and bargaining type' (Anderson, 1969, p. 345) for the purpose of achieving better quality care and reducing waste. And, finally, in countries where public spending on health accounts for a large proportion of total health expenditure, health service planning becomes a political signal for accountability: by the end of 1970s, most developed nations had produced and commenced implementation of national health plans (Anderson, 1969; Gage, 1979).

Health service planning can be triggered when a particular health problem emerges as a public concern, when periodic strategic planning is performed in an organisation or when new funds have become available – or a new willingness to release them has emerged (Issel et al., 2021). It can also be triggered on the emergence of new evidence in relation to a particular service or program.

In recent years, breast-cancer screening services have attracted a great deal of debate among researchers, politicians and consumers. It might be expected that a screening program would reduce the overall mortality associated with this cancer; otherwise, it might produce the unnecessary burden of overdiagnosis and potentially unnecessary treatment to consumers (Gotzsche & Jorgensen, 2013). Although the World Health Organization acknowledges the effectiveness of mammography screening for a 25 per cent reduction of mortality in breast cancer (Weedon-Fekjær, Romundstad & Vatten, 2014), this was challenged by some researchers in a Cochrane Review (Gotzsche & Jorgensen, 2013). Two research articles about mammography for reduction of mortality due to breast cancer were published in the *British Medical Journal* in 2014, with one claiming no effect (Miller et al., 2014) and the other claiming a significant effect (Weedon-Fekjær et al., 2014). Meanwhile, consumer demand for breast-screening services remains high, especially with the advent of high-profile celebrity disclosures increasing demand (Evans et al., 2014) and with breast screening being one of the most successful of all cancer-screening programs (Sullivan et al., 2003). This has led to a potentially awkward situation for managers in deciding whether resources allocated to breast-cancer screening should continue unchanged or perhaps should be diverted to other services. The debate continues (Román et al., 2019), prompting a call for a personalised approach (Canelo-Aybar et al, 2021). A recent systematic review found that from 2010 to 2021, 23 guidelines were issued for breast-cancer screening worldwide, all from developed countries. Although they all recommend mammography as the primary screening modality, the recommended frequency and target populations vary (Ren, Chen, Qiao & Zhao, 2022).

Management and health service planning

Health service planners

Health service plans ought to reflect the needs of target populations; they require planners to consider and balance the often-disparate interests of various stakeholders (Gagliardi, Lemieux-Charles, Brown, Sullivan & Goel, 2008). Constantly evolving models of service delivery add complexity (Gauld, 2002). Issel and colleagues (2021) argue that at least three areas of expertise are critical to health service planning: expert knowledge and experience of the health problems; research skills in epidemiology, social and behavioural science; and skills in fostering agreement across diverse constituents, capabilities and interests.

Consumer participation is essential in health service planning (Eagar et al., 2001; Issel et al., 2021; Thornicroft & Tansella, 2005), because it is an opportunity to foster effective provider–recipient interaction, with ideas and energies flowing towards the services, and results and respect from the services. Such two-way interaction facilitates implementation and, it might be hoped, contributes to ultimate consumer acceptance and satisfaction.

Participation of frontline health workers in planning processes is increasingly valued (Dyck, Tiessen & Lee, 2013; Thornicroft & Tansella, 2005). Medical practice in the Western setting has a long tradition of individual-based decision-making (Liu, Bartram, Casimir & Leggat, 2014). Since the very inception of health service planning, the failure of 'government authorities' to include frontline health providers has attracted criticism, because ultimately these personnel provide the services. Richards (1981) argues that general practitioners are best placed to participate in local health planning. General practice can help reduce inequalities in health and health services through a participatory approach to services planning and coordination (Gkiouleka et al., 2023). There are many barriers to engaging consumers and frontline health workers in a meaningful way. A lack of trust, skill, time and effective mechanisms for provider participation is common in many health systems (Gagliardi et al., 2008; Liu, Liu, Wang, Zhang & Wang, 2013).

Community and stakeholder engagement strategies may vary across different systems and cultural contexts. Nevertheless, all should adhere to the key principles recommended by the WHO – trust, accessibility (geographic, linguistic, cultural and socioeconomic), contextualisation, equity, transparency and autonomy (WHO, 2020) – and, preferably, adopt a co-design approach (Grindell, Coates, Croot & O'Cathain, 2022). There are five levels of participation: inform, consult, involve, collaborate and empower (WHO, 2020). A co-design approach endorses the highest level of participation – empowerment – which involves equal partnership and collective action (Grindell et al., 2022). Effective community and stakeholder engagement requires adequate governance, strong leadership, decentralised decision-making, mutual understanding, strong communication, collaboration and partnership and resources (WHO, 2020). They are critical in addressing concerns related to behavioural, cultural and social conditions, health system determinants, prerequisites and upstream driving forces for health (Grindell et al., 2022; Haldane et al., 2019; WHO, 2020), including in conflict-affected countries (Durrance-Bagale et al., 2022).

Decision-making

Health service planning often requires difficult decisions: priorities must be identified, with limited resources directed towards established priorities or needs. These decisions should reflect previously agreed core values and principles to guide the overall planning processes. Those core values usually include accessibility, equity, efficiency, quality and effectiveness, although some (e.g. efficiency versus accessibility) may come into conflict in planning (Eagar et al., 2001).

The pattern of stakeholder participation in planning processes dictates the values and principles adopted by planners. Issel and colleagues (2021) summarise six approaches to stakeholder participation in decision-making (see Table 32.1). Although these are not mutually exclusive, it is not uncommon for a responsible authority to favour one more than others, leading to a particular approach in the manner in which planning exercises are conducted.

Table 32.1 Comparison of various approaches to decision-making in health service planning

Approach	Description	Advantages	Disadvantages
Comprehensive rational	A textbook-written idealistic planning approach, with a systematic and logical sequence of thought processes and actions	Obtaining information from all stakeholders; considering all contingencies and peripheral influences; addressing issues facing the entire service delivery system	Failure to consider individual values; separation of planners from political reality; heavy reliance on planner's understanding of means and ends that may not be substantiated or endorsed by others
Incremental	Isolated and disjointed efforts addressing small and immediate concerns, with a hope that accumulated effect will eventuate	Strong tolerance of uncertainties and knowledge gaps; rapid response to concerns	Lack of coordination and integration that is likely to lead to conflicting or mismatched programs
Apolitical	An evidence-based practice that is built on best available scientific knowledge	Strong focus on technical aspects for high efficacy; dependence on objective information	Ignoring of political aspects and subjective experience of those with the health problem; difficulties in dealing with evidence bias and knowledge gaps
Advocacy	A planning approach that is pushed by experts who speak for or on behalf of those with certain health problems	Raising awareness and acting on behalf of those disadvantaged who are not empowered to convey their concerns	Likelihood of misinterpretation of the problem of those concerned and of conflicts and confrontations with other interested parties
Communication action	An approach of working in partnership with those with the concerned health problem through communication and empowerment	Interactions between those who are affected and those who are managing and delivering services, with a hope of achieving consensus through mutual adaptation of attention, beliefs and trust	Time-consuming; high requirement of communication and negotiating skills in those involved in the planning
Strategic planning	A service-planning process that is guided by and aligned with a strategic plan of the organisation	Consideration of organisational contexts, both internal and external; services aligned with the vision and future direction of the organisation	Lack of flexibility to respond to new environmental opportunities or threats

Various stakeholders are given different opportunities to voice their concerns within these six approaches. For example, a comprehensive rational approach pays particular attention to the balance and equality of stakeholder participation in planning. In contrast, both the communication action and advocacy approaches place significant weight on the concerns of those who experience the problems targeted by the planning, although the latter often depends on planning experts, who may misunderstand their constituents. Health professionals generally shape the incremental and apolitical approaches, whereas collective interests of health professionals are addressed in the strategic planning approach.

There is a consensus that governments should not intervene in the internal management decisions of service providers (Liu et al., 2014); however, it is hard, if not impossible, to avoid political influence, especially if the government is the primary funder of the service. Governments often want service providers to align their planning with a set of unified goals (Department of Health, State of Victoria 2011). Political agenda may also shape priority settings; for example, in the late 1990s, the Clinton administration in the United States put racial and ethnic disparities on the public agenda, leading to increased service programs aiming at eliminating ethnic disparities (Issel et al., 2021).

Cultural values shared by dominant sectors of the population often have a significant influence on decision-making in health service planning. For example, medical care services are more likely to be seen as an individual responsibility by people residing in the United States, whereas in Australia, Canada and many European nations, people would regard the provision of health services as a universal and therefore public good. The Global Burden of Disease Study reported that people of workforce age were valued higher than the others (Sabik & Lie, 2008). This has since been abandoned (AIHW, 2014) because of opposition from some countries arguing that human dignity and social solidarity should not be displaced by economic productivity (Rosen, De Fine Licht & Ohlsson, 2014).

Frameworks for health service planning

Before detailed planning commences, a working group, often in the form of a consortium, needs to be established which ideally comprises five to seven people (Issel et al., 2021). The group is responsible for devising a set of principles and core values to guide the planning process. This is perhaps the most important and most often overlooked step, because failure to adequately define the scope will ultimately lead to a quagmire of a well-intentioned but ultimately useless plan.

The goal of health service planning is to assure that finite resources available to various health programs achieve the best possible outcomes with the greatest efficiency (Eagar et al., 2001; Gaston, 2005); however, defining outcomes in isolation is often difficult. Internationally, there is a trend to incorporate ideas generated from the public and communities into health planning goals (Issel et al., 2021).

Once desired outcomes are defined, prospective measurement indicators are developed. Each indicator offers a certain perspective by quantifying the effectiveness of the interaction aimed at the health problem. Common indicators used in health service planning measure frequency (prevalence and incidence) of problems, severity and duration of problems, and cost and frequency of use of services (Fazekas, Ettelt, Newbould & Nolte, 2010;

Department of Health, State of Victoria 2011). Qualitative measures such as consumer acceptability in health service planning are often assumed yet are critical to overall effectiveness.

Health service planning is usually conducted in a cyclical manner, involving assessment of problems, prioritisation and implementation decisions (Fazekas et al., 2010; Gaston, 2005). Evaluation also forms an integral part of planning. It not only demonstrates the effectiveness of planned actions but also feeds into a new cycle of service planning (see Figure 32.1).

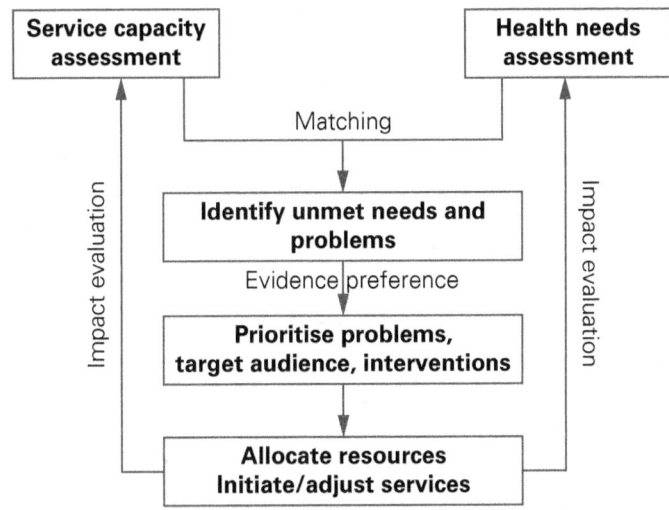

Figure 32.1 Health service planning cycle

Assessment of health needs and health service capacity

The health service planning process must commence with the clear identification of existing resources, programs and known problems or gaps in service provision. Occasionally, targeted problems have been determined, usually by funders, prior to the planning. Three types of assessment may be involved, though not necessarily all at once, in health service planning: needs assessment, organisational assessment and marketing assessment.

Needs assessment

A needs assessment defines the gaps, lacks and wants relative to a predetermined health problem or a certain population (Issel et al., 2021). Perhaps the most used definition of needs (Asadi-Lari, Packham & Gray, 2003) is Bradshaw's (1972), according to which there are four types of needs: normative, felt, expressed and comparative. Service data and administrative records usually capture normative, expressed and comparative needs, but they have often failed to reveal the felt or perceived need, which may be obtained from sources such as qualitative population surveys. Benchmarking and spatial analysis (e.g. geographic information systems) are two commonly used tools that identify comparative need (Brijnath, Ansariadi & de Souza, 2012; Eagar et al., 2001). From a summary perspective:

- **Normative need** is defined by professionals using scientific concepts and notions.
- **Felt need** examines what consumers want, wish and desire.
- **Expressed need** describes vocalised needs or how people use services.
- **Comparative need** indicates gaps between groups of people.

Organisational assessment

An organisational assessment determines the willingness and capacity of the organisation to provide the defined health services. A SWOT analysis offers a useful framework to guide organisational assessment (but is by no means the only tool available). Internal strengths (S) and weaknesses (W), as well as external opportunities (O) and threats (T), are assessed in comparison with other providers through staff consultation and use of existing organisational records (Eagar et al., 2001; Issel et al., 2021). The purpose of this process is to elicit potential strategies to create strengths from weaknesses, and opportunities from threats.

Marketing assessment

A marketing assessment intends to understand to what extent the target audience is interested in the service program and how it can be drawn into the program. Pricing and packaging design may be involved in a marketing assessment.

Set priorities

Priority-setting is an exercise involving both rational and political processes. The initial concern of the planners should be to satisfy themselves that they fully understand, firstly, what health needs should be considered and how they should be ranked, according to the size and seriousness of the problem, and, secondly, the likelihood of the problems being solved using effective interventions open to the providers. To assist with prioritisation of these issues, a scoring system can be developed to rank health problems. Bigger problems with higher levels of seriousness and those that are more likely to be solved are given higher scores. For example, a formula (Issel et al., 2021) has been adopted by the United States Centers for Disease Control and Prevention for its planning process:

Priority score = [(score of problem size) + 2 (score of problem seriousness)] × (score of effectiveness of intervention)

Many indicators have been developed to assist with decision-making in health service planning. The magnitude of a health problem is usually assessed using incidence (magnitude of newly occurring cases) and prevalence (quantity of cases in the community). The seriousness of a problem can be assessed from physical perspectives (morbidity and mortality) and functional impacts (activities of daily living) or using a combination such as burden of disease (quality-adjusted life years and disability-adjusted life years) and health-related quality of life (Price, 1999; Snow, Walker, Ahern, O'Brien & Saltman, 1999).

Effective interventions in relation to a defined health problem are usually predicated upon robust research evidence that tests outcomes (Greenhalgh, Howick & Maskrey, 2014). Cost–benefit and cost-effectiveness analyses are often used to compare alternative options. In resource-poor settings, additional indicators beyond the normal measures might be needed to rank priority populations according to need (Gherunpong, Sheiham & Tsakos, 2006). The evidence-based medicine movement has developed an increasing influence over recent decades because this provides planners with an independent and impartial defence against charges of favouritism or discrimination (Greenhalgh et al., 2014).

The next step moves from a focus on the problem to a focus on people and clients. A priority score does not provide an answer to the question of who should be looked after by society. Certain population groups often bear disproportional burdens of ill-health. Responsible planners will ensure they understand and quantify the distribution of health problems among peoples of differing age, sex, racial identity, socioeconomic status and any other differentiation relevant to the target population. From a political, cultural and economic perspective, it is important that resources and services are allocated to the right people by the right providers at the right time in the right amount in the right frequency at the right geographic location for the right outcome in a culturally acceptable manner and at the lowest possible delivered cost. Unfortunately, considerations from these differing perspectives do not always result in consensus; for example, it is difficult to argue for extra resources to treat prisoners, who commonly exhibit the lowest levels of health in any society, if this might mean the diversion of resources from other, more 'politically worthy' interests.

Issel and colleagues (2021) argue that five dimensions are likely to be considered by politicians, planners and co-planners, managers and consumers:

1. **Propriety** refers to the role of planners: whether the planners are obligated to address those problems and look after those affected.
2. **Economic feasibility** considers costs associated with actions.
3. **Acceptability** describes the willingness and frequency of use of potential services from the cultural and financial perspectives of consumers.
4. **Resources** refers to the capacity and availability of resources that are needed to deliver services.
5. **Legality** examines obligations imposed by laws, or regulatory conditions.

However, there exists a serious challenge in developing a well-accepted tool to aid multi-criteria decision-making (Oliveira, Mataloto & Kanavos, 2019).

Implement decisions

Management arrangements have been proven to be associated with quality of healthcare and patient outcomes (Aiken et al., 2014). It is naive to consider technology as a silver bullet that can bring an automatic end to a problem. Resource commitment and adequate incentive mechanisms are equally important for realising the desired goals of any service plan. Recent studies have revealed that an increase in nursing workload is associated with increased mortality and adverse events of hospital patients (Aiken et al., 2014; Ross, Howard, Ilic, Watterson & Hodgson, 2023). Over the past decade, high-performance work systems – a series of participative measures of human resource management – have attracted increasing attention from healthcare managers arising from evidence that supports the link between these systems and improved patient care (Leggat, Bartram & Stanton, 2011; Liu et al., 2014). Health service planning standards (e.g. doctors, nurses and beds per 1000 of the population) and role delineation of services (e.g. levels of qualification) may assist managers in ensuring that services are provided safely (Eagar et al., 2001).

Evaluate impact

The outcome of health service planning through the delivery of services ought to be demonstrated by impact evaluation. The term 'impact' means, in this case, the desired outcomes of a health service plan, such as the changed health status of the target audience, the changed service capacity of the provider, or both (Eagar et al., 2001), but it could, conceivably, also include unintended or negative outcomes. The potential impact of a service on non-users should not be ignored.

Since the target audience is deliberately selected and biased to those who most need the service through health service planning, the health impact on those receiving the service is often greater than on an average population (Lance, Guilkey, Hattori & Angeles, 2014). For example, restricting varieties of medicines in the provision of primary care may reduce the pharmaceutical expenditure of individuals who seek medical attention from primary care providers at that instance; however, it may encourage some patients to bypass primary care in favour of tertiary providers such as hospitals, resulting in more expensive care (Yang, Liu, Ferrier, Zhou & Zhang, 2013).

Appropriate evaluation design is critical for demonstrating the effectiveness of a service program. Theoretically, the impact of a planned service program can be confirmed only through a comparison of changes between those who are randomly assigned to a group of intervention (exposed to the service) and a group of control (not exposed to the service). Unfortunately, such randomisation is not intrinsically possible in health service planning, because service recipients often self-select or are selected into a service program. Furthermore, the effects of service may not be straightforward: it may in some respects interact with many other health determinants, such as education and income. As a result, complicated statistical analyses (such as multiple regression, matching and propensity score estimation) may be required to estimate the impact and enable adjustment due to the possibility of confounding influences of factors other than the designed service on the outcome indicators (Lance et al., 2014).

Finally, those responsible for evaluation may also influence how evaluation is conducted and impact on the results. Evaluators may be internal or external: internal evaluators are more likely to be biased in favour of a particular process; but they cost less and can facilitate the implementation of the plan (Issel et al., 2021). Health managers need to be aware of the potential bias of the different approaches to evaluations (Gopal, Chetty, O'Donnell, Gajria & Blackadder-Weinstein, 2021).

Technology use in health service planning

Planners have increasingly employed modern technologies, such as big data, social media platforms and artificial intelligence (AI), to assist in health service planning. Widespread access to the internet presents an opportunity to enhance public communication and consultations. Researchers have explored the potential for use of social media data to improve planning and responses to public health emergencies (Terry, Yang, Yao & Liu, 2023). Big data enable deeper insights into people's health needs and how healthcare services meet these needs (Bajpai & Sharma, 2018). AI-driven health interventions are also expected to help address health challenges in low-income and middle-income countries, such as workforce shortages and weak public health surveillance (Bajpai & Sharma, 2020). However, it is crucial for health services planning to remain vigilant regarding emerging technologies and the healthcare technology cycle, in order to maximise their health value while minimising potential risks, such as ethical concerns, social bias and the digital divide (Bajpai & Sharma, 2020; Berrio, Ibarra & Galeano, 2020).

Summary

- Health service planning has become an important instrument for improving quality and efficiency of healthcare. It is also seen as a core component of health system governance (Fazekas et al., 2010).
- Plans need to be well executed. The increased use of planning has attracted concerns about coordination and coherence among the plans (Hall, 1981; Wright & Sheldon, 1985).
- Things do not always happen as planned. Contingency plans are needed in case emergencies or disastrous events occur, whether natural or human-induced (Lees, 1981).

Reflective questions

1. What are the differences between population-based planning and institutional-based planning?
2. What is the goal of health service planning?
3. Who should be involved in health service planning, and what roles can they play?
4. What would you do if consensus were hard to reach among key stakeholders?
5. What dimensions are usually considered in determining priorities, and how are they measured?

Self-analysis questions

What are the key values (in terms of funding, availability and accessibility) associated with the provision of healthcare that Australians have endorsed? As a manager, how do you ensure that those values guide the practice of health service planning?

References

Aiken, L. H., Sloane, D. M., Bruyneel, L., Van den Heede, K., Griffiths, P., Busse, R. ... Sermeus, W. (2014). Nurse staffing and education and hospital mortality in nine European countries: A retrospective observational study. *Lancet, 383*(9931), 1824–1830. https://doi.org/10.1016/s0140-6736(13)62631-8

Anderson, K., Gall, A., Butler, T., Ngampromwongse, K., Hector, D., Turnbull, S., Lucas, K., Nehill, C., Boltong, A., Keefe, D. & Garvey, G. (2022). Development of key principles and best practices for co-design in health with first nations Australians. *International Journal of Environmental Research and Public Health, 20*(1), 47. https://doi.org/10.3390/ijerph20010147

Anderson, O. W. (1969). Planning health services, American style. *Medical Care, 7*(5), 345–347. https://doi.org/10.1097/00005650-196909000-00001

Asadi-Lari, M., Packham, C. & Gray, D. (2003). Need for redefining needs. *Health and Quality of Life Outcomes, 1*(34). https://doi.org/10.1186/1477-7525-1-34

Australian Institute of Health and Welfare (AIHW). (2023). *Life expectancy*. AIHW.

——— (2014). *Assessment of global burden of disease 2010: Methods for the Australian context*. AIHW.

Bajpai, A. & Sharma, S. (2018). Big data analysis in health care domain: A systematic review. *International Journal of Engineering Technologies and Management Research*, 5(2), 1–8. https://doi.org/10.29121/ijetmr.v5.i2.2018.605

Berrio, P., Ibarra, A. G. & Galeano, B. (2020). Chapter 30 – Healthcare strategic planning using technology assessment. In E. Iadanza (ed.), *Clinical engineering handbook* (*2nd edition*) (pp. 181–185). Academic Press. https://doi.org/10.1016/B978-0-12-813467-2.00030-4

Brach, C. & Fraserirector, I. (2000). Can cultural competency reduce racial and ethnic health disparities? A review and conceptual model. *Medical care research and review, 57*(1_suppl), 181–217. https://doi.org/10.1177/1077558700057001S09

Bradshaw, J. (1972). A taxonomy of social need. In G. Mclachlan (ed.), *Problems and progress in medical care: Essays on current research* (7th series, pp. 69–82). Nuffield Provincial Hospital Trust.

Brijnath, B. P., Ansariadi, M. & de Souza, D. K. P. (2012). Four ways geographic information systems can help to enhance health service planning and delivery for infectious diseases in low-income countries. *Journal of Health Care for the Poor and Underserved, 23*(4), 1410–1420. https://doi.org/10.1353/hpu.2012.0146

Buxbaum, J. D., Chernew, M. E., Fendrick, A. M. & Cutler, D. M. (2020). Contributions of public health, pharmaceuticals, and other medical care to us life expectancy changes, 1990–2015. *Health Aff (Millwood), 39*(9), 1546–1556. https://doi.org/10.1377/hlthaff.2020.00284

Canelo-Aybar, C., Ferreira, D. S., Ballesteros, M., Posso, M., Montero, N., Solà, I., Saz-Parkinson, Z., Lerda, D., Rossi, P. G., Duffy, S. W. & Follmann, M. (2021). Benefits and harms of breast cancer mammography screening for women at average risk of breast cancer: A systematic review for the European Commission Initiative on Breast Cancer. *Journal of Medical Screening, 28*(4), 389–404. https://doi.org/10.1177/0969141321993866

Commonwealth of Australia, Department of Health and Aged Care. (2021). *National Aboriginal and Torres Strait Islander health plan 2021–2031*. Retrieved from: https://www.health.gov.au/sites/default/files/documents/2022/06/national-aboriginal-and-torres-strait-islander-health-plan-2021-2031.pdf

Cooper, L. A., Hill, M. N. & Powe, N. R (2002). Designing and evaluating interventions to eliminate racial and ethnic disparities in health care. *Journal of General Internal Medicine, 17*, 477–486. https://doi.org/10.1046/j.1525-1497.2002.10633.x

Department of Health, State of Victoria. (2011). *Victorian health priorities framework 2012–2022: Metropolitan health plan*. Retrieved from: https://www.health.vic.gov.au/publications/victorian-health-priorities-framework-2012-2022-metropolitan-health-plan

Durrance-Bagale, A., Marzouk, M., Tung, L. S., Agarwal, S., Aribou, Z. M., Ibrahim, N. B. M., Mkhallalati, H., Newaz, S., Omar, M., Ung, M., Zaseela, A., Nagashima-Hayashi, M. & Howard, N. (2022). Community engagement in health systems interventions and research in conflict-affected countries: A scoping review of approaches. *Glob Health Action, 15*(1), 2074131. https://doi.org/10.1080/16549716.2022.2074131

Dyck, K. G., Tiessen, M. & Lee, A. M. (2013). Integrating health care providers' opinions into mental health service planning for underserved populations. *University of Toronto Medical Journal, 90*(4), 143–149.

Eagar, K., Garrett, P. & Lin, V. (2001). *Health planning: Australian perspectives*. Allen & Unwin.

Edwards, D. (2012). Local public health planning as a form of social action to achieve better health outcomes: What can be learned from the Victorian experience? [Doctoral dissertation]. La Trobe University. Retrieved from: https://opal.latrobe.edu.au/articles/thesis/Local_public_health_planning_as_a_form_of_social_action_to_achieve_better_health_outcomes_what_can_be_learned_from_the_Victorian_experience_/21844779

Evans, D., Barwell, J., Eccles, D., Collins, A., Izatt, L., Jacobs, C. … Murray, A. (2014). The Angelina Jolie effect: How high celebrity profile can have a major impact on provision of cancer related services. *Breast Cancer Research, 16*(442). https://doi.org/10.1186/s13058-014-0442-6

Fazekas, M., Ettelt, S., Newbould, J. & Nolte, E. (2010). *Framework for assessing, improving and enhancing health service planning*. Rand.

Gage, R. W. (1979). Planning for health services. *Journal of the American College Health Association, 27*(6), 279–280. https://doi.org/10.1080/01644300.1979.10392870

Gagliardi, A. R., Lemieux-Charles, L., Brown, A. D., Sullivan, T. & Goel, V. (2008). Barriers to patient involvement in health service planning and evaluation: An exploratory study. *Patient Education & Counseling, 70*(2), 234–241. https://doi.org/10.1080/01644300.1979.10392870

Gaston, C. (2005). *Health service planning and policy-making: A toolkit for nurses and midwives.* World Health Organization.

Gauld, R. (2002). From home, to market, to headquarters, to home: Relocating health services planning and purchasing in New Zealand. *Journal of Management in Medicine, 16*(6), 436–450. https://doi.org/10.1108/02689230210450990

Gherunpong, S., Sheiham, A. & Tsakos, G. (2006). A sociodental approach to assessing children's oral health needs: Integrating an oral health-related quality of life (OHRQoL) measure into oral health service planning. *Bulletin of the World Health Organization, 84*(1), 36–42. https://doi.org/10.1590/S0042-96862006000100012

Gkiouleka, A., Wong, G., Sowden, S., Bambra, C., Siersbaek, R., Manji, S., Moseley, A., Harmston, R., Kuhn, I. & Ford, J. (2023). Reducing health inequalities through general practice. *The Lancet Public Health, 8*(6), e463–e472. https://doi.org/10.1016/S2468-2667(23)00093-2

Gopal, D. P., Chetty, U., O'Donnell, P., Gajria, C. & Blackadder-Weinstein, J. (2021). Implicit bias in healthcare: Clinical practice, research and decision making. *Future Healthcare Journal, 8*(1), 40. https://doi.org/10.7861/fhj.2020-0233

Gotzsche, P. C. & Jorgensen, K. J. (2013). Screening for breast cancer with mammography (review) [Intervention review]. *Cochrane Database of Systematic Reviews, 6*(Cd001877). https://doi.org/10.1002/14651858.CD001877.pub5

Greenhalgh, T., Howick, J. & Maskrey, N. (2014). Evidence based medicine: A movement in crisis? *British Medical Journal, 348.* https://doi.org/10.1136/bmj.g3725

Grindell, C., Coates, E., Croot, L. & O'Cathain, A. (2022). The use of co-production, co-design and co-creation to mobilise knowledge in the management of health conditions: A systematic review. *BMC Health Services Research, 22*(1), 877. https://doi.org/10.1186/s12913-022-08079-y

Haldane, V., Chuah, F. L. H., Srivastava, A., Singh, S. R., Koh, G. C. H., Seng, C. K. & Legido-Quigley, H. (2019). Community participation in health services development, implementation, and evaluation: A systematic review of empowerment, health, community, and process outcomes. *PLOS One, 14*(5), e0216112. https://doi.org/10.1371/journal.pone.0216112

Hall, T. L. (1981). The planning of health services: Studies in eight european countries [Book review]. *Health Services Research, 16*(1), 103–105.

Issel, L. M., Wells, R. & Williams M. (2021). *Health program planning and evaluation: A practical systematic approach to community health* (5th ed.). Jones & Bartlett.

Kelaher, M., Sabanovic, H., La Brooy, C., Lock, M., Lusher, D. & Brown, L. (2014). Does more equitable governance lead to more equitable health care? A case study based on the implementation of health reform in Aboriginal health Australia. *Social Science & Medicine, 123*, 278–286. https://doi.org/10.1016/j.socscimed.2014.07.032

Klaic, M., Kapp, S., Hudson, P., Chapman, W., Denehy, L., Story, D. & Francis, J. J. (2022). Implementability of healthcare interventions: An overview of reviews and development of a conceptual framework. *Implementation Sci, 17*(1), 10. https://doi.org/10.1186/s13012-021-01171-7

Kullar, R., Marcelin, J. R., Swartz, T. H., Piggott, D. A., Macias Gil, R., Mathew, T. A. & Tan, T. (2020). Racial disparity of coronavirus disease 2019 in African American communities. *The Journal of infectious diseases, 222*(6), 890–893. https://doi.org/10.1093/infdis/jiaa372

Lance, P., Guilkey, D., Hattori, A. & Angeles, G. (2014). *How do we know if a program made a difference? A guide to statistical methods for program impact evaluation.* Measure Evaluation.

Lees, W. (1981). Health service planning for war. *British Medical Journal (Clinical Research Edition), 282*(6273), 1401–1402.

Leggat, S. G., Bartram, T. & Stanton, P. (2011). High performance work systems: The gap between policy and practice in health care reform. *Journal of Health Organization & Management, 25*(3), 281–297. https://doi.org/10.1108/14777261111143536

Liu, C., Bartram, T., Casimir, G. & Leggat, S. G. (2014). The link between participation in management decision making and quality of patient care as perceived by Chinese doctors. *Public Management Review*, (September). https://doi.org/10.1080/14719037.2014.930507

Liu, C, Liu, W., Wang, Y., Zhang, Z. & Wang, P. (2013). Patient safety culture in China: A case study in an outpatient setting in Beijing. *BMJ Quality and Safety*, *23*, 556–564. https://doi.org/10.1136/bmjqs-2013-002172

Loutfi, D., Law, S., McCutcheon, C., Carlin, R., Torrie, J. & Macdonald, M. E. (2018). Health planning for Indigenous populations: A rapid evidence review. *The International Indigenous Policy Journal*, *9*(1). https://doi.org/10.18584/iipj.2018.9.1.7

Miller, A. B., Wall, C., Baines, C. J., Sun, P., To, T. & Narod, S. A. (2014). Twenty five year follow-up for breast cancer incidence and mortality of the Canadian National Breast Screening Study: Randomised screening trial. *British Medical Journal*, *348*. https://doi.org/10.1136/bmj.g366

Oliveira, M. D., Mataloto, I. & Kanavos, P. (2019). Multi-criteria decision analysis for health technology assessment: addressing methodological challenges to improve the state of the art. *The European Journal of Health Economics*, *20*, 891–918. https://doi.org/10.1007/s10198-019-01052-3

Price, E. (1999). Functional status and health service planning. *Journal of Quality in Clinical Practice*, *19*(4), 224–225.

Ren, W., Chen, M., Qiao, Y. & Zhao, F. (2022). Global guidelines for breast cancer screening: A systematic review. *The Breast*, *64*, 85–99. https://doi.org/10.1016/j.breast.2022.04.003

Richards, B. W. (1981). Health service planning [Letter]. *Journal of the Royal College of General Practitioners*, *31*(232), 694.

Román, M., Sala, M., Domingo, L., Posso, M., Louro, J. & Castells, X. (2019). Personalized breast cancer screening strategies: A systematic review and quality assessment. *PLOS One*, *14*(12), p.e0226352. https://doi.org/10.1371/journal.pone.0226352

Rosen, P., De Fine Licht, J. & Ohlsson, H. (2014). Priority setting in Swedish health care: Are the politicians ready? *Scandinavian Journal of Public Health*, *42*(3), 227–234. https://doi.org/10.1177/1403494813520355

Ross, P., Howard, B., Ilic, D., Watterson, J. & Hodgson, C. L. (2023). Nursing workload and patient-focused outcomes in intensive care: A systematic review. *Nursing & Health Sciences*, *25*(4), 497–515. https://doi.org/10.1111/nhs.13052

Sabik, L. M. & Lie, R. K. (2008). Priority setting in health care: Lessons from the experiences of eight countries. *International Journal for Equity in Health*, *7*(4). https://doi.org/10.1186/1475-9276-7-4

Saeed, S. A. & Masters, R. M. (2021). Disparities in health care and the digital divide. *Current psychiatry reports*, *23*, 1–6. https://doi.org/10.1007/s11920-021-01274-4

Semple, A. B. (1977). Health service planning [Book review]. *British Medical Journal*, *1*, 1342. https://doi.org/10.1136/bmj.1.6072.1339

Snow, L., Walker, M., Ahern, M., O'Brien, E. & Saltman, D. C. (1999). Functional status and health service planning. *Journal of Quality in Clinical Practice*, *19*(2), 99–102. https://doi.org/10.1046/j.1440-1762.1999.00309.x

Sullivan, S. G., Glasson, E. J., Hussain, R., Petterson, B. A., Slack-Smith, L. M., Montgomery, P. D. & Bittles, A. H. (2003). Breast cancer and the uptake of mammography screening services by women with intellectual disabilities. *Preventive Medicine*, *37*(5), 507–512. https://doi.org/10.1016/S0091-7435(03)00177-4

Terry, K., Yang, F., Yao, Q. & Liu, C. (2023). The role of social media in public health crises caused by infectious disease: A scoping review. *BMJ Glob Health*, *8*(12). https://doi.org/10.1136/bmjgh-2023-013515

Thornicroft, G. & Tansella, M. (2005). Growing recognition of the importance of service user involvement in mental health service planning and evaluation. *Epidemiologia e Psichiatria Sociale*, *14*(1), 1–3. https://doi.org/10.1017/S1121189X00001858

Timmermans, S. (2020). The engaged patient: The relevance of patient-physician communication for twenty-first-century health. *J Health Soc Behav*, *61*(3), 259–273. https://doi.org/10.1177/0022146520943514

Vayda, E. (1977). Health services planning [Book review]. *Canadian Medical Association Journal*, *116*, 847.

Weedon-Fekjær, H., Romundstad, P. R. & Vatten, L. J. (2014). Modern mammography screening and breast cancer mortality: Population study. *British Medical Journal*, *348*. https://doi.org/10.1136/bmj.g3701

Windle, A., Javanparast, S., Freeman, T. & Baum, F. (2023). Evaluating local primary health care actions to address health inequities: Analysis of Australia's Primary Health Networks. *Int J Equity Health*, *22*(1), 243. https://doi.org/10.1186/s12939-023-02053-8

World Health Organization (WHO). (2020). *Community engagement: A health promotion guide for universal health coverage in the hands of the people*. WHO. Retrieved from: https://www.who.int/publications/i/item/9789240010529

Wright, J. & Sheldon, F. (1985). Health and social services planning. *Social Policy and Administration*, *19*(3), 258–272. https://doi.org/10.1111/j.1467-9515.1985.tb00238.x

Yang, L. P., Liu, C. J., Ferrier, J. A., Zhou, W. & Zhang, X. P. (2013). The impact of the National Essential Medicines Policy on prescribing behaviours in primary care facilities in Hubei province of China. *Health Policy and Planning*, *28*(7), 750–760. https://doi.org/10.1093/heapol/czs116

Index

3D objectives, 222
7-S framework, 364
ability model, 58
acceptability, 379
accessibility, 324
accommodating, 282
accountabilities, 191–2, 211
　See also holding to account
accounting equation, 234
accounting processes, 234
accreditation, 132, 136, 191
active listening, 116–17
activity-based budgets, 236
acuity, 237
adaptability, 59, 92
adaption, 81
adhocracy culture, 290
ADKAR model, 308
advisory committees, 230
advocacy, 374
aged-care services, 237
agreements, 252
alchemical effect, 143
alignment, 174
ambiguity
　and communication, 112
　and healthcare organisations, 79–80
　and leadership, 82, 83–5
　and management, 81–3
　definition, 78
　managing, 83
anchoring, 205–6
anchors, 251
anticipatory grief, 305
apolitical approach, 374
appeals
　inspirational, 171
　upward, 162, 163, 171
appraisal methods, 196–7
appraisement, 171
arbitrators, 252
arguments, 201, 204
articulation, 84
artificial intelligence (AI)
　and clinicians, 138
　described, 333
　implications, 337–8
　use of, 331, 334
arts-based approaches, 94
aspirations, 48
assertiveness, 162, 163
assets, 234
assistance, 172
assumptions, 202
Australian Charter of Healthcare Rights, 161

Australian Commission on Safety and Quality in Health Care, 132, 321, 359
Australian Council on Healthcare Standards, 191
Australian Health Professional Regulatory Agency, 197
Australian National Aged Care Classification (AN-ACC) funding model, 237
Australian Primary Care Collaboratives Program, 184
Australian Refined Diagnostic Related Groups, 237, 238
Australian Society for Telehealth, 338
authentic leadership, 20
authority, 156–7, 162, 163, 202
automation, 354
availability, 205
avoidance, 282
awareness, 308

balanced scorecard, 365
bargaining, 252
BATNA (best alternative to a negotiated agreement), 249–50
behaviourist theories, 17
behaviours, 213
below the line behaviour, 195
benchmarking, 238, 245
biases
　assessing, 203
　in decision-making, 205–6, 272
big data, 331, 333, 335–6
boards, 138
breast cancer screening services, 373
buddy systems, 196
budgets
　and costs, 240
　controlling, 245
　development, 241–5
　monitoring, 245
　nursing, 241–5
　types of, 234–6
bullying, 197
burnout, 295–6
business skills, 9

capability, 215, 351
capacity, 351
capital, 159
capped funding, 237
career-planning, 92–3

caregivers, 146
casemix, 237–9
cashflow, 245
centrality, 161
change
　and communication, 304, 308
　and staff, 304–6
　in organisations, 81, 302
　resistance to, 334
change fatigue, 305
change management
　and coaching, 310–11
　and First Nations peoples, 311–12
　and mentoring, 309–10
　approaches, 81–2
　described, 302–4
　frameworks, 306–8
charisma, 82
charismatic leadership, 19–20
checklists, 321
chief executive officers, 9
clan culture, 290
clarity, 78
clarity in negotiations, 251
climate, 71
clinical communication, 114
clinical governance
　and healthcare professionals, 133
　and leadership, 137–8
　Australian system, 136
　definition, 132
　evolution, 135
　genesis, 132–3
　responsive regulation, 136–7
　turning point, 133–4
clinical governance frameworks, 133, 137–8
clinical management, 333
clinical managers, 183–4
clinicians
　and artificial intelligence (AI), 138
　compared with managers, 125–6
closed questions, 116
coaching, 214, 310–11
coalitions, 162, 163, 171
co-creation, 180
codes of conduct, 32
codes of ethics, 32, 33
coercive power, 158
cognitive moral development (CMD) model, 34
collaboration, 143, 169, 172, 178, 214, 282
collaborative approaches, 120

386

collaborative partnerships, 146–7
collective action, 163
commitment, 194
communication
  and ambiguity, 83
  and change, 304, 308
  and conflict, 280
  and Culturally and Linguistically Diverse (CALD) groups, 119–20
  and ethics, 113
  and First Nations peoples, 119
  and healthcare, 114–16
  and leadership, 116–18
  and learning, 118
  and people with impaired physical or mental ability, 119–20
  and stakeholder partnerships, 148
  definition, 111–12
  digital, 332
  elements of, 112–14
  empathetic, 56
  responding to, 113
  types of, 114–16
communication action, 374
communities of practice and interest, 118
community engagement, 374
comparative needs, 377
compassion, 101
compassionate care, 100, 101–2, 104
competence, 74
competencies, 214
competing, 283
competing values framework, 289–90
competitive advantage, 363
competitive culture, 290
competitiveness, 186
comprehensive rational, 374
compromise, 282
conceptual skills, 8
confidentiality, 197, 336
confirmation, 205
conflict
  and culture, 283
  definition, 277
  functional, 278–9
  prevention, 280–1
  types of, 277–9
  workplace, 277
conflict management, 61, 215–16, 277, 279–84
conflict resolution, 56, 281–4
consequences, 194
consistency, 324
consortium, 376
consultations, 171
consumers
  as stakeholders, 145
  participation, 374
contingency approach, 24

continuous quality improvement, 318, 325
control culture, 290
controlling, 10, 82
conversations, difficult, 117
cooperation, 178
cooperative culture, 290
coordination, 178
corporate governance, 132
cost-benefit analysis, 378
cost-effectiveness analysis, 378
costs, 240
counselling, 296
countercultures, 288
COVID-19, 23–4, 303–4
creative culture, 290
creativity
  and organisations, 259–61
  converting, 263–4
  definition, 259
  See also innovation
creativity approaches, 94
critical questioning, 94
critical reflection, 89, 93–4
critical reflective leadership, 93
critical reflective practice
  and leadership, 91–3
  benefits, 91–2
  characteristics of, 90
  critics of, 94–5
  definition, 89
  developing, 93–4
critical thinking
  barriers to, 202–3
  described, 45–6, 201
  developing skills, 203–4
criticism, 195
cultural awareness, 119
cultural capital, 159
cultural intelligence, 149, 213
cultural load, 312
cultural safety, 312
cultural safety training, 119
culturally and linguistically diverse (CALD) groups, 119–20
culture
  and conflict, 283
  and innovation, 260, 261
  and organisational behaviour, 212–13
  subcultures, 288
  types of, 289–90
  See also workplace culture
customs, 293

data
  analytics, 335–7
  and continuous improvement, 325
  and decision-making, 337
  big, 331, 333, 335–6
  collection, 138, 173, 284
  integrity, 336
  sharing, 336
  standards for, 120, 334

data-based conflict, 278
decision-making
  and data, 337
  and evidence, 269–70, 272–3
  and information, 84
  biases and errors in, 205–6, 272
  definition, 36
  ethical, 31–2
  evidence-based, 206–7
  frameworks, 36–7
  health service planning, 374–6
  implementation, 379
  influential factors, 32–5, 37
  process, 204
deductive reasoning, 201
deliverables, 226
demand and supply gap analysis, 352
Deming, W. Edward, 317
demographics, 351
demotions, 197
deontology, 33
descriptive information, 89
descriptive reflection, 89
desire, 308
development reviews, 196
dialogic reflection, 89
difficult conversations, 117
difficult workers, 215–16
digital emotional intelligence, 55
digital health, 331
  See also technology
digital innovation, 331–2
  See also technology
digital literacy, 334
direct groups, 10
discipline processes, 196–7
distortion, 112
distributive approach, 249
documentation, 227
dominating, 283
downward communication, 114
dyad leadership models, 124–5

economic evaluation, 228
economic feasibility, 379
effectiveness, 84, 194, 321
efficiency, 322, 332
egoism, 33
Eisenhower matrix, 49
e-leadership, 20–1
electronic communication, 115–16, 117–18
electronic medical records, 332, 337
emails, 116
emergency departments, 80, 339
emotion, 112
emotion artificial intelligence, 56
emotional awareness, 56
emotional intelligence
  and healthcare, 61–2
  and leadership, 61
  and patient care, 59–61
  characteristics of, 56–7
  described, 55–6

emotional intelligence (cont.)
  gender differences, 56–7
  importance of, 45
  improving, 57
  models of, 58–9
emotional regulation, 56
emotional resilience, 292
emotional support, 103, 104
empathic leadership, 103
empathy, 56, 59
employees
  See staff
empowerment, 214, 307
engagement, 174
environment, 173–4
environmental scanning, 351, 361–2
environments
  and stress, 296
  learning, 261
episodes of care, 238
equity, 234
ERRO (Economic Relevance of Relational Outcomes), 249
errors in decision-making, 205–6
ethical climate, 71
ethical decision-making, 31–2, 36–7
ethical factors, 33–4
ethics, 113
ethnocentricity, 202
evaluation
  effectiveness, 194
  of health services, 82–3
  of impact, 379–80
  of projects, 226–9
evaluation logic model, 82–3
evaporating cloud approach, 283–4
evidence
  and decision-making, 269–70, 272–3
  appraise, 272
  sources of, 271–2
  use of, 269–70
evidence-based decision-making management, 206–7
evidence-based management
  described, 269–70
  frameworks, 270–3
evidence-based medicine, 378
evidence-based practice, 320
exchange, 162, 164, 171
executive groups, 10
expectations, 193, 194
  See also holding to account
expenses, 234
experience, 262, 271
expert power, 7, 158
exploration, 92
expressed needs, 377
external factors, 35

failure, fear of, 82
Fair Work Act 2009 (Cth), 113

families, 146
feedback, 48, 103, 113, 192, 194, 195–6
felt needs, 377
financial accounting, 234
financial burdens, 132
financial management
  described, 234
  variance analysis, 240–1
  See also budgets
financial penalties, 197
financial performance, 240
financial sustainability, 173
First Nations peoples
  and change management, 311–12
  and communication, 119
  and health service planning, 370–1
  partnerships with, 147–8
flexible budgets, 235
force field analysis, 306
formal communication, 114
frame of reference, 202
frameworks
  change management, 306–8
  clinical governance, 133, 137–8
  competing values, 289–90
  definition, 18
  ethical decision-making, 36–7
  evidence-based management, 270–3
  health service planning, 376–80
  holding to account, 193–7
  negotiation, 249–52
  projects, 223–4
  strategic influence, 170–4
  strategic planning, 360–5
  workforce-planning, 348–54
framing, 84–5, 205, 206, 251
functional conflict, 278–9
funding
  allocation systems, 238
  healthcare, 237
  reforms in, 239

gap analysis, 352
gender differences, 56–7
general managers, 9
generational differences, 215
generations, 215
global budgets, 235
globalisation, 111
Goal Setting Theory, 48
goals, 48–9, 194, 225, 241, 376
Gold Coast University Hospital, 353–4
governments, 146–7, 372, 376
graduate retention, 348
gratification, 205
great man theories, 17
grief, 305–6
ground rules, 250–1
group failure, 205
group pressure, 202

group reflection, 94
group thinking, 202, 272
guiding coalition, 307

harassment, 197
Hawthorne effect, 22
Health and Disability Services Standards, NZ, 133
health context, 351
health expenditure, 132, 372
health inequity, 371
health leadership
  See leadership
health literacy, 119
health management, 4–5
  See also management
health service evaluation, 82–3
health service planning
  and First Nations peoples, 370–1
  and management, 373–6
  and technology, 380
  cycle, 377
  definition, 370
  frameworks, 376–80
  in Australia, 372
  reasons for, 372–3
health systems
  definition, 4
  managers of, 5, 8–9
health workforce
  demand and supply, 346–8
  described, 214
  statistics, 346–8
  sustainability, 348
healthcare
  and communication, 114–16
  and emotional intelligence, 61–2
  in digital age, 334
  stakeholder groups, 145–8
healthcare funding, 237
healthcare organisations
  and ambiguity, 79–80
  foci of, 11
  levels of management, 8–9
healthcare professionals
  and clinical governance, 133
  and consumers, 145
  and families, 146
  hierarchies of, 7
  self-management, 41
  See also teams
healthcare quality
  definition, 317
  dimensions of, 319–25
  history of, 317–18
heuristics, 32, 37
hierarchy culture, 290
high-performance work systems, 216–17
historical budgets, 235
holding to account
  and leadership, 192–3
  frameworks, 193–7
  understanding of, 191

hospital boards, 138
hospital-acquired adverse events, 132, 133
hospitals, 23–4
human capital, 351
human relations movement, 22–3
human resource frames, 84
human resource management, 211
human resources
    described, 211
    shortages, 212
    skills utilisation, 212
Human Resources for Health (HRH) Action Framework, 349–53
human skills, 8, 9
humour, 82

illegal behaviour, 158, 197
impact evaluation, 227, 379–80
implementation of decisions, 379
incidence, 378
incremental approach, 374
Independent Health and Aged Care Pricing Authority, 238
Independent Hospital Pricing Authority, 239
indicators, 227, 376, 378
Indigenous leadership, 119
Indigenous peoples
    See First Nations peoples
individual accountability, 192
inductive reasoning, 201
influence
    definition, 162, 168
    frameworks, 170–4
    tactics, 162–4
    using, 169–70
    See also strategic influence
informal communication, 114
information
    and communication, 111
    and decision-making, 84
    descriptive, 89
    processing, 36
    sharing, 180
information-rich, 323
ingratiation, 162, 163, 171
innovation
    and critical reflection, 92
    and leadership, 263, 264–5
    and management, 261–4
    challenges, 262–4
    definition, 259
    digital, 331–2
inspirational appeals, 171
institutional-based planning, 371
integrated care, 127
integration, 282, 323
integrative approach, 249
intelligence, 44–5, 55
intelligence quotient, 55
interagency partnerships, 146
interdisciplinary teams, 124

interest-based conflict, 278
interorganisational networking, 184–6
Interorganisational Relations Theory, 184
interpersonal skills, 9, 59
interprofessional teams
    definition, 124
    leadership of, 126–7
    management of, 127–9
    working in, 124
interviews, 227
intraorganisational networking, 186
intrapersonal skills, 59
ISBAR model, 115

James, Brent, 317
Janusian thinking, 82
judgement, 271
justify in negotiations, 251

knowledge, 36
knowledge alliances, 185
knowledge management, 273
Kotter's theory of organisational change, 306–8

language, 69, 117
leaders
    compared with managers, 6, 10
    power and skills, 7–9
leadership
    and ambiguity, 80, 82, 83–5
    and clinical governance, 137–8
    and communication, 116–18
    and critical reflective practice, 91–3
    and emotional intelligence, 61
    and holding to account, 192–3
    and innovation, 263, 264–5
    and management, 213–16
    and networking, 181
    and reflection, 93
    and stakeholder partnerships, 150
    and values, 70–4
    and virtual teams, 340
    and workplace culture, 293–4
    challenges, 7
    definition, 3, 6, 16, 123
    effective, 264
    empathic, 103
    evidence-based, 270–3
    in learning organisations, 260
    Indigenous, 119
    of interprofessional teams, 126–7
    spiritual, 100, 103
    styles, 192
    values-based, 71–2
    within partnerships, 150
leadership theories
    evolvement,
    in healthcare, 18–21
leading, 10

learning, 91, 118
learning circles, 94
learning organisations, 260–1
leave entitlement, 242
legality, 379
legislation, 191
legitimate power, 157
legitimation, 171
Lewin's field theory, 306
liabilities, 234
listening, 114, 116–17, 203

machine learning, 333, 337–8
management
    and ambiguity, 81–3
    and difficult workers, 215–16
    and financial performance, 240
    and health service planning, 373–6
    and innovation, 261–4
    and leadership, 213–16
    and negotiation, 252
    and stakeholder partnerships, 148–9
    and workforce-planning, 354–5
    and workplace culture, 292–3
    definition, 3, 4, 16
    evidence-based decision-making, 206–7
    functions of, 21
    of budgets, 245
    of conflict, 61, 277, 279–84
    of interprofessional teams, 127–9
    of projects, 229–30
    skills for, 8–9
    See also change management
management theories
    approaches, 21–4
    evolvement, 21
managerial craftsmanship, 149
managers
    capabilities, 11
    compared with clinicians, 125–6
    compared with leaders, 6, 10
    functions of, 10–11
    health, 213–14
    in digital age, 339–40
    of health systems, 5, 8–9
    power and skills, 7–9
mandates, 361
map-building, 82
marginalised groups
    and communication, 118–20
    partnerships with, 147–8
market culture, 290
market mechanisms, 136
marketing assessment, 378
Maslow's hierarchy of human needs, 46–7
measurement, 194, 290, 294, 365
mediators, 252
medical records, 332
medication management, 338
mental health, 295–6

Mental Health Professionals Network (MHPN), 185–6
mentor systems, 196
mentoring, 309–10
mentoring programs, 214
mentors, 50
mentorship, 93
messages, 112–13
meta-regulation, 137
microsystems, 211
Mid Staffordshire NHS Foundation Trust Public Inquiry, 134–5
migrant workers, 345
Millennial workers, 215
mindfulness, 296
mission statements, 361
mix variance, 241
mixed models, 59
monitoring tools, 334
mood, 59
moral courage, 34
moral judgements, 202
morality, 33
morals, 33
motivation, 46–7, 56, 59, 70, 158
Motivation–Hygiene Theory, 47
multidisciplinary teams, 124
My Health Record, 332

National Health Reform Agreements, 239
National Health Service, United Kingdom, 133
National Safety and Quality Health Service Standards, 136–7
National Weighted Activity Unit (NWAU), 238
natural world, 68
needs, 46–7, 377
needs analysis, 224
needs assessment, 377
negotiating in bad faith, 252
negotiation
  and conflict, 284
  and management, 252
  described, 170, 249
  frameworks, 249–52
  skills improvement, 253
  unethical, 252
networking
  and leadership, 181
  definition, 178
  described, 179, 180
  examples, 179, 180
  types of, 181–6
networks, 162, 163, 178
New Zealand Health Quality & Safety Commission, 133
NHMRC Partnerships for Better Health, 180
noise, 112
non-verbal communication, 113, 116
normative needs, 377

norms, 33, 263
not-for-profit organisations, 259
nursing budgets, 241–5
nursing hours per patient day, 241–5

objectives, 48, 225, 241
obliging, 282
open questions, 116
operational accountability, 191
operational networking, 181, 183
organisation ambiguity, 79
organisational assessment, 378
organisational behaviour, 22, 212–13
organisational change, 302
organisational creativity, 263
organisational culture
  and innovation, 260, 261
  and spirituality, 103–4
  changing, 293
  definition, 100
  described, 71, 212–13
  See also workplace culture
organisational factors, 35
organisational structures, 3, 213, 229, 262–3
organisational values, 68
organisations
  and creativity, 259–61
  and evidence, 271
  and workplace culture, 291–2
  change in, 81
  described, 3–4
  future, 363
  governance, 359
  learning, 260–1
  levels of management, 8–9
  management of, 5
  managing, 364–5
organising, 10
outcome evaluation, 228
outcomes, 7
overconfidence, 205
over-prudence, 205

partnership-based public policies, 143
partnerships
  definition, 143
  examples, 144–5
  leadership within, 150
  structures, 148
  use of, 173
  with caregivers, 146
  with consumers, 145
  with families, 146
  with First Nations peoples, 147–8
  with marginalised groups, 147–8
  See also collaborative partnerships
patient care, 59–61
patient engagement, 332, 334
patient-centred care, 318, 332

patient-centredness, 319
peer pressure, 202
peer reviews, 191
penalties, 197
penalty rates, 242
people with impaired physical or mental ability, 119–20
perception, 156, 205
performance, 193
performance appraisals, 294
performance appraisals and development (PA&D), 196
performance improvement processes, 196–7
performance management, 216–17
performance reviews, 217
performance systems, 104
personal factors, 35
personal networking, 181–3
personal power, 7
personal values, 68–9
persuasion, 171
planning, 10, 360–1
  See also workforce-planning; strategic planning; health service planning
plans for projects, 225–6
plunging in, 205
policies, 192
political frames, 84
politics, 156
population health management, 172
population-based planning, 370
positional power, 7
power
  and skills, 7–9
  definition, 156
  dynamics, 159, 160
  increasing, 164
  sources of, 157–60
  types of, 7
  use of, 160–1
practitioners
  See healthcare professionals
prejudice, 203
pressure, 170
prevalence, 378
priorities, 84, 378–9
prioritisation, 49
privacy, 336, 338
problem-finding, 82
problems, wicked, 144, 149
problem-solving, 252
process evaluation, 227
processes, 4
professional boundaries, 124–5
professional identity, 128
professional values, 69–70
progresses, 365
project committees, 230
project management
  definition, 222
  described, 222, 229–30
  tools, 230–1

projects
   case studies, 228–9
   core components, 224–6
   definition, 222
   evaluation, 226–9
   frameworks, 223–4
   goals, 225
   key steps, 223
   objectives, 225
   plans, 225–6
   strategies, 225
   teams, 230
propriety, 378
public health planning, 372
public inquiries, 133–5

quality improvement
   described, 173
   dimensions of, 319–25
   history of, 317–18
Quality in Australian Health Care Study, 133
questions, 94, 116, 202, 204

randomness, 205
rational persuasion, 171
rationality, 162, 164
receivers, 114
recognition programs, 280
records, 227
re-creation, 81
recruitment, 214–15, 294, 345
referent power, 7, 158–60
reflection
   and leadership, 93
   critics of, 94–5
   described, 88
   reasons for, 88–9
   types of, 89–90
reflective practice, 50
reflective teaching, 89
reflective writing, 93
reflexivity, 149
regulation, 136–7
regulatory compliance, 334
relationship-based conflict, 277, 284
relationship-building, 174
re-orientation, 81
representation, 205
reprimands, 197
research, 146, 271
research collaborations, 146
resilience, 56, 149
resource allocation, 73, 280, 294
resources, 379
respect, 148, 192
responsibilities, 191, 192
responsive regulation, 136–7
responsiveness, 149
retention, 214–15, 354
revenues, 234
reviews
   development, 196
   external, 191
   peer, 191
   performance, 217
revitalisation, 149
reward power, 157–8
right to disconnect from work, 113
risk management, 173
rituals, 293
role ambiguity,
role-modelling, 70, 294
role-related boundaries, 125–6
roles, 351
Royal Commission into Aged Care Quality in Australia, 134, 292
rule of thumb, 205

safety, 321
safety culture, 271–2
sanctions, 162, 163
scenario-building, 362
scientific management, 21–2
security, 336, 338
self-awareness, 56, 59, 91
self-control, 42
self-help strategies, 295
self-leadership, 42
self-management
   aids for, 49–50
   definition, 41, 42
   tools, 332
self-reflection, 194
self-regulation, 42, 56, 59, 136
senders, 112–13
senior managers, 8
sense making, 85
servant leadership, 18
service improvement, 317, 319–25
service managers, 9
Shewhart, Walter, 317
silo effect, 115
SIMPLE framework, 192, 194–5
situational leadership, 17
situational management, 24
skills, 212
   acquisition of, 41, 253
   and power, 7–9
   critical thinking, 203–4
   for management, 8–9
   utilisation,212
SMART frameworks, 192, 194–5
SMART goals, 48
SMART targets, 364
smartphones, 113
SMARTT targets, 364
social capital, 159
social learning, 47–9
social skills, 56, 59
social world, 69
specialist managers, 9
spiritual horizons, 69
spiritual leadership, 100, 103
spirituality
   and compassion, 100
   and organisational culture, 103–4
spirituality theory, 102–4

sponsors, 230
staff
   and change, 304–6
   and stress management, 295–6
   difficult, 215–16
   empowering, 307
   in learning organisations, 260
   motivation, 158
   See also healthcare professionals; workforce planning
staff-mix, 212
stakeholder partnerships
   and leadership, 150
   and management, 148–9
   importance of, 143–5
   success factors, 148
stakeholders
   and evidence, 271
   definition, 143, 334
   engagement, 173, 374, 376
   identifying, 149
   in healthcare, 145–8
   projects, 229–30
standardisation, 79
standards, 136, 359
statement of values, 361
statements, 201
statistical process control, 317
stereotypes, 202
stewardship, 211
strategic accountability, 191
strategic influence, 168, 170–4
strategic issues, 362
strategic management, 359
strategic networking, 181, 183–4
strategic planning
   frameworks, 360–5
   use of, 359, 374
strategic skills, 9
strategies
   confirming, 363–4
   for strategic influence, 172–4
   projects, 225
stress management, 59, 295–6
structural frames, 84
structured communication, 115
structure-driven conflict, 278
subcultures, 288
subsidies, 237
substitutability, 161
sunk-cost bias, 205, 273
supervision, 93, 296
supply chains, 304
support groups, 10
support systems, 280
surveys, 227
sustainability, 325, 362–3
SWOT analysis, 361, 378
symbolic capital, 159
symbolic frames, 84
synergy, 143
systems, 23
systems approach, 23–4
systems of action, 11
systems-based approach, 259–60

tactics, 162–4
targets, 169–70, 364
teaching, 89
team dynamics, 126, 128
teams
    and professional identity, 128
    effective health, 216–17
    projects, 226, 230
    virtual, 339–40
    with professional boundaries, 124–5
    with role-related boundaries, 125–6
    See also interprofessional teams
teamwork, 216–17
technical skills, 8, 9
technology
    advances, 331–2
    and change, 303
    and health service planning, 380
    benefits, 332
    challenges, 334
    use of, 317, 318, 322
telehealth, 333, 338–9
telemedicine, 338–9
temporal space, 69
terminations, 197
theories, 16
theory X, 23
theory Y, 23
theory–practice gap, 47
timeliness, 322
tone, 116
tools for project management, 230–1
Toyota, 186
trait model, 58–9
trait theories, 17
transactional leadership, 17, 18–19
transdisciplinary teams, 124
transferable learning, 91
transfers, 197
transformational leadership, 17, 19, 172, 264–5
transitions, 304–5
triangulation, 227

triple bottom line (TBL) reporting, 362–3
trust, 148, 180, 211, 284
tuning, 81

uncertainty, 78, 79, 82, 160
understanding, 92
unethical behaviours, 31
unethical negotiation, 252
unprofessional behaviour, 197
unreasonableness, 204
upward appeals, 162, 163, 171
upward communication, 114
urgency, 306
utilisation variance, 241
utilitarianism, 33

vagueness, 78
value-based care, 318, 321, 322
values
    agreed, 213
    and ethics, 33
    and leadership, 70–4
    and spirituality, 103–4
    awareness, 72–3
    commitment, 74
    competing, 289–90
    cultural, 376
    definition, 67–8
    practice, 74
    recognition, 72
    statements, 361
    types of, 68–70
values systems, 68
values-based conflict, 278
values-based leadership, 71–2
variance analysis, 240–1
Victorian Virtual Emergency Department, 339
virtual teams, 339–40
virtue ethics, 33
vision, 259, 264, 265, 289, 293, 307, 361
visioning, 259
volume variance, 241
voluntarism, 136

whistleblowing, 34
whole-of-government collaborations, 146–7
wicked problems, 144, 149
wins, 249, 284, 293, 307
work breakdown structure, 226
work engagement, 214
work, right to disconnect from, 113
workers, difficult, 215–16
workforce
    demand and supply, 346–8
    described, 4
    projections, 351–2
    self-sufficiency, 345
    See also health workforce
workforce planning
    and management, 354–5
    described, 345–6
    frameworks, 348–54
    strategies, 352
workforce planning cycle, 349
workforce plasticity, 355
workforce strategies, 345
working from home, 291
working hours, 340, 355
working smarter, 354
workload, 296
workplace
    conflict, 277
    spirituality theory, 102–4
    stress in, 295–6
workplace culture
    and leadership, 293–4
    and management, 292–3
    and organisations, 291–2
    building positive, 292–4
    definition, 288–9
    measuring, 290, 294
    negative, 292
    types of, 289–90
World Health Organization, 345
writing, reflective, 93

zero-based budgets, 235
zone of possible agreement, 250

For EU product safety concerns, contact us at Calle de José Abascal, 56–1°, 28003 Madrid, Spain or eugpsr@cambridge.org.

www.ingramcontent.com/pod-product-compliance
Lightning Source LLC
LaVergne TN
LVHW081523060526
838200LV00044B/1981